Basic Bioethics
Arthur L. Caplan, editor

A complete list of the books in the Basic Bioethics series appears at the back of this book.

Vaccination Ethics and Policy

An Introduction with Readings

edited by Jason L. Schwartz and Arthur L. Caplan

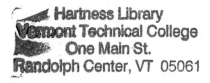
The MIT Press
Cambridge, Massachusetts
London, England

This book was set in Stone Serif and Stone Sans by Toppan Best-set Premedia Limited. Printed and bound in the United States of America.

Library of Congress Cataloging-in-Publication Data

Names: Schwartz, Jason (Jason Lee), editor. | Caplan, Arthur L., editor.
Title: Vaccination ethics and policy : an introduction with readings / edited by Jason L. Schwartz and Arthur L. Caplan.
Other titles: Basic bioethics.
Description: Cambridge, MA : The MIT Press, [2017] | Series: Basic bioethics | Includes bibliographical references.
Identifiers: LCCN 2016019369 | ISBN 9780262035330 (hardcover : alk. paper)
Subjects: | MESH: Vaccination—ethics | Health Policy | Collected Works
Classification: LCC RA638 | NLM QW 806 | DDC 614.4/7—dc23 LC record available at https://lccn.loc.gov/2016019369

10 9 8 7 6 5 4 3 2 1

Contents

Series Foreword

Glenn McGee and I developed the Basic Bioethics series and collaborated as series coeditors from 1998 to 2008. In Fall 2008 and Spring 2009, the series was reconstituted, with a new Editorial Board, under my sole editorship. I am pleased to present the forty-eighth book in the series.

The Basic Bioethics series makes innovative works in bioethics available to a broad audience and introduces seminal scholarly manuscripts, state-of-the-art reference works, and textbooks. Topics engaged include the philosophy of medicine, advancing genetics and biotechnology, end-of-life care, health and social policy, and the empirical study of biomedical life. Interdisciplinary work is encouraged.

Arthur L. Caplan
Basic Bioethics Series Editorial Board

Joseph J. Fins
Rosamond Rhodes
Nadia N. Sawicki
Jan Helge Solbakk

Introduction

Vaccination has been a prominent and effective component of medicine and public health for more than two centuries.[1] Its fundamental principles can be seen in the medical practices of various cultures for nearly a millennium. Long before the human immune system was well understood or the germ theory of disease helped to explain the infectious character of many diseases, generations of healers, scientists, and physicians recognized that the prophylactic administration of harmless or mild disease-related substances could, in many cases, prevent subsequent illness or death from that same disease.

Edward Jenner's work on smallpox and cowpox in the late eighteenth century led to his coinage of the terms "vaccine" and "vaccination," and so began the modern era of vaccination. Smallpox vaccination programs employing an approach fundamentally similar to Jenner's continued into the late twentieth century and culminated in the certification of the global eradication of smallpox in 1979. By then, researchers around the world had understood and seized on the potential of vaccines to immunize against a broad array of other viruses and bacteria, and vaccination programs were longstanding priorities of national and international health agencies. In the decades since that signal achievement in the history of global health, the pace of innovation in vaccine science, development, and implementation has only increased, and the list of potential future vaccine candidates continues to grow.

Today, vaccination can provide a lens into virtually every important aspect of contemporary biomedical science, medicine, and public health. Medical research and the role of private industry, the design and conduct of clinical trials in humans, the regulation of medical technologies, the cost of health care and efforts to ensure broad access to it for all, and the scope of government programs to promote health and to narrow U.S. and global health disparities are among the most prominent—and at times contested—areas of present-day health and medicine. All of these topics and others are directly relevant to current vaccination activities in the United States and around the world.

Although vaccination can offer insights on these frequently discussed general topics in contemporary health and medicine, it also possesses several unique features. These attributes may help to explain, in part, why vaccination receives so much attention and at times is the subject of intense controversy despite being a longstanding, familiar, and routine aspect of pediatric medicine and public health. Vaccination is at its core an individual medical intervention, one that typically occurs in the context of a doctor–patient relationship. Questions about communicating an adequate understanding of risks and benefits, the importance of informed consent, and other issues common to individual medical care are therefore highly relevant, all the more so because children are a primary focus of many vaccination efforts.

But unlike most individual medical interventions, vaccination is also a central component of public health efforts. This is due, in part, to how high vaccination rates within communities confer additional benefits against vaccine-preventable diseases to all through herd protection. This melding of medical and public health objectives, the focus on children in many vaccination programs, and the near impossibility of identifying the specific individuals who would have been harmed by vaccine-preventable diseases if not for vaccination makes vaccine policymaking and programs uniquely challenging to design and administer.

As a form of prevention, vaccination requires juxtaposing individual autonomy against societal best interests. These values are often in alignment for vaccine decision making, but in some cases, they may provide competing arguments regarding the decision to vaccinate. For a limited number of parents or patients, the benefits of vaccination may be seen as being outweighed by the associated risks and costs, however small or unlikely they may be. This is a particularly possible scenario for vaccines against diseases that have virtually disappeared in wealthy countries ironically due in part to successful vaccination programs. Those choosing not to be vaccinated would still benefit at least somewhat through herd protection, creating the potential ethical problem of benefitting as a "free rider."

Free riders are those who knowingly share in the benefits of social programs such as vaccination without personally assuming any risks, burdens, or costs, such as the risk of adverse events or the time and expense required to receive vaccines. Numerous vaccine-preventable disease outbreaks that disproportionately affect unvaccinated persons suggest that personal reliance on herd protection is often inadequate.

For all of these reasons—its common and unique features—policy and programmatic considerations for vaccines and vaccination programs are inseparable from the corresponding ethical considerations they also raise. Questions about where to invest scarce research dollars in vaccine development, how to optimally design clinical research studies, how to adequately evaluate and monitor vaccine safety and effectiveness, how to ensure vaccines are available and affordable to all who could benefit from them, and how to achieve the greatest benefit from vaccines in individuals and communities are all questions of science, business, law, policy, and public health.

But these questions and others like them are also unmistakably questions of ethics, as answers to them reflect the values and value judgments of those in positions of authority and—it is to be hoped—of the individuals and communities whose health and well-being stand to benefit. It is this perspective regarding the embedded, essential character of ethical considerations throughout vaccine science, regulation, and policy in the United States and internationally that animates this volume.

Ethical and Policy Issues Throughout the Vaccine Life Cycle

Recent events such as outbreaks of measles and other vaccine-preventable diseases, increases in parental vaccine hesitancy and refusal, and the 2014–2016 Ebola and Zika outbreaks have demonstrated the value and importance of a comprehensive and sustained examination of vaccine ethics and policy. Such an approach holds the potential to offer important insights into all aspects of the vaccine life cycle, from the earliest stages of research through deployment in national and global immunization programs. Below we identify critical moments in the life of a vaccination program and other prominent topics in contemporary vaccination policy. Multiple perspectives on all of these areas and others appear beginning in part II of this volume, following attention to major themes in vaccine history and ethics in part I.

Vaccine Research and Development

The successful development of new discoveries increasingly relies on collaborations among academic scientists, government researchers, small biotechnology firms, and large, multinational vaccine manufacturers. Although financial support for this work has traditionally come from a combination of commercial investment and government-sponsored research awards, philanthropic groups and public–private partnerships have become increasingly active supporters of vaccine development in recent years, particularly for disease targets that lack large potential markets (and thus profitability) in wealthy countries.

Such a diverse group of research entities and funders all but ensures a collection of differing research priorities, objectives, and measures of success. Although all contributors share the general aim of developing safe and effective vaccines, conflicts may arise regarding how best to achieve this goal. Research partnerships become even more ethically complex when they include clinical research in developing countries.

Vaccine development can never be immune from the twin pressures of personal advancement and corporate profitability. Nevertheless, the world community is best served by vaccine research programs that match these concerns with a continued acknowledgment of the enormous suffering that can be averted by vaccines and respect for the individuals and communities volunteering to assist in clinical research. Topics related to priority setting, research collaborations, and the design and conduct of vaccine clinical trials are examined in part II.

Vaccine Regulation and Safety

Vaccines are subject to oversight and regulation by a variety of entities in every country where they are available. It is initially determined whether a new vaccine should be licensed, and if so, the populations for whom it should be recommended. In the United States, these responsibilities belong to groups within the Food and Drug Administration (FDA) and the Centers for Disease Control and Prevention (CDC), respectively. For the life of the vaccine thereafter, activities are undertaken by these groups in collaboration with its manufacturer to monitor its safety and efficacy. These processes have generated considerable controversy in recent years, threatening public confidence in vaccination. Because the success of vaccination programs depends on earning and maintaining public trust, there are several points at which ethical considerations are relevant to regulation.

A primary concern of critics of vaccine policy in the United States is the potential for conflicts of interest among government advisors and researchers who have ties, financial or otherwise, to vaccine manufacturers. Most advisory bodies have clear policies regarding the disclosure of potential conflicts of interest.[2,3] Even when confident that financial relationships would have no impact on their actions, all those participating in vaccine policymaking need to remain highly attentive to how such interests might affect the manner in which the decisions to which they contribute may be perceived. Transparency, minimization of personal gain, divestiture, and disclosure are crucial principles that work to counteract the perception of conflict of interest influencing decision making.

Public attention to conflicts of interest among policymakers and their expert advisors is often linked to reports of vaccine safety concerns. With a majority of vaccinations in the United States and other countries recommended for children in the first 24 months of life, vaccine recipients are typically among the most ethically vulnerable of populations. Attention by vaccine stakeholders to vaccine-related risks, whether confirmed or alleged, is understandably heightened with respect to children, as is the importance of the potential benefits of routine, on-time vaccination. While striving to make decisions that are in a child's best interests, parents and guardians must navigate a sea of at times conflicting information related not only to vaccines, but also to all aspects of their child's medical care.[4-6] Widely publicized claims by critics of vaccines questioning the safety and value of vaccinations have added to the challenges faced by parents striving to make responsible and informed decisions about their children's health.

The public health and regulatory communities should respond vigorously to reports of vaccine-associated adverse events, even if they initially seem unlikely. Even when evidence suggests that a reported safety concern is unfounded, experience has shown it is unlikely that any such assurance will allay the worries of all. This has been readily apparent in the context of alleged but unsupported allegations linking childhood vaccines with autism since the 1990s. Open, expeditious, and objective examinations of possible vaccine-associated safety concerns are widely viewed as essential to maintaining overall confidence in vaccination programs and their oversight. The authors of chapters in part III consider these and related topics in vaccine regulation and safety monitoring activities.

Vaccination Requirements and Vaccine Hesitancy
Governments worldwide use a variety of approaches to promote high vaccination rates among their citizens. The United States is generally unique in its reliance on federal recommendations coupled with state school-entry vaccination requirements as central contributors to the success of vaccination efforts. Although specific requirements vary among states, all require that children receive a series of vaccinations as a condition of attending public schools or state-licensed day-care facilities. Every state allows for exemptions based on medical grounds, and most also accept religious or philosophical reasons, although not every state includes all three.

The often heated debate over vaccination school entry requirements in the United States reflects not only the common tension in public health policy between individual (or parental) autonomy and the public good but also questions over the role and scope of government intervention to protect the well-being of children. Requirements promote vaccination for individual children while also striving to limit the potential transmission of diseases among communities. School-entry requirements have long been seen by public health officials as essential to maintaining vaccination rates sufficiently high to preserve herd protection, particularly when other vaccine education and promotion efforts have failed.[7] The high vaccination rates associated with herd protection offer benefits against vaccine-preventable diseases to all members of a community, including those too young to receive vaccines, those unable to do so because of medical contraindications, and those who were vaccinated but did not generate a sufficient immune response to confer personal protection.

For those whose views on medical ethics are guided by the primacy of patient autonomy, it is understandable why U.S. vaccination requirements are so contentious. However, few ethical models place autonomy absolutely above all other considerations. Instead, respect for autonomy is typically one of several factors that shape ethical deliberation and decision making. There is a compelling argument that the lives saved and suffering prevented by vaccination outweigh the potential infringement on personal autonomy created by school vaccination requirements, as several authors of chapters in part IV propose.

A related issue is how physicians and other healthcare providers should respond to parents who desire an alternate approach to vaccination than the evidence-based recommendations developed by public health and medical authorities, such as adhering to the schedule in the United States developed by the CDC, the American Academy of Pediatrics (AAP), and other medical professional organizations. At issue has been whether physicians should decline to care for children whose parents wish to delay or omit some or all recommended vaccines. Advocates of this view believe it would clearly signal physicians' unambiguous position on the importance of on-time vaccination, and it would reduce the theoretical risk unvaccinated children pose to other patients in waiting rooms. Critics, including the AAP in a longstanding policy statement included in part IV, believe such dismissal of patients in this context should be reserved for very rare circumstances when conflicts between the views of the physician and parents present a profound impediment to the provision of care to the child.

Vaccines, Pandemics, and Bioterrorism

Concerns about anthrax or smallpox bioterror attacks in the aftermath of September 11, 2001; preparedness efforts in the early 2000s for an avian influenza pandemic coupled with the subsequent pandemic caused by a novel strain of H1N1 influenza in 2009–2010; and a series of emerging or reemerging infectious diseases including SARS, Zika, and Ebola have all called attention to the critical role that the development and deployment of vaccines can play in responding to public health and global health emergencies.

The 2009–2010 H1N1 influenza pandemic and vaccination program provided a real-time test of global preparedness and planning for a potential influenza pandemic.

Despite having overall impacts well below some of the most dire forecasts, it was still a significant cause of infection, illness, and death worldwide, particularly among children. The flu pandemic thereby provided valuable knowledge and experience that should inform subsequent planning and response activities for public health emergencies for which vaccines may be available, including potential pandemics and acts of bioterrorism.

As demonstrated in 2009, the urgency that follows the arrival of public health threats makes thoughtful discussion of these topics in real-time all but impossible, making it all the more important to engage in public deliberation and planning well in advance of public health emergencies. In particular, it is necessary to achieve and maintain public consensus on the rules that will govern allocation and rationing of vaccines and other related scarce resources. Unless the rules are widely perceived as fair—arrived at by reasonable, open procedures—and just—helping persons at greatest risk while maximizing the public good—response plans are highly unlikely to gain acceptance. The role of vaccines in planning for and responding to pandemics and bioterrorism and some of the ethical and policy questions they raise is the focus of part V.

Global Vaccination and Eradication Programs

Special ethical considerations related to vaccines in the developing world extend beyond the research issues discussed previously. A particular challenge is ensuring that new vaccines are available against diseases that are most prevalent or most severe in those nations but uncommon or mild in wealthy countries. Owing to the limited profitability of vaccines against such diseases, manufacturers are often reluctant to invest in these efforts, with occasional exceptions when potential connections exist to national security or biodefense.[8] Much of the remaining work, at both early and late stages of development, is therefore supported by private philanthropies, nonprofit entities, and public–private partnerships.

In addition to pursuing the development of new vaccines that hold particular potential for citizens in developing countries, concurrent efforts underway seek to use available vaccines to reduce or even eliminate other diseases. The successful eradication of smallpox in the 1970s generated enthusiasm for other eradication campaigns against vaccine-preventable diseases. This enthusiasm has continued despite as yet insurmountable challenges in adding additional human diseases to the list of those eradicated.

In recent years, most attention in this area has been directed toward the potential eradication of polio, a goal that has seemed tantalizingly close to proponents of eradication for many years but has encountered many setbacks and challenges. A debate over the wisdom of the continued pursuit of polio eradication has emerged among scientists, ethicists, and global health scholars. The symbolic significance of disease eradication carries an allure that may not necessarily coincide with evidence-based approaches to global health policy, critics of ongoing eradication activities suggest. Because global health resources are limited, policymakers and funding sources should ensure that attention is directed to the prevention and treatment strategies that will prevent the most suffering and thereby do the most good, whether those strategies include eradication efforts or other priorities. Part VI of this volume focuses on general issues in global vaccination activities and specific questions related to disease eradication programs of the past, present, and future.

The Future of Vaccination Ethics and Policy

Despite the challenges, questions, and ethical and policy debates raised throughout this volume, the current state of global vaccination programs is extremely strong, and its future is bright. Some of the most promising directions in vaccination science and technology are discussed in part VII. Ongoing, proactive attention to issues emerging from their development and, looking ahead, to their potential introduction can only be helpful as these and other new directions are pursued.

Throughout its long and remarkably successful history, advances in vaccination have been attributable to gains in scientific knowledge, breakthroughs in research, and the creation of sound public health policy, among many other factors. Ultimately, however, the success of vaccination depends on maintaining widespread public trust in the value, safety, and importance of vaccines and confidence in the policymakers, health officials, and healthcare providers overseeing and recommending them. Without this foundation of trust, vaccination programs cannot succeed.[9] Despite the concerns of a small but vocal minority of vaccine critics and opponents, this trust remains intact, as reflected in the overwhelming majority of parents in the United States who choose to vaccinate their children on time and long before any school vaccination requirements would apply.[10]

Preserving trust in vaccines in the United States and internationally requires an unwavering awareness that the remarkable societal benefits of vaccination ultimately involve individuals who are entitled to respect, in a broad sense, that manifests itself at every point in the vaccine life cycle. By remaining sensitive and responsive to the consideration of ethical challenges throughout vaccination policy and the design and implementation of vaccination programs, vaccines will be best positioned to add to their impressive history of public health triumphs.

This volume has its origins in a small working group on the ethics of vaccines created in 2005 at the University of Pennsylvania Center for Bioethics. What was envisioned as a short-term inquiry into a topic that at the time had received almost no attention in bioethics quickly grew into a much broader project, and it has remained a primary research interest of both of us throughout the past 11 years. We are fortunate to have worked with and learned from national and international leaders in vaccine science and policy, many of whom are authors of chapters included in this volume.

We are also grateful to our students, first at the University of Pennsylvania and more recently at New York University, Princeton University, and Yale University. Our courses on vaccination ethics and policy provided us with valuable insights on all of the topics explored here, as well as "field-testing" to help identify the specific issues and papers best suited to this volume. We extend particular gratitude to the Greenwall Foundation and their former president, the late William Stubing, for project and research funding that supported the early development of this book. We also thank William Berkley, chair of the New York University Board of Trustees, for his generous support of vaccine policy programs at NYU and Clay Morgan and Philip Laughlin, our editors at the MIT Press, for their belief in the importance of this project and their patience throughout the development of this volume. Finally, we thank our spouses, Margaret Andrews and Meg Caplan, for their boundless love and support.

Notes

1. Portions of this introduction have been adapted from Arthur L. Caplan and Jason L. Schwartz. Forthcoming 2017. "Ethics," In Plotkin SA, Orenstein WA, Offit PA, Edwards K (eds.) *Vaccines, 7th ed.* Philadelphia, PA: Saunders.

2. United States Office of Government Ethics. *Special Government Employees.* Available at: http://www.oge.gov/Topics/Selected-Employee-Categories/Special-Government-Employees/. Accessed February 2, 2016.

3. Department of Health and Human Services Office of Inspector General. *CDC's Ethics Program for Special Government Employees on Federal Advisory Committees.* Available at: https://oig.hhs.gov/oei/reports/oei-04-07-00260.pdf. Accessed February 2, 2016.

4. Schwartz, Jason L., and Arthur L. Caplan. 2011. Vaccination Refusal: Ethics, Individual Rights, and the Common Good. *Primary Care* 38:717–728.

5. Serpell, Lucy, and John Green. 2006. Parental Decision-Making in Childhood Vaccination. *Vaccine* 24:4041–4046.

6. Davis, Terry C., Doren D. Fredrickson, Connie L. Arnold, et al. 2001. Childhood Vaccine Risk/ benefit Communication in Private Practice Office Settings: A National Survey. *Pediatrics* 107:17–28.

7. Malone, Kevin M., and Alan R. Hinman. 2007. Vaccination Mandates: The Public Health Imperative and Individual Rights. In *Law in Public Health Practice*. 2nd ed., ed. R. A. Goodman, R. E. Hoffman, W. Lopez, et al., 338–360. Oxford, England: Oxford University Press.

8. Batson, Amie. 2005. The Problems and Promise of Vaccine Markets in Developing Countries. *Health Affairs* 24:690–693.

9. Schwartz, Jason L. 2009. Unintended Consequences: The Primacy of Public Trust in Vaccination. *Michigan Law Review* 107:100–104.

10. Hill, Holly A., Laurie D. Elam-Evans, David Yankey, et al. 2015. National, State, and Selected Local Area Vaccination Coverage Among Children Aged 19–35 Months — United States, 2014. *Morbidity and Mortality Weekly Report* 64 (33): 889–896.

I   Enduring Themes in Vaccination History and Ethics

Attention to vaccines and vaccination programs typically focuses on their many novel characteristics. New vaccines, new evidence regarding their benefits and risks, new allegations concerning vaccine safety, new policies under consideration by lawmakers, and newly emerging diseases for which vaccines may contribute to response efforts typically dominate popular and media discussions of vaccination.

Despite so much novelty, contemporary vaccination activities reflect their rich, remarkable, and at times controversial history—more than 200 years of programs, advances, and debates in science, public health, policy, law, and ethics. Questions such as how governments can and should promote the development and use of vaccines, what obligations—moral, legal, or otherwise—individuals have to accept vaccination for themselves or their children, and what responsibilities citizens, corporations, and governments have to support global vaccination efforts have been present (and often contested) throughout this history. These timeless questions have undoubtedly been amplified since the 1960s, and especially in the past few decades, by increased attention and investment in vaccination efforts from public and private sources and by scientific advances that have greatly expanded the vaccination toolkit.

We begin with several chapters that explore the historical foundations that underlie contemporary vaccination efforts and the tightly interwoven issues of science, policy, law, and ethics that vaccination has raised throughout its long history and continues to do today. Alexandra Minna Stern and Howard Markel offer a concise account of the history of vaccination, mapping throughout their discussion the many continuities between earlier chapters of vaccine history and present-day concerns. James Colgrove looks at efforts to promote vaccination in the United States from the nineteenth century to the present, tracing how public health advocates have employed numerous strategies and faced even more challenges in their efforts to introduce new vaccines as broadly as possible. Gregory Poland and Robert Jacobson reflect on past and present-day "antivaccinationists," implicitly rejecting in their analysis the efforts of vocal opponents of contemporary vaccination policy to distance themselves from this characterization. Finally, Chris Feudtner and Edgar Marcuse provide a framework intended to assist in the evaluation of contested ethical and policy considerations by policymakers and diverse groups of professionals and citizens.

Together, these readings remind us from the outset that vaccination efforts since their inception in the late eighteenth century have invariably both shaped and been shaped by larger scientific developments, political forces, cultural considerations, and perennial ethical and religious debates. The implications of these relationships in specific cases, in specific locations, and at specific times will be evident throughout this volume.

Further Reading

Allen, Arthur. 2007. *Vaccine: The Controversial Story of Medicine's Greatest Lifesaver*. New York: W.W. Norton & Company.

Biss, Eula. 2014. *On Immunity: An Inoculation*. Minneapolis, MN: Graywolf Press.

Colgrove, James. 2006. *State of Immunity: The Politics of Vaccination in Twentieth-Century America*. Berkeley, CA: University of California Press / Milbank Memorial Fund.

Conis, Elena. 2015. *Vaccine Nation: America's Changing Relationship with Immunization*. Chicago: University of Chicago Press.

Kass, Nancy. 2001. An Ethics Framework for Public Health. *American Journal of Public Health* 91 (11): 1776–1782.

1   The History of Vaccines and Immunization: Familiar Patterns, New Challenges

Alexandra Minna Stern and Howard Markel[*]

Human beings have benefited from vaccines for more than two centuries. Yet the pathway to effective vaccines has been neither neat nor direct. This chapter explores the history of vaccines and immunization, beginning with Edward Jenner's creation of the world's first vaccine for smallpox in the 1790s. We then demonstrate that many of the issues salient in Jenner's era—such as the need for secure funding mechanisms, streamlined manufacturing and safety concerns, and deep-seated public fears of inoculating agents—have frequently reappeared and have often dominated vaccine policies. We suggest that historical awareness can help inform viable long-term solutions to contemporary problems with vaccine research, production, and supply.

If we could match the enormous scientific strides of the twentieth century with the political and economic investments of the nineteenth, the world's citizens might be much healthier.

The gasping breath and distinctive sounds of whooping cough, the iron lungs and braces designed for children paralyzed by polio, and the devastating birth defects caused by rubella: To most Americans, these infectious scourges simultaneously inspire dread and represent obscure maladies of years past. Yet a little more than a century ago, the U.S. infant mortality rate was a staggering 20%, and the childhood mortality rate before age five was another disconcerting 20%.[1] Not surprisingly, in an epoch before the existence of preventive methods and effective therapies, infectious diseases such as measles, diphtheria, smallpox, and pertussis topped the list of childhood killers. Fortunately, many of these devastating diseases have been contained, especially in industrialized nations, because of the development and widespread distribution of safe, effective, and affordable vaccines.

* Copyrighted and published by Project HOPE/*Health Affairs* as: Alexandra Minna Stern and Howard Markel. 2005. The history of vaccines and immunization: Familiar patterns, new challenges. *Health Affairs* 24 (3):611–621. The published article is archived and available online at www.healthaffairs.org.

Indeed, if you asked a public health professional to draw up a top-ten list of the achievements of the past century, he or she would be hard pressed not to rank immunization first.[2] Millions of lives have been saved and microbes stopped in their tracks before they could have a chance to wreak havoc. In short, the vaccine represents the single greatest promise of biomedicine: disease prevention.[3]

Nevertheless, the story is more complicated than it might appear at first glance. Even as existing vaccines continue to exert their immunological power and new vaccines offer similar hopes, reemerging and newly emerging infectious diseases threaten the dramatic progress made. Furthermore, obstacles have long stood in the way of the production of safe and effective vaccines. The historical record shows that the development of vaccines has consistently involved sizable doses of ingenuity, political skill, and irreproachable scientific methods. When one or more of these has been lacking or perceived to be lacking, vaccination has engendered responses ranging from a revised experimental approach in the laboratory to a supply shortage and even insurrection in the streets. In short, vaccines are powerful medical interventions that induce powerful biological, social, and cultural reactions.

Edward Jenner, Cowpox, and Smallpox Vaccination

We begin our history of vaccines and immunization with the story of Edward Jenner, a country doctor living in Berkeley (Gloucestershire), England, who in 1796 performed the world's first vaccination.[4] Taking pus from a cowpox lesion on a milkmaid's hand, Jenner inoculated an eight-year-old boy, James Phipps. Six weeks later, Jenner variolated two sites on Phipps's arm with smallpox, yet the boy was unaffected by this as well as subsequent exposures.[5] Based on twelve such experiments and sixteen additional case histories he had collected since the 1770s, Jenner published at his own expense a volume that swiftly became a classic text in the annals of medicine: *Inquiry into the Causes and Effects of the Variolae Vaccine*. His assertion "that the cowpox protects the human constitution from the infection of smallpox" laid the foundation for modern vaccinology.[6]

How did Jenner, a country doctor, formulate the vaccine concept? To begin with, his discovery relied extensively on knowledge of the local customs of farming communities and the awareness that milkmaids infected with cowpox, visible as pustules on the hand or forearm, were immune to subsequent outbreaks of smallpox that periodically swept through the area. Moreover, a learned man immersed in the secular and rational doctrines of the Enlightenment, Jenner applied the scientific methods of observation and experimentation to this parochial wisdom, ultimately conducting one of the world's first clinical trials. He thus was able to devise an alternative to variolation (the controlled transfer of pus from one person's active smallpox lesion to another person's arm, usually subcutaneously with a lancet), which had been practiced in Asia since the 1600s and in Europe and colonial America since the early 1700s.[7]

Jenner also profited from his training as a wide-ranging generalist with a broad knowledge of science and medicine. For example, before devoting himself to private practice, Jenner focused on natural history, penning well-respected studies of the cuckoo and the dormouse.[8] In fact, Jenner was so skilled a naturalist that he was invited (although he declined) to join Captain Cook's second voyage to the South Seas to classify flora and fauna.

Jenner's interest in natural history and animal biology sharpened his medical understanding of the role of human–animal transspecies boundaries in disease transmission. He experienced the proverbial "Eureka"-like moment sometime during the 1770s, after hearing a Bristol milkmaid boast, "I shall never have smallpox for I have had cowpox. I shall never have an ugly pockmarked face."[9] Two decades later, he translated that farming lore into the guiding principle of his cowpox inoculation hypothesis. His cognizance that animals were implicated and necessary for vaccine production was truly prescient; it foreshadowed later use of cows, guinea pigs, rabbits, and even chicken eggs in vaccine production. However, this breach of the species barrier also made many people wary of and sometimes hostile to the idea of consciously introducing foreign animal products into their own bodies. During the early 1800s, for example, there was no shortage of cartoons mocking Jenner and depicting the transmogrification of the recently vaccinated into sickly cows and fantastical beasts.[10]

Beyond Cowpox

Although Jenner's milkmaid experiments may now seem like quaint fables, they provided the scientific basis for vaccinology. This is all the more striking given that our current conceptions of vaccine development and therapy are now much more encompassing and firmly rooted in the science of immunology. Until the brilliant French chemist Louis Pasteur developed what he called a rabies vaccine in 1885, vaccines referred only to cowpox inoculation for smallpox. Although what Pasteur actually produced was a rabies antitoxin that functioned as a postinfection antidote only because of the long incubation period of the rabies germ, he expanded the term beyond its Latin association with cows and cowpox to include all inoculating agents.[11] Thus, we largely have Pasteur to thank for today's definition of vaccine as a "suspension of live (usually attenuated) or inactivated microorganisms (e.g., bacteria or viruses) or fractions thereof administered to induce immunity and prevent infectious disease or its sequelae."[12]

Changing Terminology, Constant Challenges

Although vaccination and immunization are often used interchangeably, especially in nonmedical parlance, the latter is a more inclusive term because it implies that the administration of an immunologic agent actually results in the development of adequate immunity.

As the definitions of vaccine, vaccination, and immunization have changed over time, becoming more scientifically precise, many of the basic patterns and problems of vaccinology have remained constant. In particular, issues of funding have been central to the steady development and distribution of vaccines, as have concerns with contamination and safety. Furthermore, public reactions to vaccines are usually quite strong, even as they have varied from awe of a seeming scientific miracle to skepticism and outright hostility. Beyond the far-reaching microbiological and immunological discoveries that have transformed vaccinology over the past century, vaccinology has been shaped increasingly by regulations governing human-subjects research and the enforcement of sterilization and safety standards. Especially after World War II, as exemplified by the exacting standards demanded by Thomas Francis Jr. in the polio field trials of 1954, the ethical design and execution of vaccine research has become a core concern for many stakeholders.[13]

Funding and Patronage

As acceptance of his discoveries grew, Jenner was praised and feted by the British aristocracy and quickly became a celebrity in the cosmopolitan town of Cheltenham, where he had moved his family in the 1790s.[14] In the first decades of the nineteenth century, the British Parliament awarded Jenner the equivalent of more than a million dollars in today's currency, and Oxford, Cambridge, and Harvard Universities, as well as many scientific societies, bestowed honors on him.[15]

As Jenner became a celebrated figure across Europe, "Jennerian inoculation" became the sine qua non for burgeoning national health programs. Kings and presidents seized on mass-scale vaccination campaigns in an effort to demonstrate their forward-looking stance toward science and their commitment to the health of their citizenry. By 1800, for instance, 100,000 people had been vaccinated in Europe, and vaccination had begun in the United States, spearheaded by Harvard professor Benjamin Waterhouse and President Thomas Jefferson.[16] From Spain, King Charles IV sent the

Balmis Expedition to the Americas in 1803 to introduce smallpox vaccination to its colonies. Before disembarking on the Royal Expedition of the Vaccine, Francisco Xavier de Balmis rounded up five Madrid orphans for the voyage. They served as an arm-to-arm transfer chain to keep the vaccine fresh until they arrived at the Caribbean.[17]

International Investment

Since Jenner's discovery, governments have often invested, albeit unevenly and incompletely, in vaccines. Initially vaccines were considered a matter of national pride and prestige. They quickly became integral to utilitarian and public health notions of societal security, productivity, and protection. In Europe and North America during the nineteenth century, for instance, smallpox vaccination was made compulsory under state laws. In the twentieth century, as the standard battery of childhood immunizations, including diphtheria, measles, mumps, and rubella, was developed, vaccination was frequently managed or adjudicated by governmental entities (from the municipal to the federal) and eventually was required for public school attendance.

After the founding of the World Health Organization (WHO) and related organizations such as the United Nations Children's Fund (UNICEF), vaccine programs went global. In 1974, for example, the WHO launched the Expanded Programme on Immunization (EPI), with the goal of dramatically increasing vaccination rates among children in developing countries. For more than three decades, the EPI has functioned through the WHO's regional offices to meet target immunization rates for almost every disease with a corresponding immunologic agent.[18] Perhaps the WHO's most spectacular achievement was the smallpox campaign of the 1960s and 1970s. Directed by Donald Henderson, this massive effort culminated in the last naturally occurring case of smallpox in Somalia in 1977.[19] Today, this example of success serves as a beacon of encouragement for international health workers involved in ongoing and challenging immunization campaigns against polio, measles, and other diseases. For more than fifty years, similar efforts—both immunization campaigns and vaccine trials—have been supported by global health organizations and major philanthropies such as the Rockefeller Foundation and the Bill and Melinda Gates Foundation.[20]

Ironically, as vaccines have become more commonplace, they have lost some of their allure, particularly to public funding agencies. One might argue that vaccines have worked so well that many people now take them for granted. In this sense, scientific success has paradoxically contributed to the current problems with adequate funding mechanisms. In a similar twist, the triumph of the polio vaccine in 1955 fostered the idea that it was possible to obtain sufficient funding without the primary support of government, instead relying on contributions from philanthropic groups (the National Foundation for Infantile Paralysis or March of Dimes) and the pocket-books of millions of Americans.[21]

Financial and Regulatory Barriers

Ideally, the migration of vaccine production away from governmental entities, as seen in the nineteenth century, and increasingly into commercial hands could result in the positive benefits of competition, superior production, and lower cost.[22] Sadly, this has not been the case. Today, many pharmaceutical companies avoid the vaccine business because it is economically prohibitive and encumbered by regulatory barriers.[23] For example, in 1998, Warner Lambert (now Pfizer) stopped making Fluogen vaccine for influenza because of regulatory obstacles and financial loss. It sold its Fluogen factory to King Pharmaceuticals, which soon threw in the towel after determining that bring-ing its new plant into federal compliance was too costly. Clearly, this pattern greatly contributed to the Fall 2004 flu vaccine shortage in the United States.[24] The situation is similar for the ten basic childhood vaccines, the majority of which, including mea-sles-mumps-rubella (MMR) and chickenpox vaccines, are manufactured by just one company.[25]

The critical questions to ask are: If this company experiences a business or sud-den production failure, how would we vaccinate millions of American children? What backup plans do we have in case of such an event? To avoid this scenario, in 2003, the National Vaccine Advisory Committee listed an increase in funds for vaccine stockpiles at the top of its list of recommendations.[26] Nevertheless, capital infusions have not been immediately forthcoming from either the public or private sector. Given our cur-rent predicament, we could learn a great deal from the enthusiastic financial support granted to Jenner and early smallpox vaccination efforts. Although royal patronage is no longer an option, financial incentives, whether through tax relief or guaranteed purchase, may be needed to ensure an adequate and steady vaccine supply.

Manufacture, Distribution, and Safety

Jenner's initial experiments were carried out in a pre-germ theory era that lacked mod-ern methods of quality control and sterilization. Hence, the prospect of contamination constantly loomed over smallpox vaccine development, and many people were rightly wary of contracting another dreaded disease via inoculation. With a method that often involved extracting lymph from pustules on the arms of those recently vaccinated, it was not uncommon for existing microorganisms to accompany the vaccine from arm to arm, spreading diseases such as erysipelas, syphilis, and scrofula.[27]

Unlike most drugs, which are essentially chemical agents, vaccines are biologic agents that can be compromised during processing. Whether killed-virus, whole-cell, bacterial, or live-attenuated, vaccines can be disrupted at various points along the journey from the laboratory to the vial. Not surprisingly, quality control, sterilization, and monitoring have become non-negotiable for vaccine production. Even with strict standards, however, the possibility of contamination remains (although it is far less likely today than several decades ago). In addition, vaccine production must be closely supervised to ensure that vaccines induce immunity and do not produce serious infection. For example, the optimism about the polio vaccine in Spring 1955 was temporarily muted after 200 children contracted the disease (fatal for five children) from a vaccine containing active wild-type polio virus that was manufactured by Cutter Laboratories in California.[28]

Debates over virulence, killed versus live virus, and antigenic strains have played a critical role in setting the parameters of the production and manufacture of safe and effective vaccines for more than 100 years. The controversy between Jonas Salk, who advocated a killed polio vaccine, and Albert Sabin, who preferred a live polio vaccine, characterizes this divide, although there are many more examples.[29] For instance, as measles immunization was becoming widely accepted in the United States in the 1960s, a formalin-inactivated vaccine licensed in 1963 was withdrawn because it induced short-lived immunity and predisposed recipients to atypical measles syndrome if they were exposed to the wild-type measles virus. Ultimately, safe and reliable vaccines were developed from the original Edmonston B strain (initially isolated by John Enders and Thomas Peebles in human and monkey cell cultures in 1954).[30] One of these attenuated vaccines, the Moraten strain, is the only measles vaccine used in the United States today, while two additional strains—the Schwarz and Edmonston-Zagreb—are employed in worldwide immunization campaigns against a disease that infects approximately thirty million children per year, killing approximately 750,000 of them.[31] In the case of bacillus Calmette-Guérin (BCG) vaccination against tuberculosis, developed in France in 1921, concerns about efficacy and safety led to different patterns of vaccine acceptance. In Scandinavia, BCG was mass-distributed as part of the emergence of a comprehensive social welfare program. Conversely, in the United States and Britain, acceptance was much slower because of greater confidence in the long-term benefits of tuberculosis testing and treatment and apprehension that mass BCG vaccination might misconstrue the results of mass-scale tuberculin Mantoux purified protein derivative (PPD) testing by delivering large numbers of false positives.[32]

Protesting Vaccines

Especially in the 1830s, after an initial generation had been vaccinated and the incidence of smallpox had declined markedly in the United States and Europe, a vociferous antivaccination movement emerged.[33] Sometimes antivaccinationists were protesting what they considered the intrusion of their privacy and bodily integrity. Many working-class Britons, for example, viewed compulsory vaccination laws, passed in 1821, as a direct government assault on their communities by the ruling class.[34] In addition, by the mid-eighteenth century, the rise of irregular medicine and unabashed quackery encouraged antivaccinationism. For instance, irregulars generally viewed vaccination as a destructive and potentially defiling procedure of heroic medicine, akin to blood-letting.[35] In addition, antivivisectionists, who abhorred animal experimentation, sometimes joined forces with antivaccinationists.[36]

To a great extent, nation-states responded by articulating that they possessed the right to immunize for the "common good." In 1905, for example, the U.S. Supreme Court ruled in Jacobson v. Massachusetts that the need to protect the public health through compulsory smallpox vaccination outweighed the individual's right to privacy.[37] Barring exceptions for personal beliefs, which exist in all but three U.S. states, this tenet has been consistently reiterated and is lent scientific muster by the concept of "herd immunity," whereby a certain target of the population—approximately 85%–95%, depending on the disease—must be immunized for protection to be conferred on the entire group.[38]

Until quite recently, historical studies frequently depicted all antivaccinationists as irrational and antiscientific. This characterization was misguided. If we interpret antivaccinationists on their own terms and by applying historical context, we can see that many behaved as rational actors who were weighing the pros and cons of inoculation. Although nineteenth-century fears of vaccination might have been based on anecdotal horror stories of other infections, the statistical risks of vaccine-induced infection from that era would not be medically acceptable today.

In addition, many vaccine critics do not reject immunization outright but instead emphasize issues of safety and efficacy or are opposed to specific, but not necessarily all, vaccines. The passage of the 1986 National Childhood Vaccine Injury Act (NCVIA), spearheaded by parents troubled by a putative link between vaccination and neurological problems, illustrates that legislators and scientists alike continue to be exceedingly concerned with the issue of vaccine safety.[39] In the past decade in particular, parents and their watchdog groups have raised important questions about the purported link between a noticeable rise in autism and the preservative thimerosal (previously used in diphtheria, tetanus, pertussis, *Hemophilus influenzae* type b, or Hib, and hepatitis B vaccines). Although a series of scientific studies have demonstrated that there is no causal connection between thimerosal and autism, in 1999, the U.S. Food and Drug Administration (FDA), in conjunction with the U.S. Public Health Service and the American Academy of Pediatrics, ceased to license thimerosal-containing vaccines. Similar claims about a causal link between MMR and autism have also been alleged and sometimes sensationalized by the media. Not surprisingly, the suggestion that vaccinating one's child might lead to developmental disorders has fostered unease among many parents. Clearly, American parents need better access to and clearer explanations of the recent findings published in medical journals that confirm the lack of a link between thimerosal or MMR and autism or other neurological conditions.[40] However, as indicated by recent political and medical debates about the need for Americans, especially first responders, to be vaccinated against smallpox in case of a bioterrorism attack, and the hundreds of Gulf War soldiers who have rejected anthrax vaccinations, antivaccinationism will not fade away any time soon.

Elusive Vaccines and the Ethics of Vaccine Research

It took more than eighty years after Jenner's discovery for scientists to develop new vaccines. With the bacteriological revolution, which began in the 1880s, came high hopes that the identification of specific disease-causing microbes would lead directly to the development of specific inoculating agents. Although spectacular vaccines have been produced since that time, changing the course of human history, vaccines for many diseases remain elusive.

Malaria

One of the most frustrating quests has been for a malaria vaccine. The most common parasites responsible for malaria (plasmodia) have demonstrated an impressive ability to circumvent eradication efforts by becoming drug-resistant. The fact that the WHO recently announced that it was exceedingly pleased with a new vaccine that protects just 30% of those immunized indicates the immense difficulty of producing a malaria vaccine. Although this percentage is low compared with other vaccines, given the severity of malaria worldwide and the fact that it kills more than one million and infects more than 300 million children a year, even such limited coverage could save thousands if not millions of lives in the hardest-hit areas of the globe.[41]

HIV

No discussion of vaccines is complete without assessing the potential of an HIV vaccine in the twenty-first century. Like plasmodium, the HIV retrovirus is a wily and insidious microbe. Most attempts to develop an HIV vaccine have ended in failure. Recently, the Gates Foundation launched an initiative aimed to develop and eventually distribute effective TB and HIV vaccines.[42] As with other global health endeavors, there are crucial cultural and ethical questions to consider.[43] Because some of the most promising vaccines are being tested on vulnerable and impoverished populations in sub-Saharan Africa, organizations such as the HIV Vaccine Trials Network (HVTN) and the International AIDS Vaccine Initiative (IAVI) emphasize the importance of heeding the ethical guidelines promulgated in documents such as the 1947 Nuremberg Code and 1979 Belmont Report.[44] In this sense, immunization has been deeply affected by changing historical contexts and norms; especially since the 1970s, it has not been possible to launch vaccine trials and campaigns involving human subjects without clear-cut protections against human experimentation and medical abuse.

Lessons Learned

Our struggle with germs is endless and can be neither completely halted nor assuaged by vaccines, no matter how great their immunological power. Sadly, effective vaccines for two of the world's leading killers, HIV and malaria, remain in the research stage. Furthermore, even the most knowledgeable scientist cannot precisely predict the strain of next year's influenza, nor can an expert epidemiologist always explain why certain diseases rise and burn out at particular rates. Molecular biology, genomics, and proteomics will certainly reveal a great deal about similar antigens and foster the development of vaccines through cellular manipulation rather than animal experimentation.

Nevertheless, this historical overview of vaccines and immunization since Jenner's great cowpox discovery suggests we can anticipate several of the key issues that could hinder and complicate the future of vaccinology. Clearly, without adequate funding and fluid funding mechanisms, vaccine shortages will persist, and lives throughout the world will remain at risk. Closely linked are the issues of vaccine safety and the strict maintenance of sterilization standards. Even as these have improved greatly over time, the fact that vaccines are biological agents often makes them much more difficult than drugs to produce. Jenner and his peers faced this problem, and history has shown that the production of safe, efficacious vaccines will require persistent vigilance. Although antivaccinationists are still often portrayed as an annoying thorn in the side of medical progress, their concerns for safety and willingness to perform the duty of civic over-sight have had some positive effects, especially in terms of popular health education.

As this chapter has shown, there are important continuities in the history of vac-cines and immunization. There have been shifts as well; unfortunately, one of the most pronounced shifts has been the divestment of public agencies in vaccine research and production. If we could match the enormous scientific strides of the twentieth century with the political and economic investments of the nineteenth century, the world's citizens might be much healthier.

In closing, we suggest that Americans take advantage of the flu shortage hysteria of Fall 2004 to learn from the historical record. We need to transform our anxieties and energies into concrete steps to ensure a comprehensive vaccine supply in 2005 and beyond. It would be exceedingly foolish to squander one of preventive medicine's greatest assets because of a neglected public health system and an inability to ade-quately coordinate market forces and regulatory demands with basic health needs.

References

1. Meckel, R. A. 2004. Levels and Trends of Death and Disease in Childhood, 1620 to the Present. In *Children and Youth in Sickness and Health: A Handbook and Guide*. Ed. J. Golden, R. A. Meckel, and H. M. Prescott, 3–24. Westport, Conn.: Greenwood Press.

2. U.S. Centers for Disease Control and Prevention. Ten Great Public Health Achievements in the Twentieth Century, 1900–1999. Available at: www.cdc.gov/od/oc/media/tengpha.htm. Accessed February 8, 2005.

3. Markel, H. Taking Shots: The Modern Miracle of Vaccines. *Medscape*. Available at: www .medscape.com/viewarticle/481059. Accessed June 23, 2004.

4. Baxby, D. *Jenner's Smallpox Vaccine: The Riddle of Vaccinia Virus and Its Origin*. London: Heine-mann Educational Books, 1981; D. Baxby, *Smallpox Vaccine, Ahead of Its Time*. Berkeley, U.K.: Jenner Museum, 2001; and D. Baxby. *Vaccination: Jenner's Legacy*. Berkeley, U.K.: Jenner Educa-tional Trust, 1994.

5. N. Barquet and P. Domingo. 1997. Smallpox: The Triumph over the Most Terrible of the Min-isters of Death. *Annals of Internal Medicine* 127 (8):635–642.

6. Jenner, E. 1798. *Inquiry into the Causes and Effects of the Variolae Vaccine, 45*. London: Sampson Low.

7. Saunders, P. 2001. *Edward Jenner: The Cheltenham Years, 1795–1823*. Hanover: University Press of New England, 1982; and E. A. Fenn. 2002. *Pox Americana: The Great Smallpox Epidemic of 1775–82*. New York: Hill and Wang.

8. Saunders. *Edward Jenner.*

9. Quoted in Barquet and Domingo, Smallpox, 639.

10. Fulford, T., and D. Lee. 2000. The Jenneration of Disease: Vaccination, Romanticism, and Revolution. *Studies in Romanticism* 39 (1): 139–163.

11. Hansen, B. 1998. America's First Medical Breakthrough: How Popular Excitement about a French Rabies Cure in 1885 Raised New Expectations for Medical Progress. *American Historical Review* 103 (2): 373–418.

12. Advisory Committee on Immunization Practices and the American Academy of Family Physicians. 2002. *General Recommendations on Immunization. Morbidity and Mortality Weekly Report 51* (no. RR02): 34.

13. Lambert, S. M., and H. Markel. 2000. Making History: Thomas Francis Jr., M.D., and the 1954 Salk Poliomyelitis Vaccine Field Trial. *Archives of Pediatrics & Adolescent Medicine* 154 (5): 512–517.

14. Saunders. *Edward Jenner*; and Fulford and Lee. "The Jenneration of Disease."

15. Barquet and Domingo. Smallpox.

16. Ibid.

17. Rigau-Perez, J. G. 1989. The Introduction of Smallpox Vaccine in 1803 and the Adoption of Immunization as a Government Function in Puerto Rico. *Hispanic American Historical Review* 69 (3): 393–423.

18. Henderson, R. H. 1995. Vaccination: Successes and Challenges. In *Vaccination and World Health.* Ed. F. T. Cutts and P. G. Smith, 3–16. Chichester, U.K.: John Wiley and Sons.

19. Henderson, D. A. 1988. Edward Jenner's Vaccine, *Public Health Reports* 112 (2): 116–121; and G. Williams. "WHO—The Days of the Mass Campaigns. *World Health Forum* 9 (1): 7–23.

20. World Health Organization. 2004. Global Polio Eradication Initiative. Available at: www .polioeradication.org. Accessed February 8, 2005.

21. Lambert and Markel. Making History.

22. Galambos, L., with J. E. Sewell. 1995. *Networks of Innovation: Vaccine Development at Merck, Sharp, and Dohme, and Mulford, 1895–1995.* New York: Cambridge University Press.

23. National Vaccine Advisory Committee. 2003. Strengthening the Supply of Routinely Recommended Vaccines in the United States: Recommendations from the National Vaccine Advisory Committee. *Journal of the American Medical Association* 290 (23): 3122–3128.

24. Grady, D. Before Shortage of Flu Vaccine, Many Warnings. *New York Times*, 17 October 2004.

25. Giffin, R., K. Stratton, and R. Chalk. 2004. Childhood Vaccine Finance and Safety Issues. *Health Affairs* 23 (5): 98–111.

26. NVAC. Strengthening the Supply, 3127.

27. Baxby. *Smallpox Vaccine.*

28. Smith, J. S. 1991. *Patenting the Sun: Polio and the Salk Vaccine.* New York: Anchor Books; J. P. Baker. 2000. Immunization and the American Way: Four Childhood Vaccines. *American Journal of Public Health* 90 (2): 199–207; and R. D. Johnston. 2004. Contemporary Anti-Vaccination Movements in Historical Perspective. In *The Politics of Healing: Histories of Alternative Medicine in Twentieth-Century North America*, ed. R. D. Johnston, 259–286. New York: Routledge.

29. Meldrum, M. L. 1999. The Historical Feud over Polio Vaccine: How Could a Killed Vaccine Contain a Natural Disease? *Western Journal of Medicine* 171 (4): 271–273; and A. Chase. 1982. *Magic Shots: A Human and Scientific Account of the Long and Continuing Struggle to Eradicate Infectious Diseases by Vaccination.* New York: William Morrow and Company.

30. Meissner, H. C., P. M. Strebel, and W. A. Orenstein. 2004. Measles Vaccines and the Potential for Worldwide Eradication of Measles; and Baker, "Immunization and the American Way. *Pediatrics* 114 (4): 1065–1069.

31. Meissner et al. Measles Vaccines.

32. Bryder, L. 1999. "We Shall Not Find Salvation in Inoculation": BCG Vaccination in Scandinavia, Britain, and the USA, 1921–1960. *Social Science & Medicine* 49 (9): 1157–1167.

33. Kaufman, M. 1967. The American Anti-Vaccinationists and Their Arguments. *Bulletin of the History of Medicine* 41 (5): 463–478.

34. Durbach, N. 2000. "They Might as Well Brand Us": Working-Class Resistance to Compulsory Vaccination in Victorian England. *Social History of Medicine* 13 (1): 45–62.

35. Kaufman. The American Anti-Vaccinationists.

36. Baker. Immunization and the American Way; and N. Davidovitch. Negotiating Dissent: Homeopathy and Anti-Vaccinationism at the Turn of the Twentieth Century. In *The Politics of Healing*, 11–28.

37. Goodman, R., et al., eds. 2003. *Law in Public Health Practice.* Oxford: Oxford University Press.

38. Ibid.

39. Johnston. Contemporary Anti-Vaccination Movements.

40. Parker, S. K., et al. 2004. Thimerosal-Containing Vaccines and Austistic Spectrum Disorder: A Critical Review of Published Original Data. *Pediatrics* 114 (3): 793–804; N. Andrews et al. 2004. Thimerosal Exposure in Infants and Developmental Disorders: A Retrospective Cohort Study in the United Kingdom Does Not Support a Causal Association. *Pediatrics* 114 (3): 584–591; and M. Meadows. IOM Report: No Link between Vaccines and Autism. *FDA Consumer* 38 (5): 18–19.

41. McNeil, D. G., Jr. Malaria Vaccine Proves Effective. *New York Times*, 15 October 2004.

42. Bill and Melinda Gates Foundation. Global Health. Available at: www.gatesfoundation.org/GlobalHealth. Accessed October 25, 2004.

43. Specter, M. 1997. The Vaccine: Has the Race to Save Africa from AIDS Put Western Science at Odds with Western Ethics? *New Yorker*, February 3, 2003, 54–65; and M. Angell. The Ethics of Clinical Research in the Third World. *New England Journal of Medicine* 337 (12): 847–849.

44. See HIV Vaccine Trials Network. Available at: www.hvtn.org; and International AIDS Vaccine Initiative, www.iavi.org.

2 Immunity for the People: The Challenge of Achieving High Vaccine Coverage in American History

James Colgrove[*]

On June 8, 2006, the U.S. Food and Drug Administration (FDA) licensed Merck's vaccine Gardasil, a product shown in trials to prevent infection with human papillomavirus (HPV), the most common sexually transmitted disease and a leading cause of cervical cancer.[1] Although the vaccine was heralded as a major breakthrough with the potential for significant public health benefits, it also raised difficult policy issues. Its expected price of approximately $360 for a full course of three injections called into question whether it would be accessible to the uninsured. It was recommended to be given to girls at 11 to 12 years of age, a time when many young people have no regular contact with a primary care provider. Some religious conservatives voiced opposition to the vaccine, arguing that offering protection against a sexually transmitted disease would undermine prevention messages that stress abstinence.[2]

The licensing of the HPV vaccine highlights both the successes and challenges of the U.S. immunization system, which is widely regarded as one of the most important public health achievements of the past 100 years. At the same time, however, critical questions have surrounded their use. How can the benefits of immunity be distributed equitably to everyone, especially people of low socioeconomic status who experience disparities in healthcare access and outcomes? Who should bear the costs of vaccination? How should responsibility for promotion and delivery be divided among federal, state, and local health agencies, medical professionals, charitable organizations, and insurers? How should resistance or opposition to vaccines be dealt with?

The urgency of these questions has heightened over the past two decades as a consequence of the success of vaccine research and development. The number of recommended pediatric vaccines doubled from seven to fourteen from 1990 to 2006.

* Originally published in *Public Health Reports*, 2007, Mar–Apr; 122 (2):248–257. Republished with permission of American Schools of Public Health. Permission conveyed through Copyright Clearance Center, Inc.

Although coverage rates for most recommended vaccines are high, there is wide agreement that the system remains vulnerable. As an analysis by three staff members of the Institute of Medicine, a nonprofit research organization that advises the government on health issues, observed, "The United States lacks a comprehensive scientific and policy approach to explore fully the ramifications of the increasing number of vaccines that will soon be available."[3]

At this critical juncture, with increasingly expensive new vaccines either licensed or set to join an already crowded schedule, it is valuable to understand the historic evolution of immunization in the United States. This chapter describes the successive introduction of new vaccines from the early nineteenth century to the present and the efforts of key stakeholders to achieve high levels of use. In particular, I focus on two broad policy areas that have been central to vaccination programs as well as repeated flashpoints for controversy.

First, what are the most effective and ethical ways of achieving high levels of acceptance among people who are indifferent, wary, or antagonistic toward vaccination? It is a widely accepted tenet of public health practice that persuasive approaches are preferable to coercive ones whenever possible. But because the failure to immunize oneself or one's children can contribute to the spread of infectious diseases, the United States has invoked compulsory measures, primarily laws requiring immunization before children may enter school. Whether such laws are appropriate and under what circumstances exemptions to them should be allowed has been the subject of extensive debate and litigation.

Second, what is the proper scope of government activity in paying for and delivering vaccines? The United States has traditionally relied on market mechanisms rather than public sector support for health care, with limited categorical programs providing some services for the poor. Yet vaccination has always fit awkwardly within this paradigm because, unlike other health interventions that benefit the individual, it also carries a societal benefit through the herd immunity it creates. Thus, some observers have analogized immunization to public health responsibilities, such as providing clean water or sewage disposal that are not left to the free market.[4]

The current challenges facing the country's immunization system, this chapter will show, have deep roots in enduring features of American politics and society. Decisions about how to achieve immunity for the people through an increasingly sophisticated and extensive vaccine regimen should be informed by this history.

Vaccination in the Nineteenth Century: Keeping the Pox at Bay

Smallpox was one of history's most feared diseases because of its gruesome symptoms, high fatality rate, and rapid spread. Its symptoms began with chills, aches, and fever; it then progressed ominously to nausea, vomiting, and difficulty breathing. About a week after infection, bright red pustules developed on the victim's face and hands, and then spread to cover the entire body. Eventually, the pustules dried and itched intensely, scabbed over, and fell off. About one out of four victims died; those who survived were usually scarred for life and often blinded. Children, who were generally more vulnerable to infectious disease, died from the condition more often than did adults, but it struck young and old alike and without regard to social class.

The fortuitous observation by the British physician Edward Jenner that milkmaids who were infected with cowpox, a disease of cattle, rarely contracted smallpox led to the introduction of vaccination to the Western world. In 1798, Jenner published his famous treatise describing how infection with cowpox, which produced only mild symptoms in humans, also provided protection against the related disease of smallpox. Within a few years, vaccination—the intentional introduction of cowpox material into the body of a healthy person to induce immunity—had been introduced in America, where its success at protecting communities from a feared killer led to its widespread adoption.

Vaccination was an improvement over inoculation, an older method of inducing immunity in which a small amount of smallpox pustular material was introduced into the bloodstream—a technique that could inadvertently induce a full-blown case of the disease and even trigger an epidemic. The new technique joined other longstanding control measures such as quarantine, removal of the sick to a local "pest house" or infectious disease hospital, and disinfection of living quarters with sulfur and steam.[5]

An outbreak of smallpox in a town provoked a severe crisis, disrupting virtually all civic and commercial activity. As a result, many localities not only provided vaccination to all residents, but compelled it by law to ensure the common welfare. Massachusetts, an early leader in the development of public health activities, enacted the country's first mandatory vaccination law in 1809, and in subsequent decades, many other states and cities followed suit. Most of these laws required vaccination for people of all ages, although some were in effect only when an outbreak of the disease had occurred nearby. As public education became common around the middle of the century, laws specifically aimed at children attending school became widespread.[6]

The severity of the threat of smallpox led to one of the few instances of federal involvement in health in the early republic. In 1813, the U.S. Congress passed "An Act to Encourage Vaccination," which, among other provisions, appointed an agent to furnish certified vaccine matter to anyone who requested it and required the postal service to ship the vaccine free of charge. The act was repealed nine years later, however, after an incident in which smallpox rather than cowpox was mistakenly shipped, resulting in several deaths.[7]

Although securing the vaccination of all citizens was clearly recognized as a public duty, it became a focal point for debate about the authority of local governments to levy taxes. In 1820, the residents of North Hero, Vermont, voted to institute a tax to pay for the vaccination of all the town's residents after cases of smallpox were diagnosed in the area. Dan Hazen, although present at the town meeting where the tax was approved, did not vote for it and refused to pay it. In response, the town constable seized Hazen's cow and sold it to raise the payment. Hazen sued, leading to a ten-year legal battle that ended when the state Supreme Court upheld the confiscation.[8]

By far the most controversial aspect of vaccination programs in the nineteenth century was not how they should be paid for—Dan Hazen's challenge notwithstanding, there was general agreement that providing it free with public funds was appropriate—but whether it should be forced on those who were reluctant to undergo it. As vaccination led to the decline of smallpox over the course of the century, success bred complacency. Many people who had never experienced an epidemic became reluctant to undergo a procedure they viewed as unpleasant and of questionable necessity. And the procedure was not without its own risks. The arm was scraped multiple times with a lancet, usually made of ivory, until the skin was broken. The vaccine matter—lymph drawn from a cow infected with cowpox, mixed with glycerin—was then applied to the wound. The procedure was uncomfortable and caused the arm to remain sore for several days, often preventing people from working. It left a small scar. There was little oversight of medical practice, and many physicians failed to exercise proper care in performing vaccination; antiseptic procedures did not become the norm until late in the century, and instances of vaccination sores becoming contaminated, leading to serious illness and even death, were not uncommon. Thus, reluctance to undergo vaccination was not entirely unreasonable.[5]

Further, many people believed that smallpox was not a contagion but was caused by miasmas or filth, and that clean living rather than vaccination was the best preventive. Others simply gambled that they would escape harm when an epidemic struck. Viewing with dismay his fellow citizens' reluctance to be vaccinated in the 1880s, New York City Health Commissioner Cyrus Edson declared, "It is easy to be bold against an absent danger, to despise the antidote when one has no experience with the bane!"[9]

Numerous anti-vaccination societies were established in the second half of the century, whose members distributed pamphlets and broadsides, lobbied legislatures for the repeal of compulsory laws, filed lawsuits, and sought to discourage the use of vaccination. Their rhetoric rested on two linked claims: that vaccination was a dangerous and unnecessary procedure, and that to compel it through law was a violation of the country's foundational belief in individual liberty.[10]

Opinions on whether compulsory vaccination was effective or ethical varied widely among public health officials and doctors. The secretary to the state board of health of Connecticut, which declined to make vaccination mandatory, explained the decision this way: "The people of this country are too thoroughly imbued with a sense of personal independence to submit patiently to personal compulsion. The attempt would excite hostility to vaccination that does not exist at present, and would hinder rather than promote the cause of vaccination."[11] In Louisiana, which also eschewed compulsion, a health official said that such a law "would probably meet the passive resistance of one-third of our people, the violent opposition of another third, the unwilling compliance of most of the remaining third, and cheerful compliance by the small fraction comprising the intelligent and law-abiding class."[12] Very different, however, was the view of Kentucky's health commissioner, who declared that compulsory vaccination "has never yet failed to bring an outbreak under quick control."[13]

Such conflicting views about compulsion among medical professionals, lawmakers, and the public resulted in dozens of challenges to vaccination laws in state courts around the country, which produced varied decisions. Most rulings upheld the laws, especially those requiring the procedure as a condition of school entry, but others limited the scope of compulsion. An Illinois court, for example, held that vaccination for the general population could be mandated only after an outbreak of smallpox had occurred.[14] The question of whether compulsory vaccination contravened the U.S. Constitution finally reached the Supreme Court in 1905 in the case of Jacobson v. Massachusetts, in which a Lutheran minister from Cambridge challenged that state's law. In a seven–two ruling, the justices declared that compulsory vaccination was a legitimate exercise of state governments' "police powers" to guard the health, welfare, safety, and morals of citizens. If duly elected legislatures had determined that smallpox was a threat and vaccination was an effective way to prevent it, then laws requiring all citizens to comply were not unreasonable. "Society based on the rule that each one is a law unto himself," the decision stated, "would soon be confronted with disorder and anarchy."[15]

During the nineteenth century, the contours of vaccination policy became clear, as medical professionals, lawmakers, and the citizenry all sought to define the rights and responsibilities of government in guarding the communal well-being and scope of individual autonomy.

Immunization in the Early Twentieth Century: "Selling" Good Health

"Will Vaccine Be the Greatest Cure in Medical Science?" asked a headline in the *New York Times* in 1914.[16] The article reflected the excitement and uncertainty in the wake of the Bacteriological Revolution of the late nineteenth century and the expansion of the pharmaceutical industry in the early twentieth, when many new products were developed and the modern vaccine era began.

The identification of many disease-causing microbes sparked attempts to create vaccines against various contagions, including tuberculosis, cholera, plague, and typhoid. Most of these vaccines remained experimental and were never widely deployed; their efficacy remained a matter of dispute, and most of the diseases they protected against were no longer significant threats in this country. Plague, for example, was a rare occurrence, but when it struck San Francisco and Honolulu at the turn of the century, vaccine was rushed to the scene.[17,18] The typhoid vaccine proved valuable in the military, where it reduced troop mortality, but advances in sanitation made its use among civilians unnecessary except in rural areas with poor sewage disposal.[19] Nevertheless, the idea that it was possible to stimulate artificial immunity to many diseases, not just smallpox, gained currency.

The most successful of the new products was a preparation against diphtheria called toxin-antitoxin, which became the second immunizing procedure to become commonplace. The vaccine was developed in the Bureau of Laboratories of the New York City Department of Health, whose director, William Hallock Park, conducted a pioneering series of trials beginning in 1913, first on children in the city's orphanages and institutions and then in the public school system. Park and his colleagues published favorable results in a series of important medical journal articles in the early 1920s, and the increasing awareness among physicians set the stage for broad campaigns to bring this breakthrough to children across the country.[20]

The first challenge was convincing the public that diphtheria immunization was safe, efficacious, and worth taking the time and effort of bringing children in for a series of three shots, two weeks apart. Efforts to stimulate interest in the new procedure were needed in part because the incidence of diphtheria, like that of most of the contagions that had been feared killers in the nineteenth century, had dwindled considerably. By the 1920s, heart disease and cancer had already surpassed infectious diseases as the country's leading causes of death.[21] Thus, immunization was no longer a crisis-control measure designed to forestall an imminent threat to the common welfare. Not only was there less urgency that might spur the public to action; the argument that providing immunization for all was a public safety function that lay with the government was less compelling.

One policy aimed at achieving high levels of vaccine coverage that was generally rejected was to require it by law. As early as 1921, some public health and medical experts suggested that immunization against diphtheria be made compulsory for school entry,[22] and such proposals continued to be advanced over the following two decades as use of toxin-antitoxin gained popularity. But only a few states took such a step. Most public health officials were wary of triggering a political and legal backlash against the new vaccine similar to the one that had developed against the smallpox vaccine. In addition, diphtheria immunization was recommended for the first years of life, and many doctors feared that a requirement tied to school entry would lead parents to postpone the procedure until it was too late.

To "sell" the importance of immunizing children against diphtheria, public health officials turned instead to the new techniques of marketing and persuasion that were becoming widespread around that time to sell consumer goods such as cars, appliances, and cigarettes: advertisements in newspapers and mass-circulation magazines, billboards, posters, publicity stunts, and short films.[23] Businesses and charitable organizations also played key roles in popularizing diphtheria immunization and making it available to the public. The Metropolitan Life Insurance Company, for example, placed full-page ads in popular magazines such as the *Saturday Evening Post* heralding the new preventive, and its staff of visiting nurses advised policy holders to take advantage of this new development in health.[24] Charities such as the Milbank Memorial Fund and the American Child Health Association provided funding to set up health clinics and pay the salaries for nurses and doctors.[25]

Yet it was clear that advertising, by itself, was insufficient to move parents to action. High coverage was generally achieved only when parents had in-person contact with a physician or nurse and when the product was made available in a free clinic.[26] Although the price of each shot varied according to region and individual practitioner, it could cost as much as $5 (about $50 in 2006 dollars).[21]

Public health activities, like government functions more generally, were carried out almost exclusively at the local level and to a lesser extent by state health authorities. Although some agencies (notably in northeastern cities such as Boston, New York, and Providence) had active public health programs, funding in most localities was paltry. Even basic functions such as the registration of births and deaths remained spotty in many parts of the United States. There was no federal department of health, and the

U.S. Public Health Service had evolved little from its origins in port control and quarantine enforcement.

City health departments that did have sufficient resources adopted contrasting strategies for making the new preventive available. Some set up free clinics for all children regardless of the financial circumstances of the parents, while others set strict limits on access by anyone who was able to afford the services of a private physician. Some cities, including Chicago, provided free toxin-antitoxin to physicians on the agreement that they would charge only for their labor in administering it.[21] Others sought to negotiate with their local medical practitioners to offer the shots at a discount rate. In New York City, the health commissioner worked out a voluntary agreement with medical societies through which members would offer the full series of three shots for $6.[27]

The political climate during the 1920s was not conducive to public provision of immunization. In the aftermath of the "Red Scare" of 1919, potential incursions of communism into American society were a source of great anxiety. Libertarian and antigovernment civic organizations lobbied against a range of developments they viewed as socialistic, including bills to ban child labor and create a federal department of education.[28] In this environment, public health professionals in local and state health departments found that efforts to provide diphtheria immunization for free were a hard sell to the tax-paying public. Efforts at public provision of immunization provoked especially sharp criticism from physicians in private practice, who accused health departments of trying to steal their patients and encroach on their professional turf.

At the same time, however, the inability of many citizens to pay for medical services emerged as a prominent political issue.[29] In 1926, the Committee on the Costs of Medical Care was formed, consisting of physicians, economists, and public health experts who studied ways that advances in medicine might be made accessible to all Americans. Underlying their mission was the question of whether the provision of medical services should remain subject to the rules of the marketplace or whether medical care was an entitlement. The committee's final report, issued in 1932, called for the promotion of group practice and group payment systems, recommendations that were profoundly threatening to many physicians who saw them as socialistic schemes. The American Medical Association denounced the recommendations in an editorial in its journal.[30]

During the Depression, as Franklin Roosevelt's New Deal rolled out a panoply of federal programs to alleviate the nation's economic distress, the notion that it was the appropriate role of the government to intervene in urgent matters of domestic policy became more accepted. But health care remained conspicuously absent from most of the federal relief programs. Although the Social Security Act of 1935 did include matching grants to states to support maternal and child health programs,[30] the provision of immunization remained firmly within the fee-for-service paradigm that dominated medical care. Some forms of relief during the Depression aided immunization efforts; for example, workers from the Works Progress Administration assisted with outreach efforts such as visiting the homes of poor families to urge them to seek immunization.[31] Such programs were curtailed, however, when funds were cut in the early 1940s.

Despite the financial barriers, public acceptance of diphtheria immunization grew steadily, as did vaccination against pertussis (also known as whooping cough), which became available in the 1930s. Because there was no systematic surveillance of immunization coverage levels, it is impossible to determine vaccination rates with any certainty, but special surveys provide some indications of moderate to high acceptance. In the late 1930s, for example, a survey in New York City found that about two-thirds of parents had their children immunized against diphtheria.[21] Parents increasingly followed the advice of pediatricians and other child-rearing experts on how best to care for children. The American Academy of Pediatrics, founded in 1930, published its first recommendations for the routine immunization of children (nicknamed the "Red Book") in 1934 and subsequently updated the volume every two years.[32] Articles by medical journalists in *Good Housekeeping* and *Reader's Digest* stimulated public demand for experimental pertussis vaccines in the 1930s and 1940s, even when scientific evidence for it was inconclusive and medical professionals were divided over its efficacy.[33]

Immunization in the first half of the twentieth century, when vaccines against diphtheria and pertussis joined smallpox vaccination as commonplace and widely used preventive measures, may be characterized as an era of limited government involvement, partnerships between the public and private sector, and a slow but steady increase in acceptance, accomplished through the increasingly influential mass media and the advice of medical and public health experts.

Immunization at Mid-Century: The Ascendance of Science, the Fight against Poverty

"For the public," an opinion pollster wrote in 1959, "the caduceus of medicine sits proudly at the top of the totem pole of science."[34] The unprecedented level of support and respect for the nation's scientific experts—and above all for its physicians—provides the backdrop for vaccination policy in the middle decades of the century. Breakthroughs such as the antibiotic penicillin, the anti-tuberculosis drugs streptomycin and isoniazid, and the blood product gamma globulin elevated medical researchers and practitioners to the status of cultural heroes. The nationwide trials of Jonas Salk's polio vaccine in 1954 and 1955 both contributed to and drew on the sense that scientific medicine was destined to banish infectious disease.[35]

Although polio imposed a relatively small burden of morbidity and mortality, it was the subject of extraordinary public fear, and its image as a crippler of children along with the excitement surrounding the trials shaped events when the vaccine was licensed in April 1955. Unlike the introduction of diphtheria and pertussis immunization, when interest had to be stimulated among an often wary and uncertain public, the demand for the Salk vaccine was instantaneous and overwhelming. The most urgent practical choices were related to getting the most vaccine into the most arms as quickly as possible.[21]

Confusion reigned over how this was to be accomplished, however. It would be impossible for the pharmaceutical companies making the vaccine to produce enough doses in time for the summer polio season. Some kind of rationing would be necessary, although how this would be carried out fairly or consistently was unclear. The Department of Health, Education, and Welfare was created in 1953, and the agency became the subject of harsh public criticism for its failure to anticipate demand for the vaccine and its hands-off response to its distribution once it became available.[36] Reflecting the country's tradition of private sector initiatives, it was not the government but a charitable organization—the National Foundation for Infantile Paralysis, later known as the March of Dimes—that funded and coordinated the Salk trials. The Foundation played a leading role in distribution, having arranged bulk purchase of the vaccine from the manufacturers to distribute it free to states once it was licensed.[34]

Rationing was carried out through voluntary agreements in each state among public health entities and medical associations. In New York State, for example, 80% of the vaccine was reserved for official health agencies, while 20% was made available through commercial distribution channels. The state and local medical societies pledged that private physicians would give the vaccine only to children in the priority age groups.[37] During the early period of temporary shortage, children 5 through 9 years of age were given first priority, with any vaccine left over going to children from the ages of 1 to 19. Priorities within this group were to be determined locally.[37]

Although members of the U.S. Congress went to great lengths to declare that public health decision making transcended politics, hearings on proposed legislation to provide financial assistance to states made it clear that programs for polio vaccination reflected an ideology about the proper role of the government in caring for the health of citizens.[38] As had been the case in the 1920s, antipathy toward "socialized medicine" loomed large over discussions of government responsibility for providing the polio vaccine. Fear of communism, which was at a high-water mark during the Cold War, had been a key factor in the defeat of Harry Truman's plan for a universal health care system in 1949. President Dwight Eisenhower's Secretary of Health, Education, and Welfare adamantly opposed suggestions to bring distribution of the vaccine under federal control.[39]

Nevertheless, Congress did pass a bill with bipartisan support that allocated federal funds to states to provide for free immunization of people younger than 20 years of age and pregnant women of all ages. Grants were awarded based on the number of children in the state and its per capita income. The act explicitly forbade use of means testing to limit eligibility of those receiving the vaccine.[40] Over the next two years, Congress appropriated almost $54 million through the act.[41]

Despite this assistance, surveys showed that rates of vaccination among the poor lagged far behind those of the middle and upper socioeconomic classes. Polio outbreaks in the late 1950s struck urban ghettoes in Chicago, Newark, Baltimore, and Providence, and rural poverty areas in Appalachia.[42] This trend prompted heightened efforts to reach out to the poor. Doctors typically paid about $2 for a dose of the Salk vaccine and in turn offered it to their patients for about $3 to $5 per shot. Many doctors charged more, however. In 1958, the March of Dimes and the American Medical Association worked out a plan through which the doctors' organization would sponsor "dollar clinics," where people could receive their shots for $1 each (about $7 in 2006 dollars).[43]

The licensing of a second polio vaccine in 1961, a live attenuated vaccine developed by Albert Sabin, further raised the visibility of vaccination and opened a window of opportunity in which immunization proponents could argue that the federal government should play an increased role. The new presidential administration of John Kennedy was more receptive to the idea of federal involvement in health than Eisenhower had been, and in 1962, Congress passed the Vaccination Assistance Act, which created a permanent home for immunization programs within the U.S. Public Health Service.[40] The Act provided grants-in-aid to states to support delivery of the diphtheria, pertussis, tetanus, and polio vaccines (smallpox had been virtually eliminated from the United States, and vaccination against it would soon be discontinued).

The passage of the Vaccination Assistance Act exposed longstanding fissures between public health entities and private practitioners over whether it was appropriate for the government to intervene in the "marketplace" of medical care. Although doctors' groups such as the American Academy of Pediatrics provided the authoritative voice that the public trusted, their vision for how vaccines should be administered was often in conflict with that of their counterparts in public health. As an example of the ways that the issue of medical care for the poor could provoke controversy, a letter from a private pediatrician to the editor of the *American Journal of Diseases of Children* called the Vaccination Assistance Act "a waste of money" that might, "in any state with a politically inclined director of health, be the beginning of removing all immunizations from the physicians' offices, into the public health clinics and health departments of that state."[44]

The licensing in quick succession of vaccines against measles (1963), mumps (1967), and rubella (1969) further reinforced the belief that immunization was a cornerstone of medical science's triumph over disease, while it stimulated political debate about the costs of medical care and concern about how the benefits of immunization would be available to all members of society. A dose of one of the two measles vaccines licensed in 1963 cost about $3; the cost to parents to have one child immunized against measles, including the doctor's fee, a possible shot of gamma globulin that was given with the live vaccine, or three doses of the killed vaccine, averaged around $10 ($60 in 2006 dollars).[45] As a result, few public clinics for the poor made the new vaccines available; middle- and upper class families who could afford the services of a private pediatrician were the main beneficiaries of the new products. Only after federal funding to states became available through the Vaccination Assistance Act in 1965 did use of the measles vaccine become more routine and coverage rates increase.

Against the backdrop of the activist social programs of Lyndon Johnson's War on Poverty, immunization activities became more explicitly focused on efforts to bring vaccination to the poor. The enactment of Medicaid in 1965 and the creation two years later of the Early and Periodic Screening, Diagnosis, and Treatment (EPSDT) program, a Medicaid benefit intended to ensure that poor children would receive preventive care, illustrated the extent to which the federal government was seen as having a key role to play in financing health care for those who could not afford it. An ambitious (although ultimately unsuccessful) campaign to eradicate measles launched in 1966 was a piece of this broad political environment.[21]

The belief that government intervention was needed to achieve high vaccination coverage lay behind the other major policy initiative of the 1960s: the enactment of laws requiring immunization for school attendance. A hodgepodge of state and local laws, many dating from the era of smallpox in the nineteenth century, existed in about half the states. In 1967, in concert with its national eradication campaign, the U.S Centers for Disease Control and Prevention (CDC) launched a push to make the laws more extensive and uniform. From 1968 to 1974, the number of states with laws requiring all or most recommended vaccinations prior to school entry increased from twenty-five to forty.[46] States without laws gradually fell in line with the national trend, and by 1981, Idaho, Iowa, and Wyoming had become the last states to enact such laws.[47]

Charitable organizations continued to play a role in vaccine promotion. The Joseph P. Kennedy Foundation, which was concerned with mental retardation, sought to promote use of the measles vaccine because complications of measles were a leading cause of retardation. The Foundation had joined the CDC in urging lawmakers around the country to enact laws requiring children to be vaccinated before they could enter school.[21] In 1971, the foundation sent a letter to the wives of governors and congressional representatives around the country, urging them to coordinate efforts by "women's groups" in the state, such as the PTA or the Junior League.[48] The foundation's proposed programs emphasized education aimed at mothers because "many mothers simply have not been educated about the benefits of and need for immunization. If they knew, they would make sure their children were protected."[49] In addition to a strong gender bias, the wording of the foundation's letter gave voice to the view that, no matter how expansive the governmental role in providing vaccines grew, getting children immunized ultimately depended on parental action.

As school laws were enacted, immunization levels among school-age children climbed, but the laws did little to improve coverage among infants and preschoolers. In the early 1970s, the nation saw repeated outbreaks of vaccine-preventable diseases. In response, the U.S. Congress created a new program (the Vaccination Assistance Act had expired in 1968) that authorized the Public Health Service to provide grants-in-aid to help states and localities deliver vaccines.[40] This assistance, so-called "317" grants for the enabling section of the Public Health Service Act, would provide an important source of funds in subsequent years. Nevertheless, support for vaccines remained highly variable and, according to most experts, inadequate to the need. Immunization programs lacked a natural constituency of political support that might have lobbied for expanded funding. Samuel Katz, chair of the American Association of Pediatrics' Committee on Infectious Diseases, chided his colleagues for "their exquisite attention to detail but detachment from concern with some basics such as immunization status."[50]

Vaccination policy during the mid-twentieth century was characterized by dramatic strides in the science of vaccine development that brought new acclaim to the power of scientific medicine to banish disease. Ironically, however, this recognition did not translate into a steady and reliable source of financial support to ensure that needed vaccines would get into the bodies of the vulnerable children who needed them most.

Immunization in the Contemporary Era: New Products, Old Challenges

"Public Health Needs a Shot in the Arm," declared a *USA Today* headline in 1991, in the wake of a measles epidemic that had spread across the country.[51] Despite the enactment of laws, many years of education and promotion, and a patchwork of public sector programs for free or low-cost immunization, the promise of vaccines remained partially unfulfilled. This point was driven home by an outbreak of measles beginning in 1989 that struck primarily among poor African American and Latino preschool children in large cities, including Los Angeles, Chicago, Houston, Milwaukee, and Washington, DC.[52] The epidemic threw into stark relief the disparities in health coverage for poor children.

As a subsequent analysis in the *American Journal of Preventive Medicine* noted, everyone agreed that immunization rates lagged far below what they should have been, and more efforts were needed to boost coverage rates, but there was no consensus on what exactly was the source of the problem. According to some observers, parental apathy or ignorance was to blame, and intensified education programs were needed. According to others, the high cost of vaccines was the problem. Because many private insurers did not cover routine immunization, even children with health insurance sometimes had to be taken to a public clinic when it was time for shots. In still other accounts, the fragmented nature of the U.S. health care system, with children's records scattered among many providers they might see during the time they were supposed to receive their shots, led to missed opportunities to vaccinate.[40]

Dissatisfaction with vaccine costs and the system through which children received their shots was part of a larger debate about whether the United States should join the world's other industrialized democracies in establishing national health care for its citizens. A window of political opportunity for proponents of universal insurance opened with the election of Bill Clinton to the presidency in 1992.[53] One of the administration's first legislative priorities was the Children's Immunization Initiative. Although the proposal was originally intended to provide free vaccines for all children regardless of family income level, it was eventually scaled back and passed as an entitlement program, called "Vaccines for Children," designed to reach young people who were eligible for Medicaid, those who lacked insurance, and Native American children. Created as an amendment to Title XIX of the Social Security Act (Medicaid), the program provided federal dollars to states to purchase vaccines from manufacturers and distribute them free to healthcare providers in the public and private sectors who served poor children.[54] For the first time, federal funds could also be used to support costs directly related to administering vaccines, such as the salaries of doctors and nurses.

The new funding stream coincided with a dramatic growth in the schedule of recommended vaccinates. During the 1990s, vaccines against *Hemophilus influenzae* type b, hepatitis B, chickenpox, and invasive pneumococcal disease joined the CDC's schedule of recommended pediatric vaccines. The number of injections children received climbed steeply, making it even more difficult to ensure that they would get all recommended vaccines in a timely manner and at an affordable cost.

Another consequence of the rising number of shots that children received was increasing anxiety about the safety of vaccines. Attention to the potential for adverse events had achieved high visibility during the 1980s, when it was alleged that the whole-cell pertussis vaccine, typically given as one component of the trivalent diphtheria-pertussis-tetanus (DPT) shot, might in rare instances cause brain damage. This controversy led to the passage in 1986 of the National Childhood Vaccine Injury Act, which created a system of compensation for those harmed by vaccine-related adverse events.[55] During the 1990s, these concerns increased, and there emerged the most vocal and politically active anti-vaccination movement since the nineteenth century.

This development grew in part out of broad social trends. The general decline in trust and respect for institutions and authority that had occurred in the 1970s afflicted doctors, while widely publicized scandals such as the U.S. Public Health Service's Tuskegee syphilis study had also damaged health professionals' credibility.[56] This transformation set the stage for open challenges to the expert judgment of immunization proponents. The growth of the Internet facilitated the spread of rumors and unproven hypotheses. Connections were alleged between vaccination and conditions as diverse as sudden infant death syndrome, multiple sclerosis, attention-deficit-hyperactivity disorder, and diabetes.[57] Most inflammatory of all were charges of a connection between vaccines and an apparent rise in rates of autism in children. A 1998 paper in the *Lancet*[58] alleged that the measles component of the measles-mumps-rubella vaccine might be causally linked to autism (the conclusion was subsequently disavowed by the majority of the paper's authors after conflict of interest charges were brought against the lead researcher).[59] A connection was also alleged between autism and thimerosal, a mercury-based preservative used in some multidose vaccine vials to prevent contamination after the vial was opened.

One consequence of the growing sense of public unease about vaccine safety was efforts on the part of vaccine skeptics to liberalize exemptions to school entry requirements. Most public health experts agreed that exemptions served as a "safety valve" that prevented backlash against the use of law to achieve compliance with vaccine recommendations. But many expressed concern that too liberal exemption policies might lead more parents to opt out, thus putting communities at heightened risk for outbreaks of vaccine-preventable illnesses. Empirical research had demonstrated that unvaccinated clusters of children could pose serious risks to the health of the community.[60,61]

The roots of exemptions lay in religious objections to vaccination. When school entry laws were enacted during the late 1960s, members of the Christian Science church successfully lobbied legislatures in many states to include exemptions for individuals whose religious tenets specifically proscribed vaccination. During the 1990s, many states expanded their exemptions to include people with secular philosophical objections as well. As of 2006, forty-eight states allowed religious exemptions to vaccination, and in twenty of those states, parents could opt out for philosophical beliefs as well. In two states, only exemptions for medical contraindications were allowed.[62]

What is perhaps most remarkable is that given many obstacles, the United States has achieved levels of vaccine coverage equal to or greater than most other industrialized democracies. Coverage rates for recommended childhood vaccines reached record high levels in 2004. But there are several caveats to this success. Reflecting the country's highly decentralized public health system, rates varied substantially among states.[63] Vaccine production remains concentrated in just a handful of pharmaceutical companies, a situation that led to repeated shortages of pediatric vaccines from 2000 to 2002 and rationing of the flu vaccine in 2004. A report of the Institute of Medicine in 2000 on vaccine financing noted that the country's system was "fragile and unstable" and called for a major federal commitment to ensure that the achievement was sustained.[64]

It is also clear that a substrate of anxiety remains among the public about the alleged harmful effects of vaccines. These fears continue to find voice in articles in the popular media charging that public health officials at the CDC and FDA have engaged in a conspiracy to conceal the evidence of a causal connection between thimerosal and autism.[65] At least seven states have passed legislation barring mercury in childhood vaccines, and another 20 are considering such bills—moves that critics claim would increase the costs of vaccines without a clear public health benefit.[66]

As immunization pioneer Samuel Katz argued in the early 1970s, "There are many complex, interacting reasons for the persistent failure to achieve optimal immunization of all children. Sociologic, economic, educational, political, and logistical factors are all involved. They do not permit any simple, immediate solutions."[67] Katz's observation remains true today. Fundamental characteristics of American political and civic culture continue to shape and often constrain efforts to achieve immunity for the people: the absence of a universal health care system; a more general preference for addressing social problems through voluntaristic, private sector solutions; devolution of responsibility for public health activities to state and local units rather than federally coordinated efforts, resulting in great regional and local variation in health outcomes; and a strongly libertarian orientation, especially toward matters of healing and bodily integrity.

The central issues that have dominated vaccination policy for the past two centuries—how to convince the unwilling or uncertain and how to meet the demand among the ready and enthusiastic—will take on new salience in the coming years as vaccines increase in price and target diseases that afflict fewer people. Among health interventions, vaccines have always had one of the most favorable cost–benefit ratios. For a relatively low price, they have prevented huge expenditures in health care as well as reduced burdens of human suffering. Although such calculations were straight-forward in the past, they are becoming more complex in proportion to the growth of the schedule of recommended vaccines. Each newly licensed product will have to be carefully weighed, not only in terms of its financial costs, but also in terms of the number of additional shots it will require children to undergo and the severity and prevalence of the disease that is prevented.[68] These calculations will also need to take into account less readily quantifiable but equally critical considerations related to the social and political climate in which efforts to create population-level immunity will be implemented.

References

1. Harris, G. 2006. U.S. approves use of vaccine for cervical cancer. *New York Times*. Jun;9:1.

2. Specter, M. 2006. Political science. *The New Yorker*. Feb;16:58–69.

3. Griffin R, Stratton K, Chalk R. 2004. Childhood vaccine finance and safety issues. *Health Affairs*. 23 (98–111):106.

4. Marcuse, E. K. 1992. Obstacles to immunization in the private sector. Proceedings of the 26th National Immunization Conference. Atlanta, GA.

5. Colgrove, J. 2004. Between persuasion and compulsion: Smallpox control in Brooklyn and New York, 1894–1902. *Bulletin of the History of Medicine* 78:349–378.

6. Duffy, J. 1978. School vaccination: The precursor to school medical inspection. *Journal of the History of Medicine and Allied Sciences* 33:344–355.

7. Hopkins, D. 1983. *Princes and peasants: Smallpox in history*. Chicago: University of Chicago Press.

8. Hazen v. Strong, 2 Vt. 427; 1830.

9. Edson, C. 1889. *A plea for compulsory vaccination in defence of Assembly Bill No. 474, entitled "An Act Regulating Vaccination in the State of New York*. New York: Trow's Printing and Bookbinding Company.

10. Kaufman, M. 1967. The American anti-vaccinationists and their arguments. *Bulletin of the History of Medicine* 41:463–478.

11. Bell, C. 1897. Compulsory vaccination: Should it be enforced by law? *Journal of the American Medical Association* 28:49–53.

12. Duffy, J., ed. 1962. *The Rudolph Matas History of Medicine in Louisiana*. Vol. 2. Baton Rouge: Louisiana State University Press.

13. McCormack, J. N. 1902. The value of state control and vaccination in the management of smallpox. *Journal of the American Medical Association* 38:1434.

14. Fowler, W. 1927. Smallpox vaccination laws, regulations, and court decisions. *Public Health Reports* 60 (Suppl): 1–21.

15. Jacobson v. Massachusetts, 197 U.S. 11 (1905).

16. Will vaccine be the greatest cure in medical science? 1910. *New York Times*. Aug 21;V–12.

17. Shah, N. 2001. *Contagious Divides: Epidemics and Race in San Francisco's Chinatown*. Berkeley: University of California Press.

18. Mohr, J. C. 2005. *Plague and Fire: Battling Black Death and the 1900 Burning of Honolulu's Chinatown*. New York: Oxford University Press.

19. Colgrove, J. 2005. "Science in a democracy": The contested status of vaccination in the Progressive Era and the 1920s. *Isis* 96:167–191.

20. Hammonds, E. M. 1999. *Childhood's Deadly Scourge: The Campaign to Control Diphtheria in New York City, 1880–1930*. Baltimore: Johns Hopkins University Press.

21. Colgrove, J. 2006. *State of Immunity: The Politics of Vaccination in Twentieth-Century America*. Berkeley: University of California Press.

22. Preventive diphtheria work in the public schools of New York City. 1921. *Medical Record* 11:34–35.

23. Colgrove, J. 2004. The power of persuasion: Diphtheria immunization, advertising, and the rise of health education. *Public Health Reports (Washington, D.C.)* 119:506–509.

24. Rothstein, W. G. 2003. *Public Health and the Risk Factor: A History of an Uneven Medical Revolution*. Rochester, NY: University of Rochester Press.

25. Kiser, C. V. 1975. *The Milbank Memorial Fund: Its Leaders and Its Work 1905–1974*. New York: Milbank Memorial Fund.

26. Godfrey, E. S. 1933. Practical uses of diphtheria immunization records. *American Journal of Public Health* 23:809–812.

27. Wynne acts to widen immunization drive. 1929. *New York Times*. May;27:20.

28. Dumenil, L. 1990. The insatiable maw of bureaucracy: Antistatism and education reform in the 1920s. *Journal of American History* 77:499–524.

29. Moore, H. H. 1928. Public health and medicine. *American Journal of Sociology* 34 (2): 107–116.

30. Starr, P. 1982. *The Social Transformation of American Medicine*. New York: Basic Books.

31. Meritorious PWA labor. 1936. *New York Times*. Apr;9:22.

32. Coriell, L. I. 1967. Recommendation and schedules for immunization. *Archives of Environmental Health* 15:521–527.

33. Baker, J. 2001. Immunization and the American way: 4 childhood vaccines. *American Journal of Public Health* 90:199–207.

34. Withey, S. B. 1959. Public opinion about science and scientists. *Public Opinion Quarterly* 23:382–388.

35. Oshinsky, D. 2005. *Polio: An American Story*. New York: Oxford University Press.

36. Smith, J. 1990. *Patenting the Sun: Polio and the Salk Vaccine*. New York: Wm. Morrow.

37. New York City Department of Health. 1955. New York State Advisory Committee on Polio Vaccine. Minutes. May 3; box 141647; folder: polio July–December.

38. Poliomyelitis vaccine hearings before the Committee on Interstate and Foreign Commerce. 1955. House of Representatives, eighty-fourth Congress, first session. Washington, DC: Government Printing Office.

39. Blair, W. M. 1955. Mrs. Hobby terms free vaccine idea a socialistic step. *New York Times*. Jun 15;A:1.

40. Extension of Poliomyelitis Vaccination Assistance Act. Hearing before a subcommittee of the Committee on Interstate and Foreign Commerce. 1956. House of Representatives, eighty-fourth Congress, second session. Washington, DC: Government Printing Office.

41. Johnson, K., A. Sardell, and B. Richards. 2000. Federal immunization policy and funding: A history of responding to crises. *American Journal of Preventive Medicine* 19:99S–112S.

42. Alexander, E. R. 1961. The extent of the poliomyelitis problem. *Journal of the American Medical Association* 175:837–840.

43. American Medical Association. Polio inoculation clinic [undated brochure]. New York City Department of Health; box 141677; folder: Poliomyelitis.

44. Kramer, J. C. 1963. An innocuous little bill. *American Journal of Diseases of Children* 105:114.

45. Goldman J. J. 1964. New measles vaccines fail to curb incidence of disease this year. *Wall Street Journal*. Jun 25;1.

46. Measles—United States. 1977. *MMWR. Morbidity and Mortality Weekly Report* 26:109–111.

47. Hale, J. L. 1981. School laws update. Proceedings from the 16th Immunization Conference. Atlanta, GA.

48. Shriver, E. K. 1971. Letter to state health commissioners and epidemiologists, Nov 20. New York State Department of Health, series 13307–82; box 42; folder: Measles 1971–72.

49. Shriver, E. K. 1971, Nov 29. New York State Department of Health, series 13307–82; box 42; folder: Measles 1971–72.

50. Katz, S. 1974. Immunization Action Month, October 1974. *Pediatrics* 54:380.

51. Friend, T. 1991. The measles crisis: epidemic grows as vaccine rate slips; public health needs a shot in the arm. *USA Today.* Mar 18;1D.

52. National Vaccine Advisory Committee. 1991. The measles epidemic: The problems, barriers, and recommendations. *Journal of the American Medical Association* 266:1547–1552.

53. Skocpol, T. 1996. *Boomerang: Clinton's Health Security Effort and the Turn Against Government in U.S. Politics.* New York: W. W. Norton.

54. Reported vaccine-preventable diseases—United States, 1993, and Childhood Immunization Initiative. 1994. *MMWR. Morbidity and Mortality Weekly Report* 43 (04): 57–60.

55. Baker, J. P. 2003. The pertussis vaccine controversy in Great Britain, 1974–1986. *Vaccine* 21:4003–4010.

56. Rothman, D. J. 1991. *Strangers at the Bedside.* New York: Basic Books.

57. McPhillips, H., and E. K. Marcuse. 2001. Vaccine safety. *Current Problems in Pediatrics* 31:95–121.

58. Wakefield, A. J., S. H. Murch, A. Anthony, J. Linnel, D. M. Casson, M. Malik, et al. 1998. Ileal-lymphoid-nodular hyperplasia, non-specific colitis, and pervasive developmental disorder in children. *Lancet* 351:637–641.

59. Murch, S. H., A. Anthony, D. H. Casson, M. Malik, M. Berelowitz, A. P. Dhillon, et al. 2004. Retraction of an interpretation. *Lancet* 363:750.

60. Outbreak of measles among Christian Science students—Missouri and Illinois, 1994. 1994. *MMWR. Morbidity and Mortality Weekly Report* 43 (25): 463–465.

61. Feiken, D. R., D. C. Lezotte, R. F. Hamman, D. A. Salmon, R. T. Chen, and R. E. Hoffman. 2000. Individual and community risks of measles and pertussis associated with personal exemptions to immunization. *Journal of the American Medical Association* 284:3145–3150.

62. Salmon, D. A., S. P. Teret, C. R. MacIntyre, D. Salisbury, M. A. Burgess, and N. A. Halsey. 2006. Compulsory vaccination and conscientious or philosophical exemptions: Past, present and future. *Lancet* 3367:436–442.

63. National, state, and urban area vaccination coverage among children aged 19–35 months—United States, 2004. 2005. *MMWR. Morbidity and Mortality Weekly Report* 54 (29): 717–721.

64. Institute of Medicine. 2000. *Calling the Shots: Immunization Finance Policies and Practices.* New York: Basic Books.

65. Kennedy, R. F. Deadly immunity. Available at: Salon.com. Accessed January 4, 2007.

66. Levin, M. 2006. Battle lines drawn over mercury in shots. *Los Angeles Times.* Apr 10;A4.

67. Katz, S. L. 1973. Immunization Action Month, October 1973. *Pediatrics* 52:483–484.

68. Temte, J. 2006. Should all children be immunized against hepatitis A? *BMJ (Clinical Research Ed.)* 332:715–718.

3   The Age-Old Struggle against the Antivaccinationists

Gregory A. Poland and Robert M. Jacobson[*]

Since the introduction of the first vaccine, there has been opposition to vaccination. In the nineteenth century, despite clear evidence of benefit, routine inoculation with cowpox to protect people against smallpox was hindered by a burgeoning antivaccination movement. The result was ongoing smallpox outbreaks and needless deaths. In 1910, Sir William Osler publicly expressed his frustration with the irrationality of the antivaccinationists by offering to take 10 vaccinated and 10 unvaccinated people with him into the next severe smallpox epidemic, care for the latter when they inevitably succumbed to the disease, and ultimately arrange for the funerals of those among them who would die (see the Medical Notes section of the December 22, 1910, issue of the *New England Journal of Medicine*). A century later, smallpox has been eradicated through vaccination, but we are still contending with antivaccinationists.

Since the eighteenth century, fear and mistrust have arisen every time a new vaccine has been introduced. Antivaccine thinking receded in importance between the 1940s and the early 1980s because of three trends: a boom in vaccine science, discovery, and manufacture; public awareness of widespread outbreaks of infectious diseases (measles, mumps, rubella, pertussis, polio, and others) and the desire to protect children from these highly prevalent ills; and a baby boom, accompanied by increasing levels of education and wealth. These events led to public acceptance of vaccines and their use, which resulted in significant decreases in disease outbreaks, illnesses, and deaths. This golden age was relatively short-lived, however. With fewer highly visible outbreaks of infectious disease threatening the public, more vaccines being developed and added to the vaccine schedule, and the media permitting widespread dissemination of poor science and anecdotal claims of harm from vaccines, antivaccine thinking began flourishing once again in the 1970s.[1]

* From *New England Journal of Medicine*, Poland, G. A., and R. M. Jacobson. The age-old struggle against the antivaccinationists. 364:97–99. Copyright © 2011 Massachusetts Medical Society. Reprinted with permission from Massachusetts Medical Society.

Little has changed since that time, although now the antivaccinationists' media of choice are typically television and the Internet, including its social media outlets, which are used to sway public opinion and distract attention from scientific evidence. A 1982 television program on diphtheria–pertussis–tetanus (DPT) vaccination entitled "DPT: Vaccine Roulette" led to a national debate on the use of the vaccine, focused on a litany of unproven claims against it. Many countries dropped their programs of universal DPT vaccination in the face of public protests after a period in which pertussis had been well controlled through vaccination[2]—the public had become complacent about the risks of the disease and focused on adverse events purportedly associated with vaccination. Countries that dropped routine pertussis vaccination in the 1970s and 1980s then suffered 10 to 100 times the pertussis incidence of countries that maintained high immunization rates; ultimately, the countries that had eliminated their pertussis vaccination programs reinstated them.[2] In the United States, vaccine manufacturers faced an onslaught of lawsuits, which led the majority of them to cease vaccine production. These losses prompted the development of new programs, such as the Vaccine Injury Compensation Program (VICP), in an attempt to keep manufacturers in the U.S. market.

The 1998 publication of an article, recently retracted by the *Lancet*, by Wakefield et al.[3] created a worldwide controversy over the measles–mumps–rubella (MMR) vaccine by claiming that it played a causative role in autism. This claim led to decreased use of MMR vaccine in Britain, Ireland, the United States, and other countries. Ireland, in particular, experienced measles outbreaks, in which there were more than 300 cases, 100 hospitalizations, and 3 deaths.[4]

Today, the spectrum of antivaccinationists ranges from people who are simply ignorant about science (or "innumerate"—unable to understand and incorporate concepts of risk and probability into science-grounded decision making) to a radical fringe element who use deliberate mistruths, intimidation, falsified data, and threats of violence in efforts to prevent the use of vaccines and to silence critics. Antivaccinationists tend toward complete mistrust of government and manufacturers, conspiratorial thinking, denialism, low cognitive complexity in thinking patterns, reasoning flaws, and a habit of substituting emotional anecdotes for data.[5] Their efforts have had disruptive and costly effects, including damage to individual and community well-being from outbreaks of previously controlled diseases, withdrawal of vaccine manufacturers from the market, compromising of national security (in the case of anthrax and smallpox vaccines), and lost productivity.[2]

The H1N1 influenza pandemic of 2009 and 2010 revealed a strong public fear of vaccination, stoked by antivaccinationists. In the United States, 70 million doses of vaccine were wasted, although there was no evidence of harm from vaccination. Meanwhile, even though more than a dozen studies have demonstrated an absence of harm from MMR vaccination, Wakefield and his supporters continue to steer the public away from the vaccine. As a result, a generation of parents and their children has grown up afraid of vaccines, and the resulting outbreaks of measles and mumps have damaged and destroyed young lives. The reemergence of other previously controlled diseases has led to hospitalizations, missed days of school and work, medical complications, societal disruptions, and deaths. The worst pertussis outbreaks in the past 50 years are now occurring in California, where 10 deaths have already been reported among infants and young children.

In the face of such a legacy, what can we do to hasten the funeral of antivaccination campaigns? First, we must continue to fund and publish high-quality studies to investigate concerns about vaccine safety. Second, we must maintain, if not improve, monitoring programs, such as the Vaccine Adverse Events Reporting System (VAERS) and the Clinical Immunization Safety Assessment Network, to ensure coverage of real but rare adverse events that may be related to vaccination, and we should expand the VAERS to make compensation available to anyone, regardless of age, who is legitimately injured by a vaccine. Third, we must teach healthcare professionals, parents, and patients how to counter antivaccinationists' false and injurious claims. The scientific method must inform evidence-based decision making and a numerate society if good public policy decisions are to be made and the public health held safe. Syncretism between the scientific method and unorthodox medicine can be dangerous.

Fourth, we must enhance public education and public persuasion. Patients and parents are seeking to balance risks and benefits. This process must start with increasing scientific literacy at all levels of education. In addition, public–private partnerships of scientists and physicians could be developed to make accurate vaccine information accessible to the public in multiple languages, on a range of reading levels, and through various media. We must counter misinformation where it is transmitted and consider using legal remedies when appropriate.

The diseases that we now seek to prevent with vaccination pose far less risk to antivaccinationists than smallpox did through the early 1900s. Unfortunately, this means that they can continue to disseminate false science without much personal risk while putting children, the elderly, and the frail in harm's way. We can propose no Oslerian challenge to demonstrate our point but have instead a story of science and contrasting worldviews: on the one hand, a long history of stunning triumphs, such as the eradication of smallpox and control of many epidemic diseases that had previously maimed and killed millions of people; on the other hand, the reality that none of the antivaccinationists' claims of widespread injury from vaccines has withstood the tests of time and science. We believe that antivaccinationists have done significant harm to the public health. Ultimately, society must recognize that science is not a democracy in which the side with the most votes or the loudest voices gets to decide what is right.

References

1. Wolfe, R. M., and L. K. Sharp. 2002. Anti-vaccinationists past and present. *BMJ* 325:430–432.

2. Gangarosa, E. J., A. M. Galazka, C. R. Wolfe, L. M. Phillips, R. E. Gangarosa, E. Miller, and R. T. Chen. 1998. Impact of anti-vaccine movements on pertussis control: The untold story. *Lancet* 351:356–361.

3. Wakefield, A. J., S. H. Murch, A Anthony, J. Linnell, D. M. Casson, M. Malik, et al. 1998. Ileal-lymphoid-nodular hyperplasia, non-specific colitis, and pervasive developmental disorder in children. [Retraction, *Lancet* 2010;375:445.] *Lancet* 351:637–641.

4. McBrien, J., J. Murphy, D. Gill, M. Cronin, C. O'Donovan, and M. T. Cafferkey. 2003. Measles outbreak in Dublin, 2000. *Pediatr Infect Dis J* 22:580–584.

5. Jacobson, R. M., P. V. Targonski, and G. A. Poland. 2007. A taxonomy of reasoning flaws in the anti-vaccine movement. *Vaccine* 25:3146–3152.

4 Ethics and Immunization Policy: Promoting Dialogue to Sustain Consensus

Chris Feudtner and Edgar K. Marcuse*

When Benjamin Franklin recalled, in the pages of his autobiography,[1] the death of his 4-year-old son in 1736 from smallpox, he rued his decision to forego inoculation for young Francis. Years earlier, when Boston was being ravaged by the 1721 smallpox epidemic that killed hundreds, Franklin and his older brother had lambasted the Reverend Cotton Mather and Dr. Zabiel Boyleston for advocating the "mischievous" practice of variolation; but decades later, the still-aggrieved father reversed his previous position and counseled parents to pursue this "safer" course of immunization.[1,2]

Franklin's inner dialogue of pro and con regarding inoculation symbolizes an enduring societal debate that has embroiled immunization programs. Edward Jenner's development of "scientific" vaccination in the 1790s culminated in an 1867 British law mandating smallpox immunization, yet by 1869, organized political opposition had arisen and persisted unchecked (with children unimmunized) for decades.[3] Louis Pasteur's immunization in 1885 of the boy Joseph Meister against rabies created an ethical uproar that turned riotous.[4] Recent concerns about the safety of whole-cell pertussis vaccines led to a disruption or cessation of national pertussis immunization programs and a resurgence of epidemic disease in the United Kingdom, Japan, Sweden, and West Germany.[5] Sustained by the media, such turmoil roils while vaccination, acknowledged to be one of the most beneficial public health interventions ever, continues to prevent epidemics.[6]

Against this historical backdrop, three recent trends have made decisions regarding immunization policies even more complicated. First, the broad cultural consensus that has enabled the United States' universal childhood immunization programs of the past 50 years shows signs of eroding. With most parents and many grandparents no longer personally acquainted with the morbidity and mortality of vaccine-preventable

* Reproduced with permission from *Pediatrics*, 107:1158–1164. Copyright © 2001 by the American Academy of Pediatrics.

diseases, many families have shifted their focus of concern to alleged vaccine reactions. Adverse events that occur in temporal association with immunization are presumed to be causally related, leading some to oppose mandatory immunization. Indeed, fifteen state legislatures in 1999 considered bills to reduce or eliminate school entry immunization requirements (J. C. Dolins, personal communication, September 29, 1999).

Second, this questioning of mandated immunization occurs just as advances in molecular biology and immunology promise to introduce an array of novel vaccines. In the coming decade, new immunizations will present many challenging policy and funding decisions for national committees that formulate immunization recommendations and determine federal entitlements, state legislatures that enact immunization laws and allocate some immunization program funds, and both public and private health plans that decide on coverage and payment or financing policies.

Third, for the past two decades, the healthcare community has improved the methods used to evaluate medical technology and make policy decisions. Cost-effectiveness studies have weighed cost against some measure of benefit, effectiveness, or usefulness in improving health.[7–15] Such analyses, however, have not formally considered ethical concerns, such as protecting individual rights or providing an equitable distribution of healthcare benefits. Because of this limitation, cost-effectiveness analyses, although necessary for policy decisions, are neither sufficient nor complete because they currently do not address differences in values and perspectives that polarize our society.[16–18]

These three trends will make immunization policy decisions more numerous and complex. Because the powers granted to public health authorities are based on the public's trust, and in democratic societies this trust is founded on broad participation in formulating policy, healthcare decision makers may well feel mounting pressure to include the diverse perspectives not only of physicians and immunization experts but also of parent groups, politicians, special-interest advocates, economists, and, perhaps, ethicists.

How can any decision-making process accommodate such a wide variety of concerns? Ben Franklin, no stranger to complex decisions, once proposed to a friend a simple method of "moral or prudential algebra" to sort through a host of competing objectives, weighing various pros and cons, to reach a good decision (B. Franklin, letter to J. Priestly, September 19, 1772). The science of decision making has subsequently refined Franklin's method greatly, but the essential value of an explicit systematic approach remains: to protect against using unexamined biases, rather than one's best knowledge and deepest convictions, to make important decisions.[19–22]

In this chapter, we propose a systematic approach to evaluate immunization policy options. Our model combines epidemiologic, economic, and ethical concerns into a unified analytic framework, thereby helping us to understand better the tradeoffs between alternative policies and assisting us to choose a course of action that most accords with our fundamental values. We believe that such a systematic method of deliberation would foster a more explicit and morally relevant dialogue about diverse policy considerations than do current U.S. policy debates and analysis.[23]

A Scenario of the Problem

To illustrate our approach, imagine that we are public health officials on a distant island where the children are plagued by an endemic infection—Franklin Fever. Few children escape infection from this highly contagious virus. Most often the disease causes only a week of fever, a cough, and an itchy red rash, but for ~1%, it results in a prolonged course of encephalitis, and ~5% of these children either die or suffer brain damage with long-term disability, generating substantial social costs. Through the collaborative efforts of the island's academic and industrial research communities, a safe and effective Franklin Fever vaccine is now available, and an expert medical committee has recommended universal immunization of the island's children, noting that the cost of immunization would be roughly comparable to total direct medical and indirect societal costs of caring for afflicted children.

As physicians with responsibility for formulating public health policy, we must choose an immunization strategy. Stung by criticism that our previous decisions paid little heed to ethical concerns, we wish to consider several issues, including equal access to the immunization for all children, fair sharing of the benefits and risks of immunization, and due respect for those families that refuse to have their children vaccinated. How might we proceed?

I. Considering the Problem

The merits of particular immunization strategies can be clarified if we start by considering three broad domains of concerns. First are the consequences of the disease: How much harm does it cause individual children and adults? How much does society fear these harms? Does the disease pose a substantial epidemic risk through person-to-person transmission? How much does the care of the acutely ill or subsequently disabled child cost the healthcare system directly as well as the family and society indirectly?

Second are vaccine considerations: How effectively does it prevent disease, both through individual and community (herd) immunity? What adverse events does the vaccine cause, how often, and how severe? Do particular immunization strategies pose other possible adverse consequences, such as altering the epidemiology of the disease and postponing infection into adult life? Might the vaccine eventually eradicate the disease, nationally or globally? Are the price of the vaccine and the costs of its administration and program implementation compatible with our valuation of other health-care goods and services?

These considerations of disease, therapy, and certain aspects of cost constitute the standard focus for cost-effectiveness analysis. As public health authorities, however, we must also weigh important ethical considerations.[24-27] Personal liberty—particularly the freedom to refuse medical intervention—may conflict with the right of vulnerable children to be protected from harm. This conflict requires authorities to strike a balance when specifying the degree of coercion the state should exercise to enforce a specific immunization policy. Achieving such balance is difficult when members of society value immunization programs quite differently.

Equally important considerations involve matters of liberty and justice. Ideally the benefits of immunization—namely, protection from disease—should be equitably distributed across the population. For instance, in the United States, we believe that no child should fail to benefit from a universally recommended immunization program because of limited access to care, poverty, or discrimination attributable to race or ethnicity. Ideally there should be a fair distribution of the burdens of immunization. No segment of society should be placed at heightened risk of suffering a vaccine-related adverse event or falling ill because of vaccine failure or disproportionately bear the costs of disease care, adverse event care, or care provided though the immunization program as a whole. This concern for fair burden-sharing typically is posed as the question of "free riders": should any child (or their family) be allowed to take advantage of a common good (in this case, community immunity against a disease) and potentially put that collective good at risk, even if at an individual level this course might make sense, albeit from a selfish perspective?[28,29] At the same time, Americans who prize individual liberty bristle or rebel whenever any authority encroaches on personal freedom, such as occurs not only with laws requiring immunization but also statutes enforcing the use of bicycle and motorcycle helmets or automobile passenger restraints.

For childhood immunization programs and safety-promoting policies, these deeper themes of liberty and justice play out through the duties that our society entrusts to parents to promote the health and safety of their children and assigns to governmental and other agencies to safeguard the welfare of children. Acrimony often erupts when parental and societal views about these duties differ, or when parents disagree with the course of action mandated by the policy. A mandatory policy with high immunization rates, to cite a well-worn example, would protect those vulnerable children for whom immunization is contraindicated or simply fails to elicit protective immunity, but it would do so by placing many individual children at a minute yet measurable risk of severe adverse vaccine events. As troubling, although less strident, is the common problem of an immunization program failing to distribute benefits equitably because of unequal access to vaccination. An optimal immunization policy process strives to minimize both the contentious conflicts and these quieter pervasive problems.

II. Specifying the Objectives

Having outlined and organized our concerns, we can now focus our thinking by transforming these concerns into the following seven objectives for our immunization policy:

- Minimize the deleterious consequences of the disease.
- Minimize the deleterious consequences of the vaccine.
- Optimize personal liberty to choose or refuse vaccination.
- Maximize the just distribution of benefits and burdens across society.
- Promote the duty of families to protect their child.
- Promote the long-term duty of society to protect all children, now and in the future.
- Use limited healthcare resources prudently.

Are these the only or the "right" objectives? Certainly other worthy objectives exist. Identifying the objectives that matter most is the first of several steps required to make any policy decision. Each of these steps requires some value judgments, either explicitly or implicitly. Making these value-laden choices explicit has the virtue of facilitating debate. For example, the set of key objectives tackled by cost-effectiveness analysis typically includes only the minimization of deleterious disease and vaccine-related consequences and the prudent use of healthcare resources: these are not merely the most important considerations, they are the only ones. Given the incompleteness of current cost–benefit analyses, our diverse society might be well served by debating the degree to which our final decision should be influenced by cost–benefit information to the exclusion of all other concerns.

III. Envisioning Alternatives

With a clearer sense of what we are seeking to accomplish with our immunization policy, we now should develop a fuller list of alternative policies. To simplify our discussion, we will consider a single characteristic of the policy—the force with which vaccination will be promoted—and envision in some detail three alternatives: immunization with the new Franklin Fever vaccine will be mandatory, recommended, or elective. The mandatory system of immunization would require that all children be vaccinated against Franklin Fever on entering school; failing to do so either unwittingly or through conscious refusal would result in the unvaccinated child being excluded from school during outbreaks (which is the prevailing practice in the United States for enforcement of other mandatory immunizations).[30] The recommended strategy would strongly encourage immunization, using public education and expert advice as the chief persuasive means of raising immunization rates. The elective policy would likewise use public education to inform parents, but it would make clear that the choice to immunize is completely at the parents' discretion.

Deciding whether the immunization policy will promote the vaccine as mandated, strongly recommended, or entirely elective is linked to other policy decisions: under each program enforcement scenario, who will pay for the vaccine: a central payer, multiple payers, or self-payment by families? Will a special fund defray costs to families unable to pay? Who will pay for vaccine-related adverse events, or for disease care among the voluntarily unimmunized? If the mandatory policy is chosen, will "philosophical" exemptions be granted under special circumstances? If so, exactly what circumstances?[31] Beyond exclusion from school (or even preschool child care), might this mandatory policy be enforced through restriction of welfare benefits to those families receiving public assistance, as some regions of the United States currently are doing?[32] Alternatively, if the recommended or elective policies were selected, could immunization rates be increased through the effective use of financial incentives for providers[33–35] or even parents? Would policy initiatives that enhanced access and reduced barriers to obtaining health care, or facilitated voluntary compliance with these recommended or elective vaccination guidelines, suffice to raise immunization rates to desired levels?[36]

The point of tracing out these interconnected considerations is this: as we proceed in our evaluation of these policy options, we may uncover issues that warrant our returning to this step of envisioning alternatives, developing new options, or refining and enhancing existing ones. This capacity to learn and improve our options in a reiterative manner is critical because the quality of our ultimate decision is limited by the best alternative we create.

IV. Linking Alternative Policies to Outcomes

Next, we need to assess how the three policy alternatives would meet, or fail to meet, our stated objectives. We can do this by gauging the impact of each immunization policy option on five classes of outcomes: health outcomes for individuals and the population, ethical outcomes for individuals and the community, and total net costs to society. Arraying these outcomes into a flow diagram helps us to see how they are interrelated, with process-oriented ethical outcomes occurring before health-related outcomes, and the collective outcomes resulting from the aggregation of individual outcomes. For example, if under an elective enforcement policy quite a few children were left unimmunized because of financial reasons, the program would not only have failed these children ethically; it also, by allowing them to remain susceptible to disease, would have failed to distribute benefits equitably and would have raised to some degree the risk of epidemic disease. Conversely, a mandatory immunization policy that coerced certain children to be immunized might lower their individual risk of disease and share more fairly the burdens of maintaining a protective level of herd immunity but violate their family's autonomy and place these children at some risk of experiencing an adverse event. These health and ethical outcomes, in turn, determine much of the healthcare and administrative cost outcomes of alternative immunization policies. (The price of the vaccine also determines the costs, but lies beyond the scope of this chapter.)

For many of these outcomes, surprisingly little data exist on which to build evidence-based answers. Considering this series of process- and health-oriented outcomes, however, draws our attention to how our decision would be better informed if we had reasonable estimates of how the rates of immunization were likely to differ among mandatory, recommended, and elective immunization strategies, and how the marginal differences in coverage rates would translate into beneficial and harmful outcomes. Let us illustrate this point by returning to our Franklin Fever scenario. Suppose we estimated that an immunization program promoted by recommendation would result in 80% of eligible children vaccinated, whereas a mandatory program would achieve 95% coverage. Immunizing this additional 15% of children, we might further estimate, would diminish the annual number of cases of Franklin Fever by 100,000 but compel immunization on 500,000 unwilling participants. We would then be able to ask—under these hypothetical assumptions—whether our society should choose to immunize five children whose families are opposed to immunization to prevent a case of disease. Such information would advance our thinking beyond simply stating qualitatively how the programs differ, enabling us to measure the amount by which they differ—a move that will help us substantially when we come subsequently to examine tradeoffs.

V. Assigning Values

Ethical analyses of healthcare programs usually wrestle with how to prioritize large overarching ethical objectives, such as whether securing the greatest good for the greatest number is to be preferred over protecting the rights of all individuals. In our scheme, however, the next step is smaller and more concrete, as we assign values to particular child health and ethical outcomes. Picking several important examples, we need to ask: How do we value differently, if at all, the loss of freedom when a family cannot afford to choose to have their child immunized (as might occur under an elective system) versus the loss of freedom that occurs when an unwilling participant is coerced into being vaccinated (because of a mandatory immunization policy)? Do "natural" illnesses caused by an infectious microbe represent the same loss of value as a precisely equivalent degree of illness caused by a vaccine-related side effect, or is the vaccine-related morbidity somehow more costly? How should we compare the value of a case of disease prevented today from one prevented a generation from now? From a societal perspective, is a dollar in immunization-generated savings that returns to the pocket of a parent of equal value to a dollar that enters an employer's corporate coffer?

Many critics decry ever assigning such values, believing the judgments required are too subjective and contentious. However, every policy decision requires us to make such evaluations; the important choice is whether these evaluations are made implicitly as they are done today or in a more transparent, explicit manner. Returning to our previous example, cost-effectiveness analyses give health status and cost full sway but largely omit concerns for respecting family decision-making autonomy and distributing benefits and burdens fairly. Combining the private evaluation made by different policymakers into one "societal" value is problematic—and in an objective formal sense perhaps even impossible.[37] Nevertheless, every policy decision ultimately depends not just on information but also on an underlying structure of values and preferences that guide choices. Even if a ruckus ensues, we believe that a public debate about such values and their relative weights should be part of policy formulation to maintain the robust consensus required to support immunization policy.

VI.   Examining Tradeoffs

We now examine how the various policy options would or would not accomplish our objectives, constructing a table that arrays the alternatives across our objectives and then considering which alternative best addresses each objective. Although judgments as to which options serve the various objects "best" are debatable (and should be the subject of research and public dialogue), our major point is that this kind of table breaks down the much larger decision of "what policy to implement" into more manageable smaller assessments, which highlight pivotal tradeoffs. Each assessment requires both factual information and value judgments. The minimization of disease-related injury versus the minimization of vaccine-related injury is one tradeoff dimension that at first glance has similar concerns, namely, the minimization of harm. Informing the debate with numbers needed to treat for benefit and for harm might help clarify and thus promote consensus on this particular tradeoff. For each vaccine, these considerations would differ, suggesting that a spectrum of policy enforcement strength is warranted, titrating the degree of coerciveness to the particular disease and vaccine-specific tradeoffs.

Underneath the debate regarding how to minimize various types of harm lies another tension, however, between promoting the just distribution of burdens and benefits and the protection of personal liberty—that is, quite specifically, for those who wish not to be immunized. Children who are left inadvertently unimmunized because of failure of poorly organized immunization programs (such as occurs under elective systems) represent instances of diminished family autonomy, not having had the chance to choose to immunize their child. Even if we wish not to call this lost opportunity a loss of freedom, certainly something of value has been lost. On the other side, compelling families to immunize their children against their wishes represents a clear loss of personal freedom. Evaluating these competing issues of justice and freedom, and striking a renewable and hence sustainable consensus, is a task as much of political dialogue as epidemiology.

These two levels of tension—one involving preferred health risks and the other involving civil liberties—raise the possibility of an additional "higher level" tradeoff between these different levels of concern. To address this tension, we should move beyond debating general philosophical questions or arguing over which objectives we care most about and instead concentrate on how much the differing programs enhance or compromise each particular objective. Focusing on the amounts of benefit and harm at stake when choosing between options, we can make our value judgments more relevant to the policy decision by titrating a set amount of good against varying amounts of bad. Is a single case prevented worth ten immunized unwillingly? Or is the threshold 100 or even 1,000? What if we consider, on the benefit side, disease prevention through community-wide immunity for immunocompromised children for whom vaccination may be contraindicated; does our tolerance toward immunizing children of unwilling families go up, so that we might tolerate immunizing 5,000 children unwillingly to prevent a case among these vulnerable children? Conversely, if we shift to consider preventing unwilling immunization as a benefit of a recommended immunization program, how many children are we willing to be left unimmunized inadvertently to prevent an instance of unwilling immunization? Breaking down broad tradeoffs between different categories of concerns into a comprehensible series of smaller judgments clarifies our values and facilitates the dialogue about how to think about and make these complex tradeoffs, promoting a discussion that is itself a fundamental task for a transparent policymaking process.

VII. Making Health Care Policy Decisions

Public health programs involve more than just issues of health. In recent decades, the medical literature has reflected a societal emphasis on economic considerations, but public health is also a morally laden medical venture. Concerns for individual liberty and social equity permeate public health policy and should be incorporated into mainstream analyses of healthcare programs. Outcomes research must encompass these moral and political concerns. Worry that special interest groups might manipulate or abuse such considerations is likely well founded; omitting moral considerations, however, will not protect against such abuses. Instead, leaving moral concerns as "gaps" in our formal analyses of such decisions merely makes the policymaking process less transparent and the abuses harder to spot. Explicitness, a virtue of clearly stated moral considerations and how they are to be measured, would help to foster constructive debate, which in turn may help to sustain the consensus required for effective public health programs.

What is the ideal immunization program? Certainly, no single answer exists. Yet our society still must decide a course of action, choose a vaccination policy, and pursue it. We intended this hypothetical case study to expose more clearly our areas of confusion and genuine disagreement. We believe that this framework, straddling the interface between moral and empirical reasoning, offers several key elements of a minimally sufficient public dialogue regarding vaccine policy. Such a dialogue must involve clinicians, public health authorities, legislators, and the public, and must therefore take place not only in the deliberations of national committees but in the scientific and lay press, in the electronic media, and on the Internet. We believe that a broad dialogue is essential to sustain the societal consensus that empowered the immunization initiatives of the past half-century, and that only through such continuing dialogue can we be enabled to take full advantage of new opportunities to enhance public health through immunization in the century ahead.

References

1. Franklin, B. *The Autobiography of Benjamin Franklin*. New York, NY: Barnes and Noble. (Originally published in 1791)

2. Blake, J. B. 1985. The Innoculation Controversy in Boston, 1721–1722. In: *Sickness and Health in America: Readings in the History of Medicine and Public Health*. 2nd ed., rev. ed., eds. Leavitt JW, Numbers RL, 347–355. Madison, WI: University of Wisconsin Press.

3. Swales, J. D. 1992. The Leicester anti-vaccination movement. *Lancet* 340:1019–1021.

4. Geison, G. L. 1995. *The Private Science of Louis Pasteur*. Princeton, NJ: Princeton University Press.

5. Gangarosa, E. J., A. M. Galazka, C. R. Wolfe, L. M. Phillips, R. E. Gangarosa, E. Miller, and R. T. Chen. 1998. Impact of anti-vaccine movements on pertussis control: The untold story. *Lancet* 351:356–361.

6. Ten great public health achievements—United States, 1900–1999. 1999. *MMWR. Morbidity and Mortality Weekly Report* 48:241–243.

7. Koplan, J. P., S. C. Schoenbaum, M. C. Weinstein, and D. W. Fraser. 1979. Pertussis vaccine—an analysis of benefits, risks and costs. *New England Journal of Medicine* 301:906–911.

8. Willems, J. S., C. R. Sanders, M. A. Riddiough, and J. C. Bell. 1980. Cost effectiveness of vaccination against pneumococcal pneumonia. *New England Journal of Medicine* 303:553–559.

9. Patrick, K. M., and F. R. Woolley. 1981. A cost-benefit analysis of immunization for pneumococcal pneumonia. *Journal of the American Medical Association* 245:473–477.

10. Mulley, A. G., M. D. Silverstein, and J. L. Dienstag. 1982. Indications for use of hepatitis B vaccine, based on cost-effectiveness analysis. *New England Journal of Medicine* 307:644–652.

11. Riddiough, M. A., J. E. Sisk, and J. C. Bell. 1983. Influenza vaccination. *Journal of the American Medical Association* 249:3189–3195.

12. Cochi, S. L., C. V. Broome, and A. W. Hightower. 1985. Immunization of US children with Haemophilus influenzae type b polysaccharide vaccine. A cost-effectiveness model of strategy assessment. *Journal of the American Medical Association* 253:521–529.

13. Lieu, T. A., S. L. Cochi, S. B. Black, et al. 1994. Cost-effectiveness of a routine varicella vaccination program for US children. *Journal of the American Medical Association* 271:375–381.

14. Miller, M. A., R. W. Sutter, P. M. Strebel, and S. C. Hadler. 1996. Cost-effectiveness of incorporating inactivated poliovirus vaccine into the routine childhood immunization schedule. *Journal of the American Medical Association* 276:967–971.

15. Tucker, A. W., A. C. Haddix, J. S. Bresee, R. C. Holman, U. D. Parashar, and R. I. Glass. 1998. Cost-effectiveness analysis of a rotavirus immunization program for the United States. *Journal of the American Medical Association* 279:1371–1376.

16. Ubel, P. A., M. L. DeKay, J. Baron, and D. A. Asch. 1996. Cost-effectiveness analysis in a setting of budget constraints—is it equitable? *New England Journal of Medicine* 334:1174–1177.

17. Nord, E., J. L. Pinto, J. Richardson, P. Menzel, and P. Ubel. 1999. Incorporating societal concerns for fairness in numerical valuations of health programmes. *Health Economics* 8:25–39.

18. Menzel, P., M. R. Gold, E. Nord, J.-L. Pinto-Prades, J. Richardson, and P. Ubel. 1999. Toward a broader view of values in cost-effectiveness analysis of health. *Hastings Center Report* 29:7–15.

19. Keeney, R. L., and H. Raiffa. 1976. *Decisions With Multiple Objectives: Preferences and Value Tradeoffs*. New York, NY: John Wiley & Sons.

20. Zalkind, D. L., and R. H. Shachtman. 1980. A decision analysis approach to the swine influenza vaccination decision for an individual. *Medical Care* 18:59–72.

21. Kenney, R. L. 1992. *Value-Focused Thinking: A Path to Creative Decisionmaking.* Cambridge, MA: Harvard University Press.

22. Hammond, J. S., R. Ļ. Keeney, and H. Raiffa. 1999. *Smart Choices: A Practical Guide to Making Better Decisions.* Boston, MA: Harvard Business School Press.

23. Casarett, D. J., F. Daskal, and J. Lantos. 1998. The authority of the clinical ethicist. *Hastings Center Report* 28:6–11.

24. Diekema, D., and E. Marcuse. 1998. Ethical issues in the vaccination of children. In *Primum Non Nocere, Today.* 2nd ed., eds. G. Burgio and J. Lantos, 37–49. Amsterdam, The Netherlands: Elsevier.

25. Ross, L. F., and J. D. Lantos. 1995. Immunisation against chickenpox. *BMJ (Clinical Research Ed.)* 310:2–3.

26. King, S. 1999. Vaccination policies: Individual rights v community health. We can't afford to be half hearted about vaccination programmes. *BMJ (Clinical Research Ed.)* 319:1448–1449.

27. Davis, M. M., and J. D. Lantos. 2000. Ethical considerations in the public policy laboratory. *Journal of the American Medical Association* 284:85–87.

28. Hardin, G. 1968. The tragedy of the commons. The population problem has no technical solution; it requires a fundamental extension in morality. *Science* 162:1243–1248.

29. Fine, P. E., and J. A. Clarkson. 1986. Individual versus public priorities in the determination of optimal vaccination policies. *American Journal of Epidemiology* 124:1012–1020.

30. Orenstein, W. A., and A. R. Hinman. 1999. The immunization system in the United States—the role of school immunization laws. *Vaccine* 17:S19–S24.

31. American Academy of Pediatrics, Committee on Bioethics. 1997. Religious objections to medical care. *Pediatrics* 99:279–281.

32. Kerpelman, L. C., D. B. Connell, and W. J. Gunn. 2000. Effect of a monetary sanction on immunization rates of recipients of aid to families with dependent children. *Journal of the American Medical Association* 284:53–59.

33. LeBaron, C. W., J. T. Mercer, M. S. Massoudi, et al. 1999. Changes in clinic vaccination coverage after institution of measurement and feedback in 4 states and 2 cities. *Archives of Pediatrics & Adolescent Medicine* 153:879–886.

34. Hillman, A. L., K. Ripley, N. Goldfarb, J. Weiner, I. Nuamah, and E. Lusk. 1999. The use of physician financial incentives and feedback to improve pediatric preventive care in Medicaid managed care. *Pediatrics* 104:931–935.

35. Smith, S. W., P. Connery, K. Knudsen, et al. 1999. A preschool immunization project to enhance immunization levels, the public-private relationship, and continuity of care. *Journal of Community Health* 24:347–358.

36. Freed, G. L., W. C. Bordley, and G. H. DeFriese. 1993. Childhood immunization programs: An analysis of policy issues. *Milbank Quarterly* 71:65–96.

37. Arrow, K. J. 1951. *Social Choice and Individual Values*. New York, NY: John Wiley.

II Issues in Vaccine Research and Development

Although the approval of a new vaccine brings with it any number of questions and potential challenges related to implementation, promotion, long-term safety and effectiveness, and other topics, it also marks the successful culmination of a long, complicated, and exceedingly difficult process of research and development. That a substantial number of new vaccines have been introduced within the past 15 years may obscure just how much must go right in order for this to occur—from a particular disease being identified as a promising target for vaccine development, to the development of a plausible method of generating long-lasting immunity, to successful results of non-human and progressively larger human clinical trials, even before considering the enormous financial resources required to support this work over many years or even decades, in some cases.

Successful vaccine research and development typically involves collaborations among government-employed or government-supported basic scientists, other academic researchers and institutions, and large multinational vaccine manufacturers. Smaller biotechnology companies, private philanthropies, and vaccine manufacturers based in developing countries are increasingly common contributors to vaccine research and development efforts as well. This section explores issues emerging from these collaborations, their strengths and weaknesses in promoting investment in vaccine strategies with broad potential benefits to public health and global health, and some of the specific concerns that have emerged when conducting vaccine research, generally, and international research for vaccines against HIV, specifically.

R. Gordon Douglas and Vijay B. Samant begin with an overview of the vaccine industry and a few of the principal drivers of vaccine development. Adel Mahmoud continues this discussion, looking in particular at what is present and lacking from the current global vaccine enterprise. One particular strategy to stimulate attention toward novel vaccine strategies that lack obvious markets in wealthy countries has been the advance market commitment, an approach next reviewed and critiqued by Donald Light.

When research progresses to clinical trials in humans, ethical considerations are always paramount, and vaccine trials are no exception. Robert J. Levine examines ethical issues in international vaccine research and development, from granular concerns such as the specific design of trials to more fundamental questions such as whether or how ethical standards should differ depending on the location where research is conducted. This latter question is at the core of a debate over what level and duration of treatment is owed to research subjects in developing countries who become infected with HIV—through no fault of the researchers—during their participation in HIV vaccine clinical trials, as Seth Berkley and Michael Specter each discuss. As the recent guidance document from UNAIDS shows, there has yet to be consensus reached on this vexing question of ethics and clinical research, only a recognition that a preemptive, collaborative effort to determine how to proceed in each case is essential.

Further Reading

Anthony S. Fauci and Hilary D. Marston. 2014. "Ending AIDS—Is an HIV Vaccine Necessary?" *New England Journal of Medicine* 370: 495–498.

Louis Galambos with Jane Eliot Sewell. 1995. *Networks of Innovation: Vaccine Development at Merck, Sharp & Dohme, and Mulford, 1895–1995*. Cambridge: Cambridge University Press.

Paul A. Offit. 2007. *Vaccinated: One Man's Quest to Defeat the World's Deadliest Diseases*. New York: Smithsonian Books.

Mark Pauly. 2005. "Improving Vaccine Supply and Development: Who Needs What?" *Health Affairs* 24(3): 680–689.

5 The Vaccine Industry (*Excerpt*)

R. Gordon Douglas and Vijay B. Samant[*]

The vaccine industry is composed of companies that are engaged in any of the following activities: research, development, manufacture, sales, marketing, and distribution of vaccines. They receive their revenue chiefly from the sales of vaccine products or expectations thereof. The vaccine industry is relatively small but growing. We estimate that total vaccine sales in 2010 were more than $25 billion worldwide. Although components of the vaccine industry are found in 50 countries worldwide, the large vaccine companies are primarily U.S.- or European-based companies and have the dominant share of vaccine business on a revenue basis, but regional companies are gradually growing their market share on a dose basis.[1]

The United States has been extraordinarily successful in vaccine research and development (R&D).[2,3] In the past 25 years, more than two thirds of all new vaccines approved worldwide have been developed in the United States. Eighteen new vaccines were approved in the United States between 1980 and 1996.[4,5] Since then, combinations of existing vaccines have been introduced for easier pediatric vaccination, resulting in a wider adoption of acellular pertussis vaccination. A polyvalent pneumococcal conjugate vaccine for infants introduced by Wyeth (now a subsidiary of Pfizer) has been widely adopted. In 2006, four new vaccines were licensed, including a combination of MMR and varicella, and new vaccines against rotavirus, zoster, and human papilloma virus (HPV). The HPV vaccines developed by Merck and GlaxoSmithKline significantly expanded the field of adolescent vaccines and confirmed market acceptance of premium pricing. This growing success results from a "delicate fabric of public and private collaboration" that evolved in response to scientific, public health, and economic forces during the past 60 years.[6] This delicate fabric is a network of independent industrial, governmental, and academic partners engaged in vaccine R&D. It is

* Reprinted from *Vaccines*, 6th edition, Douglas, R. G., and V. B. Samant, "The vaccine industry," pp. 33–43. Copyright © 2013, with permission from Elsevier.

not controlled by a single authority. Each component makes independent decisions based on its own interest. It is important that policymakers are aware of this independence and interdependence.

Vaccine Development

Vaccine development is difficult, complex, highly risky, and costly, and it includes clinical development, process development, and assay development. The risk is high because most vaccine candidates fail in preclinical or early clinical development. Estimates of cost of development of a new drug or vaccine have risen from $231 million in 1991 to $802 million in 2003 to $1 billion in 2010.[7–9]

These estimates take into account all costs, including R&D costs on products that fail, postlicensure clinical studies, and improvements in manufacturing processes. Approximately 50% of the cost is tangible; the remainder is the cost of capital. These numbers have been debated (others estimate $100 to $200 million); however, the higher estimates have been validated in two ways. First, the number of new vaccines brought to licensure annually by a company or the industry is small and correlates with R&D expenditures of $600 to $800 million for each new product. Thus, if a company spends $100 million annually for vaccine R&D, one might expect one new product every 6 to 8 years, and this appears to hold true. Second, biotechnology companies that are focused on one vaccine and have successfully brought it to market have spent $500 to $700 million on R&D (Aviron/Medimmune).

Funding Sources for Vaccine Research and Development

Funding sources for vaccine R&D include government, profits from sales of product, risk capital, and charitable foundations. The National Institutes of Health (NIH) competes with other federal agencies and programs for taxpayer support and, in general, has been more successful than most. Similarly, vaccine R&D sponsored through the Department of Defense (DOD), the U.S. Food and Drug Administration (FDA), the Centers for Disease Control and Prevention (CDC), and the United States Agency for International Development (USAID) is competitive with other public needs as determined by the executive and legislative branches of government. Recent funding for bioterrorism vaccines (anthrax, smallpox) and emerging pathogens (Ebola, West Nile virus, pandemic influenza) could have long-reaching impact on vaccine research and manufacturing and could potentially create new players in the vaccine business.

Large vaccine companies, which are divisions of much larger pharmaceutical companies, seek a profit by selling products. Because vaccine companies are subsidiaries of large companies, vaccine R&D and manufacturing must compete with other product areas for resources. Therefore, within companies, there is an expectation that sales-to-expense ratios for vaccines will be similar to those of other pharmaceutical products and revenues will increase every year. Although some of this increase may be accomplished with sales volume, prices stabilize as vaccine products mature, and increased revenues are no longer possible, hence, the requirement for a steady rollout of new products. However, unlike pharmaceuticals, old vaccines continue to be profitable for a variety of reasons:

1. The absence of a regulatory pathway for generic vaccines deters potential entrants from engaging in a complex and expensive approval process.
2. In most cases, access to know-how, such as proprietary cell lines, virus strains, and internally developed processes, are far more valuable than patent protection.
3. The birth cohort is renewable, providing an ongoing unmet need for vaccines.

As a result, sole-sourced vaccines, manufactured in fully depreciated assets, are profitable for pharmaceutical companies. One such example is MMR, which after 40 years still has no competition in the United States. A typical vaccine company will have several vaccine candidates in basic research, defined as all R&D through phase 1 clinical testing.[1,10] Those that are most promising in terms of technical feasibility, strong patent protection, and potential market size will be taken forward into development (post-phase 1). In addition, other candidate vaccines might be licensed from small companies. Even in the largest companies, only a few products can be in development at the same time. Thus, go/no go decisions must be made, and market size is a major determinant of the choice between two candidate vaccines, otherwise equal in technical feasibility and likelihood of success.

This system has worked extremely well for vaccines with large potential markets in the developed world when technical feasibility is demonstrated. It does not work for vaccines for diseases that exist predominantly in the poorer regions of the world (e.g., TB); it works imperfectly for diseases of the developed world that affect relatively few persons because of geographic restriction (e.g., Lyme disease) or diseases limited to specific risk groups (e.g., cytomegalovirus [CMV] in transplant recipients), and it does not work when technical feasibility has not been demonstrated (e.g., HIV/acquired immunodeficiency syndrome). The last problem has to be solved by a strong basic program in vaccine-related sciences, particularly for HIV, hepatitis C, and other challenging targets. Niche vaccines for developed-world markets are much more attractive to biotech than to large pharmaceutical companies as evidenced by recent biotech vaccine efforts for West Nile virus, Japanese encephalitis virus, the CMV transplant indication, and dengue.

To involve large companies in development and manufacturing of vaccines to meet needs such as biodefense or health needs of poorer countries, incentives must be established to convince these companies that they should develop and manufacture such products. Such incentives might take the form of guaranteed purchase of certain volumes of a vaccine if specified standards are met, direct contracting by a government agency, or some other publicly funded mechanism.[11,12] Without special incentives, it is unrealistic to expect companies to engage in R&D on diseases that only or predominantly affect the poorer regions of the world.[13]

However, manufacturers in developing countries (initially in India and China, and more recently in Brazil) are playing an increasing role in meeting these needs. Indeed, they already supply the majority of doses of older vaccines for the Third World. As their expertise and capacity in vaccine R&D increase, they will perhaps evolve into major players in supplying new vaccines to the developing world. The Indian vaccine industry is the most advanced among these three developing countries and is already providing a significant portion of the world's vaccine supply as well as developing new vaccines. China is on the verge of the transition from a domestic-only provider to a vaccine exporter, and it is demonstrating solid progress in vaccine innovation. Brazil is approaching the point of supplying its own domestic needs, largely with technology transferred from the developed world. Together these emerging players from middle-income countries will have increasing influence in the global vaccine industry over the coming years.

Pricing of Vaccines

Pricing is a critical component of success for large companies and for venture funding of small companies because potential sales determine the desirability of an investment decision. The public expectation is for low vaccine prices, although this has changed somewhat in recent years with the introduction of several new, higher priced vaccines, such as varicella, rotavirus, pneumococcal conjugate vaccine, zoster vaccine, and HPV vaccine. Large companies believe that vaccines should be priced according to value to society, such as reduction in health care and related costs, relief from pain and suffering, and/or prevention of death, and that they should be rewarded for taking the enormous risks inherent in early vaccine development. Such prices far exceed manufacturing costs but are essential to produce the revenue streams that allow vaccines to be competitive for R&D and manufacturing resources within large pharmaceutical companies or that make biotech companies attractive investment opportunities.

A vigorous large-company vaccine industry is dependent on several factors:

1. A rich research environment sponsored largely by the NIH and mostly carried out in academia, as the source for new creative ideas.
2. Strong patent laws and protection of intellectual property.
3. Freedom to price products at fair levels related to value of product to society.
4. Well-implemented immunization practices.

Although the first two of these factors have been consistently present in recent years, downward pressure on price is a major threat to current companies and a disincentive to new companies. Freedom to price vaccines is restricted to the private market. Less than one half of the vaccines for children sold in the United States are sold in the private market; the rest are sold to the federal or state governments at reduced prices. Controls are even greater in Western Europe and Japan, and internationally there is strong downward pressure on prices as one moves from well-developed to less-developed regions of the world.

In addition to the burden of partial price controls, the vaccine industry is subject to intense regulation. It cannot sell products until the vaccine and the facility in which it is manufactured are approved by the FDA or other regulatory authorities; each batch must be released by the appropriate regulatory agency; and the usage, and therefore market size, is largely determined in the United States by the CDC and in Europe by national regulatory authorities. This oversight has led to the identification of manufacturing problems. Thus, the vaccine industry does not operate in a free-market environment, and its behavior reflects these constraints.

The delicate balance among innovation, government support, industrial expertise and development, and market forces has led to the establishment of a robust vaccine industry that will continue into the future. The industry is changing, however, with the growth of new markets in emerging economies and with the pressing need for new vaccines for the developing world. The current efforts of product development partnership organizations and public creation of markets in response to this need will be successful if lessons learned from the industrial vaccine effort are incorporated into these government and philanthropically driven experiments.

References

1. Warren, K. S. 1986. New scientific opportunities and old obstacles in vaccine development. *Proc Natl Acad Sci U S A* 83:9275–9277.

2. Ibid.

3. Halsted, S. B., and B. G. 1994. Immunizing children: Can one shot do it all? In: *Medical and Health Annual 1994*. Chicago, IL: Encyclopedia Britannica.

4. Cohen, J. 2002. Public health: U.S. vaccine supply falls seriously short. *Science* 295:1998–2001.

5. Peter, G., M. des Vignes-Kendrick, T. C. Eickhoff, et al. 1999. Lessons learned from a review of the development of selected vaccines. National Vaccine Advisory Committee. *Pediatrics* 104:942–950.

6. Marcuse, E. K., J. Braiman, R. G. Douglas, et al. 1997. United States vaccine research: A delicate fabric of political and private collaboration. *Pediatrics* 100:1015–1020.

7. Gregerson, J. 1987. Vaccine development: The long road from initial idea to product licensure. In *New Generation Vaccines*, eds. M. M. Levin, G. C. Woodrow, and J. B. Kaspe, 1165–1183. New York: Marcel Dekker.

8. DiMasi, J., R. Hansen, and H. Grabowski. 2003. Cost of new drug development. *J Health Econ* 22:151.

9. Adams, C. P., and V. V. Brantner. 2010. Spending on new drug development. *Health Econ* 19:130–141.

10. Pasternak A., A. Sabow, and A. Chadwick-Jones. 2006. *Structural Shift: Promising Yet Challenging New Markets for Vaccines*. New York: Mercer Management Consulting.

11. DiMasi, J., R. Hansen, and H. Grabowski. 2003. Cost of new drug development. *J Health Econ* 22:151.

12. Berndt, E. R., and J. A. Hurvitz. 2005. Vaccine advance-purchase agreements for low income countries: Practical issues. *Health Aff* 24:653–665.

13. Mercer Management Consulting. Testimony on vaccine policy before the U.S. House of Representatives Committee on Commerce.

6 A Global Roadmap Is Needed for Vaccine Research, Development, and Deployment

Adel Mahmoud[*]

At the turn of the current century, there was a renewed surge of interest in vaccines—this one of global dimension. The discovery and development of several new vaccines were both a catalyst and a result of this interest.[1] New vaccines included the pneumococcal[2] and meningococcal[3] conjugates—vaccines in which antigens are chemically bonded with proteins to make the immune responses more effective in young children. Also in this group were vaccines that targeted rotavirus, the major viral cause of childhood diarrhea;[4,5] human papillomavirus, which protects against cervical as well as anogenital and head and neck cancers;[6,7] cholera;[8] shingles;[9] and several pediatric combination products.[10] The twenty-first century also ushered in an era of pandemic influenza with H5N1 and H1N1 and concomitant efforts to develop vaccines for both.

The remarkable development of new vaccines and the rise of new epidemic threats coincided with the birth of the GAVI Alliance, originally called Global Alliance for Vaccines and Immunization. The organization, a public–private global health partnership founded in 2000, focused its efforts on vaccine use in the least developed countries.[11] Since then, the GAVI Alliance has achieved a number of early successes—most notably, the adoption of global hepatitis B vaccination.[12] The growth of the global market for vaccines also led to the rapid advent of new vaccine manufacturers and expansion of existing manufacturers located in middle-income countries, which in turn resulted in the significant enlargement of worldwide vaccine manufacturing capacity.[13]

In recent years, multiple innovative financing mechanisms for global immunization efforts also have been introduced, including the International Financial Facility for Immunization[14] and the advance market commitment.[15] These new initiatives, started by governments and philanthropic organizations, highlight how valuable vaccines are

* Copyrighted and published by Project HOPE/Health Affairs as: Adel Mahmoud. A global roadmap is needed for vaccine research, development, and deployment. *Health Affairs*, 30 (6):1034–1041, 2011. The published article is archived and available online at www.healthaffairs.org.

in the prevention and control of infectious diseases. Adding to the vaccine momentum, the 2010 United Nations Summit and the Bill & Melinda Gates Foundation launched the "Decade of Vaccines" initiative to spur progress in this field.

Despite these exciting developments and the renewed focus on vaccines and global immunization efforts, there are reasons to reflect critically on the status of the whole effort. The number and variety of discovery and development efforts means that they often compete with each other for visibility and funding. In addition, there is no real global strategy for the broad introduction of new or recently developed vaccines for rotavirus[4,5] or human papillomavirus.[6,7]

The multiple forces that shape the global vaccine map, such as international organizations, public–private partnerships, and advocacy groups, are not united in a vision. Nor are they in agreement about what steps to take to prioritize which vaccines will be rolled out in the developing world or which vaccines are urgently needed. Establishing such a priority list would help focus discovery and development efforts.

Additionally, the multiple agendas among the many vaccine players create tension. Disagreements are occurring among multiple scientific, policy, and advocacy voices on many fronts, such as which new vaccines need to be discovered or developed. The World Health Organization's Initiative for Vaccine Research Report 2008–2009 demonstrated the complexity and multiplicity of vaccine targets.[16] Although the document served as a repository of all vaccine activities, it also provided ample evidence of the struggles that are under way to sort out which vaccine targets and directions to pursue.

Debates and differences of opinion are healthy if the outcome is a clearer vision. This article analyzes the fundamental aspects of global vaccine discovery and development that will determine the shape and outcome of the totality of efforts for decades to come. My aim is to initiate a wide-ranging debate that will galvanize and possibly add a degree of concordance to conflicting views about the future of vaccine development and deployment.

Scientific Basis for Vaccine Discovery

The scientific basis of discovery of most vaccines currently available for human use is predicated on clinical or laboratory findings dating back more than two centuries.[17] The often-repeated statement that vaccine discovery and development are based on both empiricism and art, rather than on clear theoretical or scientific advances made since this earlier era, is reflected below.

Animal Pathogen

For example, the first principle for vaccine development was the use of an animal pathogen (cowpox) to immunize humans against smallpox and was introduced by Edward Jenner in 1796[17]—more than a century before the discovery of viruses. This is the same technology that was used in the early 1900s to develop the widely used vaccine against tuberculosis, bacille Calmette-Guérin (BCG), and more recently in the production of the rotavirus vaccine, which is based on a bovine rotavirus platform.[4] This technology uses the characteristic exchange of genetic materials between human and bovine viruses, allowing the bovine virus to function as a carrier for the genetic materials of the human organisms, thus inducing protection.

Live and Killed Microbes

The second principle for vaccine development, attenuation of live microbes, was first observed by sheer accident by Louis Pasteur in 1860, who then used the principle to develop vaccines against human rabies and anthrax.[18] This approach—in which a live virus is weakened or attenuated so that it is no longer capable of making a person ill but can still stimulate a protective immune response—was also used nearly a century and a half later to develop one of the newly available rotavirus vaccines.[5]

Around the turn of the twentieth century, two new principles for vaccine development were introduced. In one, the causative microbes of disease are killed. In the other, their toxins are modified to induce immunity without causing harm.[19]

Conjugates

Yet another principle of vaccine development was discovered in 1929. However, the technology of conjugation—the chemical joining of complex sugars that make up the outer cell walls of bacteria to a protein backbone—has only been used in vaccines during the last two decades. Vaccines produced this way include one for *Haemophilus influenzae* type b (Hib) in 1997, for pneumococcus in 2000, and for meningococcus in 2001.

Propagated Viruses

In 1949, scientists discovered how to propagate viruses in cell culture.[19] This advance made it possible to develop several vaccines for most childhood viral infections, such as poliomyelitis, measles, mumps, rubella, and varicella (chicken pox).[1]

Recombinant Technology

We do not intend to minimize the tremendous achievements of the vaccine community over the past decades, but it is sobering to realize that with the exception of two relatively recent vaccines for human use—hepatitis B and human papillomavirus—most other vaccines are based on scientific empiricism and discoveries of past centuries.

Both the hepatitis B and human papillomavirus vaccines were discovered and developed in the last two decades of the twentieth century.[20,21] Both are produced by recombinant technology, where a defined component of the virus is cloned in yeast or other systems for production of viral protein in vitro (meaning in an artificial environment outside of the living being). The scientific rationale for cloning these specific viral proteins was unclear at the start and remains poorly understood now. The cloned proteins of both viruses have to undergo a process of folding (internal molecular structural rearrangements) that results in what are known as virus-like particles. These are self-assembled structures similar to the whole virus but are made of only one protein component and devoid of all the other genetic materials that constitute the complete virus.

The basis for this phenomenon of self-assembly is unknown, as is why these proteins produce protection in the host when they are folded correctly. As a matter of fact, these individual viral proteins, if used prior to appropriate folding, produce no protection in animal experiments and induce poor immune responses. A realistic assessment of the basis for this realization is that it was pure serendipity—a comment that should not detract from this remarkable discovery. Multiple attempts to isolate single protective molecules from many other microbial pathogens to evaluate their ability as vaccine candidates have uniformly failed to date, despite tremendously innovative new molecular and immunological tools.[18]

Adjuvants for Human Use

One more recent and significant advance relates to the approval of two new so-called adjuvants for human use. Adjuvants are substances added to vaccines to increase their immune-producing effect. After decades of using alum salts as the only approved adjuvant for human vaccines, the approval of two new adjuvants, labeled AS047 and MF-59,17 paves the way to explore more specific and potentially more effective adjuvant molecules, which are urgently needed for new vaccine discovery.

Other New Vaccine Pursuits

The past two decades also witnessed a remarkable effort to discover and develop new vaccines, particularly against the three big infectious diseases (tuberculosis, malaria, and HIV) as well as several emerging infections such as dengue.[17] Most of these efforts have yet to result in vaccines available for human use. Despite the tremendous scientific discoveries of monoclonal antibodies, DNA sequencing, genomics, and detailed dissection of host immune responses, multiple hurdles still exist.[17] The difficulties are both scientific in nature and in planning strategies for the future.

Global Efforts for Vaccine Deployment

The second aspect of this analysis of global immunization efforts concerns the way in which international entities are organizing themselves and others to advance the discovery and deployment of vaccines. The beginning of this century marked the birth of the GAVI Alliance to expand the reach of vaccines, particularly in the least developed countries, and to address the obvious delays in introducing new vaccines such as hepatitis B and Hib.[22] Both vaccines were introduced in the developed world 15 to 20 years before being deployed in developing countries.

GAVI Alliance

Formation of the GAVI Alliance represented a major step forward in establishing a fresh set of approaches for developing and deploying vaccines. Forming the GAVI Alliance was not the choice of the global vaccine establishment; rather, it was an expression by new forces of the desire for major change. The leading roles of the Bill & Melinda Gates Foundation, the governments of several developed countries, the pharmaceutical industry, and academics were evident at GAVI's inauguration—not only in securing initial funding but also in the insistence that all of these stakeholders should have seats on the board of the organization. The GAVI Alliance board includes representatives of governments and vaccine manufacturers from developed and developing countries; the main international organizations involved in health policies (such as the World Health Organization, UNICEF, and the World Bank); and representatives of philanthropic and civil society organizations, as well as several research institutions.

Phase I of the GAVI Alliance (2000–2005) was marked by a disciplined focus on the introduction of new vaccines and enhanced basic immunization practices such as safe injections and disposal of used syringes. An example of the success of Phase I was expanding the reach of hepatitis B vaccine to a considerable percentage of children in the least developed countries. This expansion represented a landmark in global vaccination efforts.[23] In 2000, hepatitis B vaccine was barely used in the 72 low-income countries targeted by the GAVI Alliance. At the conclusion of GAVI's Phase I effort, the vaccine was administered to approximately 50% of the birth cohort in these countries.[12] As a result of this success, financial support for the GAVI Alliance tripled for the organization's next phase.

The goal of Phase II (2006–2015) is reducing mortality for children under age five, which reflects one of the key United Nations Millennium Development Goals (goal 4). These goals were articulated by the United Nations at the beginning of the twenty-first century to galvanize a major push for reducing global poverty. The specific objective of goal 4 is to reduce the mortality rate by two-thirds among children under age five between 1990 and 2015. Achievement of that goal is fundamentally dependent on the global expansion of immunizations.

To implement such a goal, the GAVI Alliance determined it will make advanced vaccine products available to the world's poorest countries and strengthen delivery systems to ensure that children in these countries derive the full benefits of immunizations.[12] Although these are important objectives, GAVI has yet to define them with any specificity: which countries, which diseases, which immunizations. Additionally, it has not declared what quantitative measures will be used to demonstrate progress. More troubling is the fact that Phase II does not give specific guidance or priorities to developing countries about which vaccines to introduce or how to phase in a sequence of vaccine introduction programs.

Role of Middle-Income Countries

In the meantime, there have been several important, but separate, developments in the global vaccine sphere as a result of the GAVI Alliance. Among the most important is the enhanced role of middle-income countries—such as India—as vaccine manufacturers.[13] These manufacturers currently produce approximately half of the vaccines procured by UNICEF for the GAVI Alliance.[12] Furthermore, this group of manufacturers is providing a basis for new vaccine formulations such as combination products that contain multiple vaccines (e.g., for diphtheria, tetanus, pertussis, Hib, and hepatitis B), which used to be the sole domain of manufacturers in industrialized countries.[13]

It is hoped that in the near future, vaccine manufacturers in middle-income countries will become involved in the development of new, effective vaccines such as the recently introduced cholera vaccine, manufactured by Shantha Biotechnics, part of the Sanofi-Aventis Group,[8] and the meningitis A vaccine, manufactured by the Serum Institute of India.[24] The continued expansion of vaccine manufacturers in middle-income counties is crucial to meet the urgent need for vaccines in many parts of the developing world.

Two Important Documents

The global vaccine expansion movement also triggered the publication of two important documents during the first decade of the twenty-first century. In 2005, the leadership of the World Health Organization and UNICEF approved the Global Immunization Vision and Strategy 2006–2015.[25] This document focused on four general areas: immunizing more people, introducing new vaccines, making vaccination a component of health interventions, and positioning vaccines globally. The document provided useful information and guidance for the global community but lacked implementation strategies and financial backing.

In 2008, the two international organizations estimated the cost of maintaining global immunization at the 2005 level through 2015 to be $19.3 billion. If expansion were attempted, they estimated, an additional $16.2 billion would be necessary.[26] These are lofty goals, and it remains unclear how such a plan may be funded.

In September 2010, the United Nations summit on the Millennium Development Goals published a document committing world leaders to a set of activities and goals to be accomplished by 2015 that included raising $40 billion for advancing women's and children's health. That commitment included an emphasis on sustaining and expanding prevention and vaccination programs.[27]

The overlap among these documents, organizations, and plans for global immunization, along with the call for a Decade of Vaccines, is considerable. The estimated costs of these efforts are tremendous, and yet there are no clear financing mechanisms. The many voices advocating for immunization, whether disease-specific or not, complicate plans for all other goals for economic and social development. It is no wonder, therefore, that a considerable degree of confusion is occurring between what developing countries perceive as their priorities and what international organizations, multiple public–private partnerships, and advocacy groups are calling for. The confusion and multiplicity of players and agendas call out for a road map that all parties can embrace and use as a coordinating mechanism.

The Missing Elements

The challenge ahead is to define how decisions are made about global deployment of vaccines and their introduction into any specific country. In developed countries, such as the United States, first new vaccines are licensed by a regulatory agency, and then recommendations for use are delegated to advisory bodies.[28] In most circumstances, the regulatory and advisory steps are followed by concurrence of professional and health care organizations. Financing may be secured by either governmental agencies or health insurance coverage.

In contrast, in most developing countries, there is no such established pathway for developing and introducing vaccines. Most developing countries rely on either the World Health Organization to approve a vaccine for global use or the recommendations of that organization's Strategic Advisory Group of Experts on Immunization. These recommendations are not country-specific. From that step, there is no clear pathway for vaccine assessment or how to plan introductions into an individual country.

Multiple reasons for these deficits, at either the national or the global level, may include inability to assess the burden of specific diseases, inability to prioritize, financial difficulties, and absence of political will. Other major deficiencies include weak infrastructures of individual countries' health systems, particularly in connection with vaccine procurement, transportation, cold-chain maintenance to preserve vaccines whose temperatures must be controlled, and general administration. Under these circumstances, it is a challenge for a developing country to prioritize specific vaccination programs.

Given the inability of most developing countries to prioritize which vaccines to introduce nationwide, the decision-making process is left to what the international community proposes and what financial support mechanisms become available. But the multiplicity of special interests, lobbyists, and advocates leads to confusion and offers little help to the leaders of most developing countries who are seeking advice and information. This puts the national leadership of developing countries in an awkward position, given the complexity of the global agenda for vaccines, mainly driven by donors, and their own perception of priorities and what they perceive as important for their own country.

Although representatives of developing countries are present in most of the global vaccine meetings and summits, the impact of the deliberations on domestic policies, priorities, and practices of these countries is unclear. Indeed, it is a tremendous challenge for these leaders to make vaccines and immunization a priority.

Global health is the concern of all national and global leaders and not simply the result of calls from outside the borders of developing countries. For example, how does a country rank-order vaccination programs amid other major global efforts to address malaria, HIV/AIDS, tuberculosis, and noncommunicable diseases? The future is directly linked to the health of children and adults in every country. If developing countries are unequipped to define and prioritize vaccination and immunization program needs, progress will be limited.

It is time to alter the debates about global health in general and vaccination specifically and move them beyond the domain of intellectuals, scientists, and policymakers in the developed world and of international organizations. World leaders have to stop behaving like the American character in V. S. Naipaul's novel *A Bend in the River*, who describes Africa as though the continent were a sick child and he were the parent.[29] The decision-making process must be placed in the hands of those in charge in individual countries, with the expertise about the national priorities of developing countries to come from their national leaders.

In most of the global discourse about immunization, leaders of the developing world either stand by or simply agree on plans devised by others. If these developing countries are not able to articulate a set of clear priorities for the health of their own people, and to demonstrate leadership and willingness to implement the necessary programs, then the struggle against poverty, ill health, and lack of development will not go nearly far enough.

The myth that global immunization programs have to be funded by donors, international organizations, and philanthropies has to come to an end. This is not callous or cruel; it is simply a plea for leaders of the developing world and their populations to shoulder the responsibility of shaping their own future. National leaders have to show commitment and the ability to use their own resources, although small, in initiating and sustaining immunization efforts before they seek global support.

There are several examples of such countries, including Ghana and Vietnam.[30,31] Rates of vaccination in both countries are remarkably high, and sizable national resources are used to partially fund these efforts. These countries have achieved successes in vaccination because of their own commitment of energy and money, not simply because some international donors handed them the cash.

Country-level leadership with a vision, determination, and persuasion is urgently needed for the global vaccine effort. There is no more room for paternalism. Maybe what is needed is reform: As Dambisa Moyo put it, the chief weapon in the "war on poverty" should not be aid but policy reform.[32] This means that we need a concerted effort that involves leaders of developing and the developed countries as well as leaders of international organizations to agree on a road map moving forward.

What Is to Be Done?

The global science and health communities also have an opportunity to propel the vaccine effort forward, but we are at a crossroads.[33] With the increased global interest in immunization manifested by the call for a Decade of Vaccines; the June 2011 Pacific Health Summit, which is to be devoted to vaccines; this issue of Health Affairs; and many other initiatives, a far-reaching debate has begun. The debate should result in a road map for global immunization efforts that includes the following objectives.

Focus on New Sciences
First, there is no alternative for the future of discovery and development of new vaccines and improving some of the currently available products than a determined focus

on basic understanding of microbes, their genes, and products. What is needed is not more of what we, the global scientific community, feel is in our comfort zone. New sciences such as genomics, structural biology, and computational understanding are reshaping our fundamental knowledge of microbes. We urgently need a new generation of specialists from developed and developing countries who are comfortable and experienced in these new sciences.

Second, we need to develop focused and quantitative measures for what we plan to implement and what outcomes are to be achieved. The global community is tired of sloganeering and lofty unrealized goals. There must be concrete objectives for whatever programs are designed, and measures are needed that can be evaluated at reasonable intervals, measures such as vaccination rate for a specific vaccine, the rate of introduction of new vaccines, and use of new vaccine technologies.

Third, national leaders must shoulder the responsibilities for using their resources in ways that benefit their country. They must provide evidence to their people and the global community that they are committed to the health of future generations.

Last, we need global activism and champions who stand up for what is right and do not hide behind politically convenient slogans.

Conclusion

This assessment of the scientific basis for vaccine discovery and development, and the extent of our achievements to date, brings the global community to a fork in the road. Repeated attempts to discover new vaccines are being pursued in vain. Instead of continuing efforts based on dated scientific methodologies, it is imperative to develop new pathways in discovery of urgently needed vaccines.

Despite the successes of the past two decades in developing several new vaccines, all of these were developed based on old principles. The recent history of vaccine development produces the inescapable conclusion that we need new ways of thinking and approaches. We need a new generation of scientific talents not beholden to futile attempts and methods.

These individuals should come from scientific disciplines such as genomics, metabolomics (metabolic changes induced in cells following infection), computational studies, and quantitative sciences—disciplines that traditionally have not been major players in vaccine discovery and development. These scientists will provide fresh eyes and possess capabilities that should address the challenge in new ways. They will be charged with following through on Joshua Lederberg's adjuration—from his 2000 masterpiece on the history of infectious disease, titled "Infectious History"—that we must match "our wit against their genes" to combat microbial diseases.[34]

This new generation will be charged with developing a more detailed and comprehensive understanding of microbes and defining the microbes' most susceptible structures to the host's immune response as the first step in the right direction. Our incomplete understanding of the forces of evolutionary biology results in a rush to use the host's immune response as a lead to define potential vaccine targets. This is a simplistic assumption based on predicting that microbes will expose their most susceptible structures to the host's immune-protective mechanisms. If that were true of the phenomenon of infection and parasitism, no infectious organism could have survived over the millennia and would have disappeared from nature many centuries back.

What is needed, therefore, is a return to basics, to examine and define microbial structures, organization, genomics, and metabolomics in an attempt to characterize their significant and crucial elements of survival in a host. Only then will the induction of protective immune responses—responses against specific susceptible components of the microbe—pave the way for the discovery and development of a new generation of vaccines.

The time is now to initiate a global effort aimed at exploring infectious diseases based on new scientific principles. The effort should be multidisciplinary and global in nature, involving new generations of scientists from developing and developed countries.

References

1. Mahmoud, A., and M. Levin. 2007. Vaccines at the turn of the 21st century: A new era for immunization in public health. *Int J Infect Dis* 11 (Suppl 2):S1–S2.

2. Centers for Disease Control and Prevention. 2010. Licensure of a 13-valent pneumococcal conjugate vaccine (PCV13) and recommendations for use among children—Advisory Committee on Immunization Practices (ACIP), 2010. *MMWR Morb Mortal Wkly Rep* 59 (9):258–261.

3. Centers for Disease Control and Prevention. 2011. Updated recommendations for use of meningococcal conjugate vaccines—Advisory Committee on Immunization Practices (ACIP), 2010. *MMWR Morb Mortal Wkly Rep* 60 (3):72–76.

4. Clark, H. F., P. A. Offit, S. A. Plotkin, and P. M. Heaton. 2006. The new pentavalent rotavirus vaccine composed of bovine (strain WC3)–human rotavirus reassortants. *Pediatr Infect Dis J* 25 (7):577–583.

5. Bernstein, D. I. 2006. Live attenuated human rotavirus vaccine, Rotarix. *Semin Pediatr Infect Dis* 17 (4):188–194.

6. Shi, L., H. L. Sings, J. T. Bryan, B. Wang, Y. Wang, H. Mach, et al. 2007. GARDASIL: Prophylactic human papillomavirus vaccine development—from bench top to bed-side. *Clin Pharmacol Ther* 81 (2):259–264.

7. Schwarz, T. F. 2009. Clinical update of the AS04-adjuvanted human papillomavirus–16/18 cervical cancer vaccine, Cervarix. *Adv Ther* 26 (11):983–998.

8. Sur, D., A. L. Lopez, S. Kanungo, A. Paisley, B. Manna, M. Ali, et al. 2009. Efficacy and safety of a modified killed-whole-cell oral cholera vaccine in India: An interim analysis of a cluster-randomised, double-blind, placebo-controlled trial. *Lancet* 374 (9702):1694–1702.

9. Kimberlin, D. W., and R. J. Whitley. 2007. Varicella-zoster vaccine for the prevention of herpes zoster. *N Engl J Med* 356 (13):1338–1343.

10. Zepp, F., H. J. Schmitt, J. Cleerbout, T. Verstraeten, L. Schuerman, and J. M. Jacquet. 2009. Review of 8 years of experience with Infanrix hexa (DTPa-HBV-IPV/Hib hexavalent vaccine). *Expert Rev Vaccines* 8 (6):663–678.

11. Sandberg, K. I., S. Andresen, and G. Bjune. 2010. A new approach to global health institutions? A case study of new vaccine introduction and the formation of the GAVI Alliance. *Soc Sci Med* 71 (7):1349–1356.

12. GAVI Alliance. 2011. *Phase II (2006–2010)* [Internet]. Geneva: GAVI. Available at: http://www.gavi.org/about/strategy/phase-ii-%282007-10%29/. Accessed May 13, 2011.

13. Jadhav, S., M. Datla, H. Kreeftenberg, and J. Hendriks. 2008. The Developing Countries Vaccine Manufacturers' Network (DCVMN) is a critical constituency to ensure access to vaccines in developing countries. *Vaccine* 26 (13):1611–1615.

14. International Finance Facility for Immunisation [home page on the Internet]. London: IFFIm. Available at: http://www.iffim.org. Accessed May 11, 2013.

15. Advance Market Commitments for Vaccines [home page on the Internet]. 2007. Geneva: AMC. Available at: http://www.vaccineamc.org. Accessed May 26, 2011.

16. World Health Organization. 2010. *The Initiative for Vaccine Research Report 2008–2009*. Geneva: World Health Organization.

17. Plotkin, S. A. 2009. Vaccines: The fourth century. *Clin Vaccine Immunol* 16 (12):1709–1719.

18. Plotkin, S. A., and S. L. Plotkin. 2008. A short history of vaccination. In: *Vaccines, eds. S. A.* Plotkin, W. A. Ornestein,, and P. A. Offit PA, 1–16. Philadelphia: Elsevier.

19. Enders, J. F., Weller, T. H., and F. C. Robbins. 1949. Cultivation of the Lansing strain of poliomyelitis virus in cultures of various human embryonic tissues. *Science* 109 (2822):85–87.

20. Valenzuela, P, A. Medina, W. J. Rutter, G. Ammerer, and B. D. Hall 1982. Synthesis and assembly of hepatitis B virus surface antigen particles in yeast. *Nature* 298 (5872):347–350.

21. Schiller, J. T., I. H. Frazer, and D. R. Lowy. 2008. Human papillomavirus vaccines. In: *Vaccines, eds. S. A.* Plotkin, W. A Ornestein, and P. A. Offit, 243–258 . Philadelphia: Elsevier.

22. Mahmoud, A. 2004. The global vaccination gap. *Science* 305 (5681):147.

23. Lydon, P., R. Levine, M. Makinen, L. Brenzel, V. Mitchell, J. B. Milstien, et al. 2008. Introducing new vaccines in the poorest countries: What did we learn from the GAVI experience with financial sustainability? *Vaccine* 26 (51):6706–6716.

24. Meningitis Vaccine Project. 2003–2011. MenAfriVac successfully introduced at large scale in Africa [Internet]. Ferney-Voltaire, France: The Project. Available at: http://www.meningvax.org/. Accessed May 13, 2011.

25. World Health Organization. 2011. Global immunization vision and strategy 2006–2015. Geneva: World Health Organization. Available at: http://www.who.int/immunization/givs/en/. Accessed May 23, 2011.

26. Wolfson, L. J., F. Gasse, S. P. Lee-Martin, P. Lydon, A. Magan, A. Tibouti, et al. 2008. Estimating the costs of achieving the WHO-UNICEF Global Immunization Vision and Strategy, 2006–2015. *Bull World Health Organ* 86 (1):27–39.

27. United Nations. 2010. UN Summit: High-level plenary meeting of the General Assembly [Internet]. New York, NY: United Nations. Available at: http://www.un.org/en/mdg/summit2010/. Accessed May 26, 2011.

28. U.S. Food and Drug Administration. 2010. Vaccines, blood, and biologics [Internet]. Silver Spring, MD: U.S. Food and Drug Administration. Available at: http://www.fda.gov/BiologicsBloodVaccines/Vaccines/default.htm. Accessed May 3, 2011.

29. Naipaul, V. S. 1989. *A Bend in the River*. New York, NY: Vintage International.

30. GAVI Alliance. 2008. *Ghana* [Internet]. Geneva: GAVI. Available at: http://www.gavialliance.org/resources/Ghana_GAVI_Alliance_country_fact_sheet_June_2008_ENG.pdf. Accessed May 13, 2011.

31. GAVI Alliance. 2008. *Viet Nam* [Internet]. Geneva: GAVI. Available at: http://www.gavialliance.org/resources/Viet_Nam_GAVI_Alliance_country_fact_sheet_June_2008_ENG.pdf. Accessed May 13, 2011.

32. Moyo, D. 2010. *Dead Aid: Why Aid Is Not Working and How There Is Another Way for Africa*. 1st ed. Toronto: Douglas and Mcintyre Ltd.

33. Mahmoud, A. 2010. Vaccines at crossroads. Global Health Magazine [serial on the Internet]. Available at: http://www.globalhealthmagazine.com/top_stories/vaccines_at_crossroads. Accessed May 26, 2011.

34. Lederberg, J. 2000. Infectious history. *Science* 288 (5464):287–293.

7 Making Practical Markets for Vaccines

Donald W. Light[*]

"In the time it takes you to read this preface, 100 people will die of diseases that can already be prevented with vaccines, and 150 more will die of malaria, HIV or tuberculosis."[1] So begins Making Markets for Vaccines, a report from the Center for Global Development (CGD) in Washington, DC that is being vigorously promoted to leaders of the G8 and foundations as a blueprint for how to spend billions of dollars in donations to end the economic and personal burdens of so much suffering and loss.

To stop children "dying at the rate of an average-sized high school every hour," the report offers a plan that is "simple and practical"—make an "advance market commitment" (AMC) to purchase the equivalent of the revenues that the big multinational firms would receive from major Western drugs once the vaccine or vaccines are discovered, tested, and brought to market. This commitment, says the report, will induce companies to start investing serious research funds and unleash the creative powers of their large research teams to discover new, effective vaccines. In return for a large buy-out of a few billion dollars, the company or companies that win the windfall contract(s) would commit thereafter to sell all doses at a very low, cost-plus price (i.e., basic cost plus a small profit margin). Contracts would also depend on poor countries participating, paying a co-payment of about a dollar a dose, and meeting other requirements. The result will be that hundreds of millions of children will get immunized against deadly diseases so that they can learn, create, and unleash the productive potential in poor nations to transform themselves.

The AMC, which is not like a market in most ways, becomes a long-term contract best aimed at late-stage and existing vaccines, not at research for nonexistent vaccines. An advanced commitment is a slower, less efficient way to incentivize research to discover an effective new vaccine than direct research support. As a complement to public

* Originally published in *PLoS Medicine* 2 (10):e271. Republished under the terms of a Creative Commons Attribution License.

and charitable funding of research and development, an advanced commitment can buy many more millions of doses, to save millions more lives, at a much lower price because the risk and cost of research and development are being borne by the funders. While advanced commitments are a good idea for overcoming long delays due to patent enforcements, what leaders need is a different kind of report on how to make a big splash and a real difference with between US$1 billion and $5 billion, a report that outlines how advanced commitments can be most effective in saving lives and how the key issues in the manufacturing, organization, and delivery of vaccines in poor regions can be addressed. I will first identify the problems in what could be called the "core draft" of the CGD model by Michael Kremer, who holds the Gates professorship at Harvard, and then comment briefly on how the final report to leaders fudges and qualifies Kremer's model with add-ons to please all readers, so that what is being proposed becomes less coherent and more difficult to pin down.

The Context

As a professor of comparative healthcare systems, I served on the "Pull" Mechanisms Working Group (the Group) that the Gates Foundation funded the CGD to manage. Over the past several years, the Gates Foundation has transformed vaccine and drug research and development (R&D) for global diseases through bold funding and institution-building. These are called "push" efforts because they use the direct force of contracts, funds, and grants to push along leading projects and programs. As a result, over a dozen promising new vaccines are entering clinical trials or soon will be. But Kremer had proposed using the "pull" of a large financial commitment as the way to induce R&D in the private sector for neglected diseases.[2] Although this is called an "advanced market commitment," it is not a market, but one or a few donors making a large purchase. The Group should have explored and assessed the pros and cons of various pull mechanisms, but I felt it increasingly became a cheering squad for Kremer's model, which then was applied to malaria as the way to supersede the many previous efforts by government- and foundation-sponsored scientists to discover an effective vaccine. The more I learned as a neophyte about how weak the evidence was that this appealing idea would work and the ways it might make things worse, the more doubtful I became.

Little Bang for Big Bucks

Two studies were featured in the report as proof that advanced commitments are a revolutionary technique to launch a new era of innovation. The study by Finkelstein provides a systematic analysis of how advanced commitment funding for vaccines has affected investments in R&D.[3] Finkelstein finds that only large firms respond to the inducement by taking an already discovered vaccine off the shelf and testing it, such as GlaxoSmithKline's (GSK's) vaccine candidate for malaria with modest, short-term efficacy.[4] Ironically, this is the only candidate mentioned in the Group's report, Making Markets—yet it was push funding for testing, not pull inducement, that apparently got GSK to take it off the shelf after 15 years and start trials. Finkelstein found that small firms, where most innovation is taking place, begin to participate later in a sustained larger market, which this advanced commitment model is not designed to create. Finkelstein concludes from her large sample that "for every \$1 permanent increase in expected annual market revenue from vaccines against a particular disease [the CGD design], the pharmaceutical industry will spend an additional 6 cents annually in present discounted value on R&D for vaccines against that disease."[3]

The other major study cited in the CGD report as evidence that a \$3 billion advanced commitment would have long, deep pull back to basic research (rather than short, shallow pull to fund clinical testing) comes to the implausible conclusion that just a 1% increase in market size leads to a 4%–6% increase in new drugs.[5] Not a four- to six-fold increase in research funding (also implausible) but a four- to six-fold increase in actual new drugs! This miraculous conclusion is stated as if it were fact, when it is based on a highly artificial econometric model. The model assumes that all individuals live indefinitely, there is only one firm at any one time with the best-practice technology, anticipated future market size (not actual size) prompts more innovation over long periods, and "new drugs" include all generics and newly approved drugs, although less than 15% of the latter are therapeutically superior to existing drugs.[6,7] Like Finkelstein, the authors sensibly note that "pharmaceutical companies may respond more to profit incentives at the later stages of the research process than at the earlier stages." Thus, both studies support using advanced commitments to encourage late-stage development, not basic research to discover new drugs or vaccines.

The studies cited to prove that donor-pull will spur companies to invest in basic research that might or might not discover an effective vaccine 10 to 15 years down the road in fact offer dubious evidence. Further, the vaccine business is technically different from drugs, and most of the big companies decided years ago to get out of it. Is an advanced commitment for one vaccine (or one disease—an ambiguity that creates further problems) enough to get them back into the vaccine business? A central problem is that the CGD model creates a one-time market and does not address sustainability. Meanwhile, the few companies that have vaccine research teams are already being funded directly or through public–private partnerships (PPPs), often by the Gates Foundation, so that an AMC for research is unnecessary. Finally, going after a big contract designed not to pay a penny until a company has invested a decade or more in discovery, development, testing, and approval is a less cost-effective way to commit billions of dollars than to do what Gates and others are doing already: funding the best basic research ideas (including from private-sector teams), creating PPPs and other bridging organizations, and bringing the best experts together in a global research community.

Market-induced basic research is still less plausible in the CGD model because the more closely one reads the text, the less clear it becomes how much a company would actually get if it were to gamble hundreds of millions so that it could discover an effective vaccine. The core Kremer model comes up with $3 billion to match the average sales of an individual top-selling drug to make investing in research as attractive as for other products. But then it makes room for second or third successful vaccines by other companies, among whom the total amount of money has to be shared. Contracts also depend on the governments of each participating poor country agreeing to terms as subsidized purchasers. Then the final report shifts the argument from an advanced commitment for a vaccine to an advanced commitment for all vaccines for a given disease. In summary, these provisions make it unclear how much a company would get after years of R&D investments.

These same provisions also make a binding contract impossible because the donor cannot specify what it would pay a company if it invests in research to discover a new vaccine. What is a company to make of the assurance that an advanced commitment will not cost the donor a penny until an effective vaccine meets the contractual criteria? If the advanced commitment requires no set-aside, why should investors and companies think it's real and not subject to executive or political change? If donors' financial commitment is real, why not save real lives by committing to make an effective vaccine available to the world's poor now, rather than possibly save hypothetical lives years from now?

The Scientific Barriers to Vaccines

Besides weak evidence that a $3 billion advanced commitment would induce basic research, nothing is mentioned about the daunting scientific barriers to developing a vaccine for either malaria or HIV-AIDS. The Kremer model assumes that creating a large purchase will induce a solution, but scientists who have done the research say that the scientific obstacles may be insurmountable because the targets are multiple and evolving. This observation leads to a more serious weakness in a global competition for a big contract: it rewards scientific secrecy rather than sharing, whereas the cooperative push efforts in recent years have fostered partnerships and sharing. Here is a stark trade-off. Which is more likely to lead to better vaccines faster: fierce competition for a big future payoff or cooperative sponsorship and PPPs? The more cooperative government, university, and nonprofit research teams will probably get nothing under the advanced commitment model.

The other big trade-off question was (and is): will committing large sums to the deep, long pull of an advanced commitment mean less money for grants and contracts to push vaccine development forward? The report asserts it would not. I find that suspect. I was told, in support of this assertion, that wealthy countries are ready to commit billions, and then billions more, to eradicating global diseases of the poor beyond the multinational scheme to buy and administer existing but underused vaccines. Is that true? If so, why have at least two studies concluded that foundations and governments (especially European) have not yet adequately funded R&D for neglected diseases?[8,9] Three billion dollars more for research will foster more innovation than $3 billion committed as an inducement for more research.

The big trade-off question gets buried by emphasizing that advanced commitments are to be added to current push efforts to "complement" them, as if committing a few billion dollars to "pull" funding has no effect on "push" funding. But if it does, the CGD report documents how much more progress has been made, for a fraction the cost, through directly funded grants and programs. Ironically, complementary uses of pull mechanisms with push ones were little discussed by the Group over the months of deliberation. Criticisms of the Kremer draft led to softening the final report but not to substantive development of synergistic combinations. Those are still waiting to be done.

To summarize, the rationale for Kremer's model, which still lies behind all the add-ons and qualifiers of the CGD final report, assumes that a large purchase will unleash innovative research to discover effective vaccines for the world's most intransigent diseases.[10] It is promoted, as Farlow notes of Kremer's book, "in much the same way that some pharmaceutical companies promote 'wonder drugs': emphasizing the positives, burying the negatives, and ending up suggesting that we now have all the answers. ..."[11] Neither evidence nor logic support the Kremer and CGD model, and advanced commitments for early stage research can crowd out faster, more effective efforts both politically and economically. The CGD model belies its president's call for a "global commons" in which the best minds and teams work together for "a global social contract" to benefit humanity.[1,7] Why is there such a discrepancy between the rhetoric and the reality of the CGD model?

Designed for Big Pharma

As drafts of the CGD report progressed, the number of contractual features and one-sided passages that favored the multinational corporations made me increasingly uncomfortable. Here are several examples.

Why is the advanced commitment contract designed so that competing firms get no money until a new vaccine is fully tested and approved? Only big Western firms have the cash reserves to sink hundreds of millions into research to discover and develop new vaccines, shutting out smaller companies in Asia, the Americas, and Africa. Interim and milestone payments were suggested but rejected as part of push grants, not pull AMCs. There are good reasons for using such payments in both initiatives. The final report keeps repeating that the process is open to all, but the contractual terms allow only cash-rich corporations to gamble for years for a possible big payoff and exclude future biotech companies that discover a vaccine after the initial contacts are signed.

Why do the winners get to keep patent rights, when these patent rights are the principal reason for the long delays in getting vaccines to poor countries at low prices? Drug companies with patent rights do not have a good record for sharing and building a global commons. Sharing and combining vaccines for malaria is especially important. A $3 billion advanced commitment is supposed to be a windfall buyout to short-cut access to poor nations, and it should include the rights and technical know-how needed for flexible capacity-building for that price. In fact, in many cases, those rights could probably be bought for a tenth of that price.

What happened to the early goal of building up technical and manufacturing capacity in each continent? Several design features of the CGD model mitigate against it.

Why were principal legal advisers to big pharma chosen to do all the legal work, rather than a more neutral source? They are now coauthors with Group members as part of the promotional push for the "one true answer." Why are the contractual term sheets drawn up by these advisers so vague in all the critical places? Innovative firms in Korea, India, China, Cuba, Brazil, or elsewhere outside the big pharma U.S.–UK club are unlikely to trust this contractual process. Finally, why launch the report in the offices of principal legal advisers to big pharma?

Why is the cost of an advanced commitment set to the sales curves of drugs rather than to the sales curves of better-selling vaccines? Why does the report draw almost exclusively on industry-supported data and studies for the "facts" on which the advanced commitment is based? The result, when combined with the other points, is a bonanza for big pharma, and the text indicates that $3 billion is only a starting price, which is likely to increase rapidly to between $5 billion and $8 billion.

After the big payoff for 200 million courses, little is said (or discussed) about how to sustain the vaccine effort. Sustainability is a major issue in vaccines for the poor, yet all the focus here appeared to be on a multibillion dollar payment to big pharma.

Almost no time was spent analyzing the organizational, regulatory, and financial causes of past delays in making new vaccines available in poor countries. Will a $3 billion buyout solve all the sources of delay? Learning from the past did not seem to be the point.

Likewise, no time was spent understanding the organizational, political, and cultural barriers to effective delivery of the vaccines, only purchasing them. Rather than actually delivering vaccines to people, is a windfall purchase the real goal here? As an expert in healthcare delivery, I could not endorse a report that ignored these issues.

Why is GSK's marginally effective vaccine candidate mentioned by name in the report, and why are the terms of contract then made loose enough that a small, hand-picked committee is permitted to lower (but not raise) the minimal thresholds for a vaccine to be acceptable?

Answers to such questions were brought into focus by the comment in Europe of a senior, international expert on vaccines and their markets. He explained that the major companies are running out of markets to sustain their rapid growth. That's why they're turning sexual performance or shyness into medical problems. They have been looking for years for a way to make a profitable market out of global vaccines, and in the CGD group's proposal, it looks as if they have found a way: "Why don't they just say they want to give GSK $3 billion for their marginally effective vaccine?"

Were members of the CGD group being used as agents for this agenda?

Making Markets for Sustainable Cheap Vaccines

The reasonable doubts here that led me to withhold my endorsement of the CGD report do not address a number of other serious concerns: how difficult, for instance, it is to get the buyout price, and especially the post-buyout price, right years in advance. There are also problems with the contracts, the oversight committee, and liability issues; problems of inequities; and problems with the increasingly confused terms of what is being proposed—issues taken up in more detail elsewhere.[12–14] The G8 finance ministers have been misadvised to write that advanced purchase commitments are a potentially powerful mechanism to incentivize research.[15] But none of these problems detracts from my thinking that advanced purchase commitments are a good idea when applied where they work best: on existing vaccines that could save millions from suffering and dying now. It seems morally dubious for a foundation or nation to do otherwise. The singular omission in the Grand Challenges in Global Health is that they do not call for the eradication of all the diseases for which effective vaccines already exist.[16,17] When millions of lives could be saved now, why give priority to future lives that might or might not be saved?

Remember the quiz show, "The Price Is Right," where contestants guessed how much things actually cost? A big problem with advanced purchase or market commitments is that guessing both the payoff price and the post-payoff price is difficult when attempted years before one even knows the kind of effective vaccine that will be discovered and how it is to be administered.

To be fair to competitors, the payoff price should be adjusted for how much R&D was paid for by governments and foundations because some risk much less of their own money, net of tax subsidies, than others. The CGD price of $15 per course and $3 billion might be much too high or too low by 2015. And no adjusters are mentioned for external subsidies and other factors.

The permanent post-payoff cost of manufacturing most vaccines in volumes above 10 million units, according to information given to our Group, is low, between one and five cents. But a new-age biologic vaccine might cost much more. The CGD price of $1 per course is quite high compared with many generic vaccines and for many poor governments. But then it might not cover the costs of a technically expensive vaccine. Both prices can be right, however, if an advanced commitment can be made for an existing vaccine to eradicate a dread disease.

An advanced commitment as a complement to paying for R&D could be designed to establish a sustainable, long-term market for an effective vaccine to eradicate a global disease. With little risk or private investment to pay off, one could commit to 600 million doses for $3 billion rather than 200 million doses. The terms should build in financial support as well as expert help to strengthen the public health delivery systems of recipient nations and their capacity to build the new vaccine into their budgets and planning. The donor could announce honestly that it is eradicating a global scourge, instead of saying that it might do so 10 years from now. Licenses for low-income markets as well as manufacturing know-how would be part of the deal, and favoring regional manufacturers would be a related goal. Through this kind of flexible, long-term contracting focused on delivery and capacity-building, an advanced commitment could create sustainable, whole-systems markets for new vaccines that current R&D efforts are pushing forward. This is one idea, but we need the kind of report I described at the beginning, which assesses this model along with other forms of advanced commitments and push–pull combinations.

References

1. Center for Global Development. 2005. *Making Markets for Vaccines: Ideas into Action*. Washington, DC: Center for Global Development.

2. Kremer, M. 2001. Creating markets for new vaccines: Parts 1 & 2. In *Innovation policy and the economy. 1*, eds. A. B. Jaffe, J. Lerner and S. Stern. Cambridge, MA: MIT Press.

3. Finkelstein, A. 2004. Static and dynamic effects of health policy: Evidence from the vaccine industry. *Quarterly Journal of Economics* 119:527–564.

4. Alonso, P. L., J. Sacarlal, J. J. Aponte, A. Leach, E. Macete, J. Milman, et al. 2004. Efficacy of the RTS,S/ASO2A vaccine against Plasmodium falciparum infection and disease in young African children: Randomized controlled trial. *Lancet* 364:1411–1420.

5. Acemoglu, D., and J. Linn. 2004. Market size in innovation: Theory and evidence from the pharmaceutical industry. *Quarterly Journal of Economics* 119:1049–1090.

6. National Institute for Health Care Management Research and Education Foundation. 2002. *Changing patterns of pharmaceutical innovation*. Washington, DC: National Institute for Health Care Management.

7. Prescrire International. 2003. A review of new drugs and indications in 2002: Financial speculation or better patient care? *Prescrire Int* 12:74–77.

8. Towse, A. 2004. *The Initiative on Public-Private Partnerships for Health: Estimates of the Medium Term Financial Resource Needs for Development of Pharmaceutical to Combat Neglected Diseases*. London: Office of Health Economics.

9. Moran, M. 2005. New EU approaches to funding R&D for neglected diseases. Available at: http://www.who.int/intellectualproperty/submissions/Mary.Moran.pdf. Accessed July 15, 2005.

10. Kremer, M., and R. Glennester. 2004. *Strong Medicine: Creating Incentives for Pharmaceutical Research on Neglected Diseases*. Princeton, NJ: Princeton University Press.

11. Farlow, A. 2004. Over the rainbow: The pot of gold for neglected diseases. *Lancet* 364:2011–2012.

12. Farlow, A., D. W. Light, R. T. Mahoney, and R. Widdus. 2005. *Concerns Regarding the Center for Global Development Report, "Making Markets for Vaccines."* Geneva: Commission on Intellectual Property Rights, Innovation and Public Health.

13. Barder, O., M. Kremer, and R. Levine. 2005. *Answering Concerns About Making Markets for Vaccines*. Geneva: Commission on Intellectual Property Rights, Innovation and Public Health (CIPIH).

14. Maurer, S. 2005. *The Right Tool(s): Designing Cost-Effective Strategies for Neglected Disease Research*. Berkeley, CA: University of California at Berkeley Goldman School of Public Policy; Available at: http://www.who.int/intellectualproperty/studies/S.Maurer.pdf. Accessed July 15, 2005.

15. G8 Finance Ministers. 2005, June. *G8 Finance Ministers' Conclusions on Development*. London: HM Treasury.

16. Gates Foundation. 2005. *Grand Challenges in Global Health: Gates Foundation*. Available at: http://www.grandchallenges.org.

17. Birn, A. E. 2005. Gates's grandest challenge: Transcending technology as public health ideology. Available at: http://image.thelancet.com/extras/04art6429web.pdf. Accessed July 15, 2005.

8 Ethical Issues in International Vaccine Research and Development

Robert J. Levine[*]

In this discussion of the ethics of multinational vaccine trials, I will refer primarily to the UNAIDS Guidance Document, Ethical Considerations in HIV Preventive Vaccine Research (hereafter, Guidance Document).[1] This document, which was developed in the mid-1990s, states that its scope is limited to multinational trials of HIV preventive vaccines. However, I suggest that it is more generally relevant to multinational trials, or development programs, for vaccines. This Guidance Document was influential in the development of another major document, which provides ethical guidance and direction for research involving humans as subjects, the CIOMS (Council of International Organizations of Medical Sciences) International Ethical Guidelines for Biomedical Research Involving Human Subjects (hereafter, International Ethical Guidelines)[2] and, indirectly, the World Medical Association's Declaration of Helsinki (hereafter, Helsinki).[3]

Ethical Universalism vs. Cultural Pluralism

When one is working to develop ethical guidelines in the international arena, one is immediately confronted with one of the classical questions in ethics: Are ethics universal or do they differ from one culture to another? One might be able to escape this question when working locally or within the confines of a relatively homogenous culture, but not in the international context.[4] Ethical universalism is a position which holds that ethics, or ethical principles, are the same in all places and in all times. Universalists note that ethics seem to be evolving over the years, but the people who have a strong commitment to universalism hold that this is just an indication that we're getting closer and closer to the universal truth. Cultural pluralism—in contrast

* Originally published in *Yale Journal of Biology and Medicine*, 2005; 78 (5):231–237. Reprinted with permission.

to universalism—notices that ethics are, after all, developed in the course of conversations within specific cultures, and they necessarily reflect the histories and traditions of those cultures. Cultural pluralists conclude that differences in ethics across cultures are both inevitable and legitimate. Cultural pluralists sometimes refer to universalists with the derisive term *ethical imperialists*. Some universalists similarly disparage pluralists by calling them *ethical relativists*.

My position is one of compromise: I believe there are some ethical principles that appear to be universal, particularly when they are stated at a highly abstract level. However, I believe that there is also a large degree of legitimacy in cultural pluralism. Even the universal ethical principles may be interpreted differently in diverse cultures. What it means to show respect for persons in the United States may be vastly different from what it means in Sub-Saharan Africa. In my own work in the development of international ethical codes and guidelines, I aspire to what I call "global applicability." That means that the guidelines are, as far as we can tell, applicable currently in all the cultures and societies in the world. There is an assumption that we will be revising these guidelines from time to time as new understandings come to the fore.

Substantive and Procedural Norms

A substantive norm is a rule that specifies what one should do because it is morally right to do so; similarly, such rules may specify what one should not do because it is morally wrong to do so. Procedural rules specify what procedures one should follow. Some define the procedures one should follow to determine what to do when substantive rules do not give clear guidance as to what specific behavior is called for in a particular situation. Other procedural rules provide support or assistance as one attempts to comply with the requirements of a substantive norm. An example of the first type of procedural rule is the requirement for review and approval of all research proposals by an institutional review board (IRB); the purpose of this procedure is to ensure compliance with ethical rules and to see to it that the requirements of ethical norms are interpreted appropriately in particular circumstances. The requirement for a consent form is a procedural norm of the second type; it helps the investigator remember all the elements of information that must be divulged during the process of informed consent. (The requirement for informed consent, itself, is a substantive norm; it is required because it is morally right to provide prospective subjects with information that will empower them to protect their own interests.)

When developing guidelines for relatively homogenous populations, one can include a relatively large proportion of substantive norms. Guidelines for heterogeneous populations, by contrast, are characterized by a higher proportion of procedural norms. It is much more difficult to specify substantive norms when dealing with the diversity of circumstances and cultural traditions that globally applicable guidelines must accommodate.

Capacity Building

The UNAIDS Guidance Document and the CIOMS International Ethical Guidelines each devote considerable attention to multinational research, in which the sponsors are located in the wealthy industrialized countries and the research subjects are in low-resource countries; the latter are referred to as "host countries." The UNAIDS Guidance Document insists that the research should be limited to countries and communities that have the capacity for independent scientific and ethical review. It specifies that "the capacity must be adequate before the research begins."[1] This, I believe, is an "aspirational" standard. An aspirational standard is one that we hope will be applicable sometime in the future; we must, however, acknowledge that this standard cannot be followed today. This requirement is not in the CIOMS document. Implicit in the CIOMS International Ethical Guidelines is an understanding that we should be striving in that direction. Meanwhile, according to CIOMS (Guideline 20), sponsors and investigators from the wealthy industrialized countries "have an ethical obligation to ensure that biomedical research projects ... contribute effectively to national or local capacity to design and conduct biomedical research, and to provide scientific and ethical review and monitoring of such research. Capacity building may include, but is not limited to ... establishing and strengthening ethical review processes/committees; strengthening research capacity; developing technologies appropriate to health-care and biomedical research; training of research and health-care staff and educating the community from which research subjects will be drawn."[2]

Capacity building is required to ensure the scientific and ethical conduct of research. It also should be designed to foster meaningful self-determination for the communities in which the research is carried out, as well as for the individuals who serve as subjects. There is in all of the international documents a strong recommendation that we should be striving to develop partnerships of equals and that the people from the wealthy industrial countries should be regarded as the moral equals of those in the host countries.

Community Engagement

Engagement of the community is designed to develop the vaccine development program as a collaboration involving the sponsors, investigators, community leaders, prospective subjects, and other stakeholders as appropriate. One major goal of community engagement is to ensure the acceptance of the research and development by the community in which the research is to be carried out. All aspects of the research program are to be discussed—even the scientific design of the protocols. Opinions of the community's members about the scientific and logistical features should be solicited, and the wishes of the primary stakeholders should be accommodated to the extent this is feasible without compromising scientific validity. There should be a discussion leading to the design of risk reduction interventions and the development of effective methods of dissemination of information about the trial. Community engagement should also be designed to develop the informed consent process, ensure equity in the choice of subjects, reach agreements regarding the standards of care for research subjects who get sick during the course of a clinical trial, and develop plans for the distribution of the vaccine in case it proves to be suitably safe and effective; the latter includes reaching agreements about the meaning of "reasonable availability" for the particular vaccine development program (see below).

Early Phase Vaccine Testing

The 1993 version of the CIOMS International Ethical Guidelines contained a requirement that the early phases of vaccine research (phase one and perhaps phase two) should be carried out in the country of the sponsoring agency.[5] This requirement was designed to protect the low-resource countries and communities from exploitation. Since the 1970s, there has been a general expectation reflected in the ethical codes and guidelines that special justifications are required to involve vulnerable populations in research programs in which there are serious risks presented by interventions or procedures that do not hold out the prospect of direct benefit to the individual subjects.[6] Among the special justifications that might be considered are that the strain or clade of virus does not exist in the country of the sponsor, and the conduct of the early phase vaccine development in the developing country could be seen as a capacity-building experience to get the people in the host country accustomed to doing this kind of research.

The requirement to conduct early phase vaccine research in the country of the sponsor was relaxed in the UNAIDS Guidance Document and the 2002 revision of the CIOMS International Ethical Guidelines. This change was in response to protests presented at the conferences that led to the development of the UNAIDS document. Participants from the low-resource countries protested that the CIOMS position on the developing countries was highly paternalistic. They noticed, in particular, that the guidelines for doing research in developing countries looked almost exactly like the guidelines for doing research involving children. They argued that they were not to be treated as children. In particular, they should be entitled to decide what sorts of research will be carried out in their countries.

Responsiveness to the Health Needs and Priorities of the Host Country

Research carried out in a low-resource country by sponsors and investigators from the wealthy industrial countries must be responsive to the health needs and priorities of the host country. This standard, which first appeared in the CIOMS International Ethical Guidelines in 1993,[5] distinguishes health needs from priorities. Health needs of a country could be determined by an outside agency. This agency could review epidemiological data and decide that because many people are afflicted by a certain disease, the country "needs" a means to treat or prevent the disease. Priorities, by contrast, are determined by the appropriate authorities within the country. Such authorities may decide that although the country has multiple "needs," they will assign a high priority to only one or two. Decisions about priority must take into account factors other than disease incidence or prevalence such as limitations in the country's resources.

Just Distribution of Benefits

The products of multinational research carried out in low-resource countries should be made reasonably available to the residents of the host country. This concept was introduced into international documents in the 1993 version of the CIOMS International Ethical Guidelines.[5] It has been included in subsequent promulgations by UNAIDS, the World Medical Association, and CIOMS.[1-3] Originally, it was designed to apply to the therapeutic, diagnostic, or preventive products of the research. Subsequently, it has been interpreted to mean as well the new knowledge developed as a result of research. The reasonable availability standard sounds fine in the abstract; however, in particular cases, it has been difficult to decide whether reasonable availability should apply only to the individuals who participate as subjects in the trials, whether it should apply more broadly to the entire host community or country, or whether it should apply to all populations at high risk for developing whatever disease is the target of the research.

Moreover, it remains to be determined whether "reasonably available" could mean simply marketing the product in the host country or making it available at a price that is within the means of the host country. Although we cannot define what "reasonable availability" means in general, there is a consensus that its meaning within a particular research context should be agreed in advance among the primary stakeholders in the research program; this agreement should be negotiated during the process of community engagement.

"Sustainability" is another criterion for ethical justification of research designed to develop a therapeutic, diagnostic, or preventive product. "Sustainability" refers to the ability of the host country to continue to make the product available to the residents of the host country after the research has been completed and the sponsors and investigators have departed, taking with them the extra funds and other resources typically made available during the conduct of the research. If the host country cannot sustain the use of the product, it is an indication that the researchers may not have been adequately compliant with the requirement for responsiveness to the health needs of the country.[7]

Placebo Controls

Placebo controls are ethically acceptable when there is no established vaccine for the indication for which the candidate vaccine is to be tested.[1-3] In some placebo-controlled vaccine trials, it may be appropriate "to provide for those in the 'control arm' a vaccine that is unrelated to the investigational vaccine" (e.g., BCG) (see [2], Guideline 11). When there is an established vaccine, one requires a compelling reason to use placebo controls in a new vaccine trial. Such reasons might be that the established vaccine is not believed to be effective against the strain of virus that prevails in the host country or convincing evidence that the biological conditions during the initial vaccine trial differ to the extent that the results cannot be applied confidently in the new host country.

Provision of Healthcare Services

According to the CIOMS International Ethical Guidelines:

External sponsors of research are ethically obliged to ensure the availability of healthcare services that are essential to the safe conduct of the research; treatment for subjects who suffer injury as a consequence of research interventions; and services that are a necessary part of the commitment of a sponsor to make a beneficial intervention or product developed as a result of the research reasonably available to the population or community concerned. ([2], Guideline 21)

In the commentary on this guideline, CIOMS states, "Although sponsors are, in general, not obliged to provide health-care services beyond that which is necessary for the conduct of the research, it is morally praiseworthy to do so. Such services typically include treatment for diseases contracted in the course of the study. It might, for example, be agreed to treat cases of an infectious disease contracted during a trial of a vaccine designed to provide immunity to that disease, or to provide treatment of incidental conditions unrelated to the study. ..."

When prospective or actual subjects are found to have diseases unrelated to the research, or cannot be enrolled in a study because they do not meet the health criteria, investigators should, as appropriate, advise them to obtain, or refer them for, medical care.

The UNAIDS Guidance Document [Guidance point 16], in its specific consideration of the development of HIV preventive vaccines, states that those who become infected with HIV during the course of a clinical trial should be treated at one of three levels: (a) the level of care that would be offered in the country of the sponsor, (b) a level to be decided by the host country, and (c) a level consistent with that available in the host country. The level to be employed in any particular trial should be agreed on during the process of community engagement before the trial is begun. It is not clear whether this guidance is applicable to clinical trials of vaccines other than those designed to prevent HIV infection.

Informed Consent

In some cultures and societies, informed consent may be problematic for any of several reasons; the following are some examples. In many cultures, informed consent is unfamiliar because it is not part of the customary interactions between healthcare professionals and patients. Many or most of the prospective subjects may be unfamiliar with such concepts as cause and effect relationships, contagion, placebos, randomization, and double-blind. In some communities, it is required that an individual must have the approval of a third party or a group before making the sorts of decisions required in the process of informed consent. These points notwithstanding, UNAIDS[1] (Guidance Points 12–15) requires individual informed consent in each case except when the subject is incompetent or incapacitated; in such cases, third-party permission may be acceptable. UNAIDS requires that the process of informed consent be monitored. CIOMS [2] similarly requires informed consent or third-party permission; however, monitoring is not required.

Selection of Subjects

UNAIDS's requirements for selection of subjects in such a manner as to ensure the equitable distribution of risks and benefits are generally harmonious with those embodied in most contemporary ethical codes and regulations. I will comment on several distinctive features of these requirements. First, as mentioned earlier, "low-resource" or "technologically developing" countries are not to be regarded as generally vulnerable. The developed/developing distinction refers primarily to economic considerations, which are not the only relevant factors in HIV vaccine research. It also establishes two fixed categories, whereas in reality countries and communities are distributed along a spectrum, characterized by a variety of different factors that affect risk. It is more useful to identify the particular aspects of a social context that create conditions for exploitation or increased vulnerability for the pool of participants that has been selected [Guidance Point 7]. "Women, including pregnant women, potentially pregnant women and breastfeeding women, should be eligible for enrolment in HIV preventive vaccine trials, both as a matter of equity and because in many communities throughout the world women are at high risk of HIV infection" [Guidance point 17]. Similarly, "Children, including infants and adolescents" should be eligible for enrollment [Guidance point 18].

Economic Considerations

Several features of these guidelines create the potential for serious economic distortions. For example, provision of free medical services may be seen as an undue inducement to subjects, as well as to the host country. Often in the course of a clinical trial of a new vaccine, subjects receive medical goods and services that they simply would not get in the absence of research. Sometimes the research sponsor develops elaborate facilities to provide health care during the course of the research; local health authorities see this as an opportunity to redirect their efforts and resources. Then when the research has been completed and the sponsors and investigators leave, the people of the community are even worse off than they were before the trial started because they do not even have what they had before the ministry of health withdrew its resources. Sponsors and investigators must be careful not to leave the host country worse off than it was before the research program began.

The requirement for reasonable availability may also be seen as an undue inducement to both the subjects and the country. How else could residents of some Sub-Saharan countries be assured of continuing access to a vaccine or a drug that costs more than the annual per capita health budget in that country? Reasonable availability may also have an effect on the sponsor. If the reasonable availability standard were interpreted to require making the developed product reasonably available to all persons residing in the country, the prudent sponsor would prefer to conduct the research program in countries with relatively small populations.

Closing Comment

The distribution of wealth among the nations of the world is clearly inequitable. There is a temptation to use international research documents as devices to correct inequities. I believe that, to some extent, this is a reasonable and constructive activity. However, I also believe that we must avoid the development of guidelines that would impede the efforts of sponsors and investigators in industrialized countries to assist countries with lesser resources in their efforts to develop treatments and preventions they can afford.

References

1. UNAIDS. 2000, May. Guidance Document: Ethical Considerations in HIV Preventive Vaccine Research. Available at: http://data.unaids.org/Publications/IRC-pub01/JC072-EthicalCons_en. pdf. Accessed May 30, 2006.

2. Council for International Organizations of Medical Sciences (CIOMS). 2002. International Ethical Guidelines for Biomedical Research Involving Human Subjects. Available at: http://www .cioms.ch/frame_guidelines_nov_2002.htm. Accessed May 30, 2006.

3. World Medical Association. 2004. Declaration of Helsinki: Ethical Principles for Medical Research Involving Human Subjects.

4. Levine, R. J. 1996. International codes and guidelines for research ethics: a critical appraisal. In: *The Ethics of Research Involving Human Subjects: Facing the 21st Century*, ed. H. Y. Vanderpool, 235–259. Frederick, MD: University Publishing Group.

5. Council for International Organizations of Medical Sciences (CIOMS) in Collaboration with the World Health Organization. 1993. *International Ethical Guidelines for Biomedical Research Involving Human Subjects*. Geneva, Switzerland: CIOMS.

6. Levine, R. J. 1988. *Ethics and Regulation of Clinical Research*, 2nd ed. New Haven, CT: Yale University Press.

7. Levine, R. J. 2000. Revision of the CIOMS International Ethical Guidelines: A progress report. In: *Biomedical Research Ethics: Updating International Guidelines: A Consultation*, eds. R. J. Levine, S. Gorovitz, and J. Gallagher, 4–15. Geneva, Switzerland: CIOMS.

9 Thorny Issues in the Ethics of AIDS Vaccine Trials

Seth Berkley[*]

At this week's U.S. National Institutes of Health AIDS vaccine meeting and the upcoming 13th International Conference on HIV/AIDS and Sexually Transmitted Infections in Africa, the need for vaccine trials in high-incidence developing countries, and associated ethical concerns, is high on the agenda.

Some bad experiences of the past must not override the need for well-designed trials that address the health needs of such populations. Through global inaction, 70 million people have already become infected with HIV-1, and 30 million have died. A concerted effort is needed to limit HIV-1 transmission, provide treatment and care to those already infected, and mitigate the effects of AIDS on communities. But equally important, a worldwide effort is needed to develop means to achieve long-term success: better, cheaper, and easier-to-take treatments; female-controlled prevention methods such as microbicides; and, most important, effective AIDS vaccines.

The most profoundly unethical course is to do nothing to prevent or alleviate such suffering. Unfortunately, the ethics of action versus inaction tend to be forgotten once the level of debate on trial-related ethical issues becomes heated. Although increased financing has been made available for HIV/AIDS prevention and treatment, the AIDS vaccine effort remains grossly inadequate;[1] less than 1% of health research and development is directed toward developing an AIDS vaccine, and only one vaccine has completed efficacy testing in the 22 years since the start of the epidemic.

Ethics and implementation issues can be addressed by adherence to global standards, and truly informed consent can be acquired with careful engagement of communities in which trials are done. This challenge is not trivial because the insufficient capacity to do ethics reviews at the local level has limited the speed at which trials can be done. Therefore, it is critical that local regulatory agencies, ethics review agencies,

* Reprinted from *The Lancet*, Berkley S., Thorny issues in the ethics of AIDS vaccine trials, 362:992, Copyright © 2003, with permission from Elsevier.

and community advisory bodies are given technical assistance and access to materials and decisions made by their counterparts in other countries.

A pressing challenge facing those involved in HIV-1 prevention trials is the provision of treatment for trial participants who, despite counseling, become HIV-1 infected during the trial. At a WHO and UNAIDS meeting on this issue in Geneva in July 2003, HIV-1 vaccine researchers supported the provision of antiretrovirals, but they could not agree on exactly how this should be done. Should we provide the best standard of care or the best available standard of care; and if we provide antiretrovirals, will it create inequities in host communities and an unreasonable inducement to participate in clinical trials?

Pragmatic solutions, such as those proposed by HVTN for setting up a fund, SAAVI for an insurance scheme, and IAVI for a baseline provision of 5 years' coverage, are useful, but what happens when coverage ends, and what should be done for family and extended family members? The argument about care, however, cannot focus solely on the availability of highly active antiretroviral therapy (HAART). In many of the countries where clinical trials are being considered, expenditures on health care remain frighteningly low at around US$10–$20 per person per year. As a result, antiretrovirals are not available, nor are basics such as antidiarrheals, antibiotics, and antipyretics. Thus, the priority is to ensure that participants in clinical trials have access to basic, comprehensive primary health care, including antiretrovirals if appropriate.

Who should provide this care? If the people responsible for AIDS vaccine clinical trials are required to provide lifetime care, it will further reduce the incentives for manufacturers and trial sponsors to do research in developing countries. Furthermore, will other less well-financed areas, such as research into improving uptake of barrier methods or microbicide research, be held to these standards? If so, who will pay for care for participants who become infected?

In the end, only governments can provide long-term-care guarantees. We need a development approach to strengthen their capacity to provide these services. It is clear that accelerating vaccine research and supporting community participation in trials requires shared responsibility. Communities participating in AIDS prevention and treatment trials, whatever the results, are contributing knowledge that is a global public good and should benefit in return. I suggest that communities which participate in this research become not only a national priority for scaled-up care but also a stated priority for multilateral programs (Global Fund to Fight AIDS, Tuberculosis and Malaria; and the World Bank's Multi-Country HIV/AIDS Program) and bilateral programs, such as the U.S. Bush administration's Emergency Plan for AIDS Relief.

The advantages of this approach are many: making care available for communities avoids difficult decisions on whether individual participants, whole families, or extended families should receive treatment; choosing communities in which to scale up care becomes less arbitrary; it rewards and provides an incentive for communities to participate in research; and, by acting at the community level, it lessens any risk that individual participation is unduly encouraged because it is no longer a qualification for receiving treatment.

In the meantime, if governments are too poor to meet their obligations, trial sponsors and donor agencies should work together to fill funding gaps. By implementing this approach, the world would not only acknowledge and reward those responsible for developing AIDS therapies, but it would also provide beneficence for the people in who they are tested. Finally, governments and multilateral and bilateral agencies should join forces to ensure that when a successful vaccine is identified, a global access plan is in place that includes adequate financing for communities unable to afford such a product.[2] Lack of attention to access would raise further horrendous ethical dilemmas and prove that, once again, we cannot learn from history.

References

1. Klausner, R. D., A. S. Fauci, L. Corey, G. J. Nabel, H. Gayle, S. Berkley, et al. 2003. The need for a global HIV vaccine enterprise. *Science* 300:2036–2039.

2. IAVI. 2001. *A New Access Paradigm: Public Sector Actions to Assure Swift, Global Access to AIDS Vaccines*. New York: IAVI.

10 The Vaccine (*Excerpt*)

Michael Specter[*]

At 41, Hala has five children and eight grandchildren. Her first husband left when their second child was born. Her second husband died of AIDS nearly 20 years ago, in the earliest days of the epidemic. Hala often tells people that she sells charcoal, doughnuts, or cooking oil on the streets, but that isn't true. She is a prostitute, who has spent nearly half her life working out of a wattle hut in Pumwani, one of Nairobi's most crowded—and violent—slums. On an average day, she might see ten men, most of them truck drivers from Tanzania. Her "office" has just enough room for a single bed, a stool, a customer, herself, and a wicker basket filled with condoms. The basket is a recent addition; only in the past year or so have her clients agreed to use condoms with any regularity.

None of these details makes Hala unusual. Despite the severity of the AIDS epidemic, Kenyans have only just begun to speak openly about the disease, and the epidemic has certainly done little to deter prostitution. As many as two and a half million people in Kenya, one in six adults, are infected with HIV. In Pumwani, more than 90% of prostitutes—and many of their clients—test positive for the virus. Hala has engaged in unprotected sex with hundreds of HIV-positive men. Her best customer—a man who visited her regularly for 17 years and never used a condom—recently died of AIDS. Remarkably, she has never become infected.

The day I was introduced to Hala, at a clinic not far from where she lives, she was draped in black robes and wore a purple shawl with gold piping down the sides. She is a handsome, businesslike woman, and she is completely baffled by her fate. "I have no idea why I of all people have been spared," she told me. "But if my luck can be useful to the doctors then I will be grateful."

Hala belongs to an increasingly famous cohort of research subjects, known by AIDS experts throughout the world as "the Nairobi prostitutes." In the late 1980s, the

* Originally published in *The New Yorker*, February 3, 2003. Reprinted with permission.

Canadian infectious-disease expert Francis Plummer noticed something startling: in a study of 2,000 Nairobi prostitutes, as many as 200 remained uninfected, despite years of constant high-risk behavior. Later, when Plummer and his colleagues examined the data more closely, they realized that if the prostitutes didn't become infected within 5 years of their first exposure to the virus, they were unlikely to become infected at all.

How, exactly, were these women protected when millions who engaged in the same behavior fell ill and died? It couldn't have been luck; nobody gets lucky a thousand times in a row. Nor was it good nutrition; the women often lived on plantains and rice, and many were weak, undernourished, and sickly. Plummer concluded that these women harbored a rare defensive weapon within their immune systems. To many vaccine researchers, the implications were thrilling: if they could identify that weapon and somehow bottle it, they might help to end the world's most devastating epidemic. "We all held our breath for a while," Job J. Bwayo, the director of the International AIDS Vaccine Initiative in Kenya, told me when I went to see him at the University of Nairobi. "Nobody expected a simple solution to come from it, but we have all kept hoping that somehow the girls will provide the key."

The search for a solution has become desperate. Twenty-one years after the first cases of "slim disease," as AIDS was initially called in Africa, appeared in a Ugandan village on the shores of Lake Victoria, scientists are only marginally closer to producing a successful vaccine than they were when they identified the virus that causes it. A great deal has changed for people with AIDS in those two decades: medicines are now routinely available throughout the developed world. But, of the 40 million people who are living with HIV, less than 5% have access to them. Because that percentage will not change dramatically in the next decade, the world has never needed a medical intervention more urgently than it needs an AIDS vaccine today.

To date, 65 million people around the world have become infected with HIV, most of them in Africa. Twenty-five million have died. In the next 20 years—as the epidemic moves swiftly through India, Russia, and China—the number could more than double. There are no scenarios for any kind of war that project the type of complete destruction, the numbers of dead, or the social collapse that can already be attributed to AIDS. The disease represents the worst disaster that we can reasonably expect to befall humanity in our lifetime.

That is why Hala and the other women of Pumwani are essential. "You do the research where the problem is," Kevin De Cock, the chief representative in Kenya for the Centers for Disease Control, told me. "Africa needs the answer, the world needs the answer. But you are not going to solve the AIDS crisis in a convent in Montana." To gauge the effectiveness of an AIDS vaccine, scientists will need to compare thousands of people who receive it with thousands who do not. That will never happen in the United States or Europe—regions where less than 1% of the population is infected, and where most patients have access to effective treatments. Only extensive human trials among groups with high infection rates will produce a vaccine. In practice, this means that tens of thousands of Africans and Asians from remote villages and overcrowded cities will have to be recruited for tests on a scale never seen before.

The scientific challenges presented by the epidemic have proved to be humbling: in laboratories across the world, researchers have thrown everything they have at HIV, but nearly every time they manage to move one step forward, the virus seems to move two. As great as the scientific and logistical hurdles are, however, the ethical problems associated with long-term vaccine trials in the developing world—funded by Western donors and designed, largely, by Western scientists—may be tougher still. In 1796, after Edward Jenner noticed that dairymaids seemed immune to smallpox, he simply inoculated a healthy young boy with cowpox and then a few weeks later exposed him to the human disease, at great risk to the child. No scientist could do such a thing today. There are rules that prohibit researchers from gambling with the lives of their subjects: they have to minimize the risks, obtain consent, and provide the volunteers with "appropriate treatment." But what, exactly, constitutes appropriate treatment? In America or Europe, such a trial would have to include the requirement that every infected participant receive the best care available today—a lifetime commitment to expensive antiretroviral medicine. Should such a promise be made to Africans? Is appropriate treatment for a community in northern Uganda the same as it would be in Manhattan?

The issue of whether Western ethics and the rules of medical care that accompany them should prevail in Africa has for many people become the central debate of the AIDS epidemic. Several prominent American physicians, led by Marcia Angell, who teaches at Harvard and is a former editor of the *New England Journal of Medicine*, have argued that medical ethics has no borders: what is morally right in America is morally right in Africa, too. They believe that international rules of medical experimentation require that volunteers in such trials receive the best treatment available, not simply the level of care typical of an impoverished community.

No country in Africa, and few countries elsewhere in the developing world, can afford Western levels of treatment. So the principal question for researchers and public-health officials is both simple and harsh: Will scientific objectives drive the search for an AIDS vaccine, or will a series of ethical imperatives imposed by the West take precedence? Because that question has gone unanswered, fear of exploitation and abuse hangs over the trials, threatening not only to impede their progress but to prevent them altogether.

Issues of equity in clinical research preoccupy Western ethicists and public-health officials. Will people used as subjects benefit from the research? (Africans served as essential participants in trials for the principal vaccine now used against hepatitis B; yet when the vaccine finally arrived, they could not afford it.) Should volunteers get better medical care than other people in their villages? Should they get better treatment than other members of their own families? Are we exploiting research subjects if we don't promise special treatment? Are we bribing them if we do?

"I am very worried about these trials," Peter Lurie, the deputy director of Public Citizen's Health Research Group, told me when we met one rainy day in the organization's offices, just off Dupont Circle, in Washington, DC. Lurie and his colleague Sidney Wolfe have long been concerned about what they regard as the cavalier attitude of American researchers toward Third World subjects. "Instead of seeing themselves as activists for better care in Africa, scientists will use the poor quality of care to justify what they want to do anyway," Lurie said. "But you are not permitted simply to use subjects in order to collect data because it is useful to you. That is exploitation and abuse. That is what Tuskegee was." In the Tuskegee experiment, which ran from 1932 until 1972, researchers allowed poor black men with syphilis to go untreated to study the long-term effects of the disease; it remains America's signature instance of research undisciplined by ethical oversight. Lurie fears that, in the name of science, doctors could again withhold treatments that they know will work. "If we aren't careful," Lurie said, "we could be in for the greatest injustice in the history of medicine."

•

The Windsor hotel, just a few miles from the center of Entebbe, has a commanding view of Lake Victoria. It sits at the end of a rutted dirt road crowded with men selling tomatoes and fresh Nile perch, not far from the Uganda Virus Research Institute.

I went to the Windsor late one afternoon at the urging of Pontiano Kaleebu, a virologist who is the Vaccine Initiative's principal investigator in Uganda. The group's community advisory board was planning its first serious discussion of the Phase III trials that the International AIDS Vaccine Initiative hopes to conduct in Uganda. Once vaccines have shown promise in the laboratory and in animals, they are generally tested on humans in three stages. In the first phase, a few people are given the vaccine simply to ensure that it causes no serious side effects. Next, scientists try to find out whether the vaccine can stimulate people's immune systems. The final phase, and the one that matters the most, requires thousands of volunteers (and several years) in order to provide reliable statistical evidence of whether a vaccine actually prevents disease. The vaccine for which Kaleebu was trying to recruit volunteers had been developed by Andrew McMichael, Tomas Hanke, and their collaborators at Oxford, based in part on immunological information gleaned from the blood cells of the Nairobi prostitutes. It is one of dozens of vaccines currently under development (and among several that the I.A.V.I. is supporting), but it has shown particular promise. The plan is to expand that trial to include thousands of people in at least three African countries. But first Kaleebu and his colleagues would have to convince a group of Ugandan civic leaders—educators, newspaper editors, and clergy among them—that the people of their country should once again subject themsel   to the inconvenience and uncertainty involved in testing a vaccine.

It was the beginning of the monsoon season, and the intense daily rain had just ended as the members of the advisory board arrived at the hotel. The scent of jasmine filled the air, and a family of monkeys played on the lawns. It is never easy to persuade people to submit to medical experiments, even in a country like Uganda—which is both enlightened about AIDS and has nearly been destroyed by it. People are instinctively wary of offering their bodies for research. Meetings like this, where risks and benefits are explained, are essential if any drug or vaccine is to succeed.

Kaleebu had confided to me that he was nervous about the meeting because without the support of community leaders, a vaccine trial could never be completed. "We have asked the people of this country to be guinea pigs before, and they have responded admirably," he told me. "But we have not been able to come back and say, 'Here is your reward.' I worry about how many times we can ask for the sacrifice. But, of course, I worry far more about what we would do if people gave up and said, 'No, go away.'"

The group gathered in a large, muggy conference room on the second floor. Fred Nakwagala, a young medical officer for the I.A.V.I. program, explained how the vaccine works. He is a thin, unprepossessing man, and at first he spoke too softly to be heard. "We need to create a world without AIDS," he said. "In order to do that, we need a safe, effective, and affordable vaccine. This is up to you. No one else can do it." Sweat poured from his brow as he began explaining, in the simplest possible terms, that a vaccine is a scientific product that prepares your body to fight infection.

Father Christopher Kiwanuka, the leader of an Entebbe Catholic parish, asked whether a vaccine was really the only thing that could eliminate the threat of HIV. "There are drugs now," he said. "They are getting cheaper. Won't they eventually be here, too?"

Antiretroviral therapies, which stop HIV from replicating, are already available to Ugandans rich enough to pay for them. When the drugs are purchased by agencies such as Doctors Without Borders, they cost no more than $300 a year, less than a dollar per day. That doesn't seem like much, but as it happens, it is Uganda's annual per-capita income. The government spends an average of about $6 a year on health care for each of its citizens; a dollar a day might as well be a thousand. Nakwagala explained that, even with falling prices, antiretroviral therapies will never resolve Uganda's AIDS crisis. "Neither will prevention," he continued. "Prevention has had limited success. Education and condoms work only up to a point. We have one million people in our country currently infected. Half a million are dead. I wish I could offer you different news, but we have run out of things we can try."

"But why us?" a prominent journalist asked. "It seems it's always us. For how many years does Uganda have to be the test case?" There were murmurs of agreement.

It is an awkward fact that the very countries where vaccine trials must take place are usually the poorest and the most politically unstable. Before researchers can invest hundreds of millions of dollars in a scientific study, they need some assurance that the government will allow it to run for years. In Africa, that is asking a lot. Earlier that day, Kaleebu told me that he had made plans to attend an AIDS conference in the Ivory Coast later that week. But, he said, as if he were passing along an unpleasant weather report, "I had to cancel because of the coup."

Nakwagala spoke frankly to the advisory board: "There are no answers right now. Only questions. There will be none tomorrow, either. But if we ever want anything to change we have to do this." After an hour, tea was served, everyone agreed that there was no real choice except to go forward, and the meeting came to an uneasy end.

The campus of the Uganda Virus Research Institute is spread across a few dozen acres, and most of the offices are housed in airy little bungalows that face Lake Victoria. After the meeting, I followed Kaleebu back to his office there. Kaleebu is an urbane and reflective man with a sad smile; a thin oval of hair surrounds his mouth. He was brought up in Kampala and finished his medical studies at Makerere University in 1986. He then moved to London, where he earned a PhD. Since returning to Uganda, he has been in charge of the U.V.R.I.'s immunology division. "I am worried that the question of how to do the trials, and whether they can be done fairly and ethically, will overshadow the science itself," he said, in a soft British accent. "There is an endless amount of talk—in the West, not here—about what kind of treatment all the volunteers should receive and whether it's fair to use them. I know people in America think this discussion is for our benefit, but they are wrong. I am Ugandan and, believe me, I have no stake in taking advantage of anyone in this country for my research. We will give people the best care they can get, the best care we can afford. That is fair. If we could distribute antiretroviral drugs, I would be thrilled. But I don't see how, and I don't see when. And the debate is a bit patronizing. We are not blind here. This is not an issue of individual rights—as American ethicists would like it to be. It is the opposite: a public-health emergency."

Kaleebu is married and has four young children. He lives near the institute so that he can walk to work. He stays at the lab until dinner, spends an hour with his family, and then returns until ten. "That's my life," he said with a shrug. "And it will be my life as long as AIDS is with us."

•

The International AIDS Vaccine Initiative has its main offices in Manhattan, high above the financial district. With money from a coalition of public and private donors—not least the Bill & Melinda Gates Foundation, which has made the discovery and distribution of an AIDS vaccine its most significant project—the initiative acts as both a medical gateway and a sort of philanthropic venture-capital firm dedicated to funding the effort to find a vaccine.

I went there one morning to talk with Seth Berkley, the man who runs the initiative. Berkley is a rangy 46-year-old physician who was trained at Brown and Harvard and worked as an epidemiologist in Brazil and Uganda during the 1980s. He was in Africa just at the time that the full horror of AIDS became clear.

Berkley is often criticized for his single-minded pursuit of this goal. But his assertions are hard to dismiss; in 2001, less than 2% of the $20 billion spent on AIDS prevention, treatment, and research across the world was devoted to the search for a vaccine. After millions of deaths, only a single vaccine has made it into the late stages of human trials.

The International AIDS Vaccine Initiative exists for a strange reason: an AIDS vaccine may be a global necessity, but it is really in no single country's or company's interest to spend the sort of money that would be necessary to find one. Most pharmaceutical firms view any such vaccine as a liability nightmare, and the demand would be greatest among the populations that are least able to pay. Making drugs, by contrast, involves a much greater financial incentive and much lower risk. "We have left vaccine development to the commercial sector as if there were an incentive for companies in the marketplace to make a product," Larry Corey, the head of the HIV Vaccine Trials Network and a professor of medicine at the University of Washington, told me. "But there is no incentive. And what is society's response? Well, society can't get it together. Remember, these trials can cost hundreds of millions of dollars. Do we use public–private partnerships? Does the government fund it all? We are just asking all these questions today. Twenty years after the epidemic began."

Much has been written about whether governments have spent enough money developing an AIDS vaccine—whether there should have been a sort of viral Manhattan Project—and whether existing resources have been used wisely. It is a difficult matter to resolve. There is no question that more money, particularly in the early years, would have helped push research forward. But scientific discovery isn't linear; it moves in unpredictable patterns. Billions of dollars have been spent on the war on cancer in the past 30 years, and, many would argue, to little avail.

"Please don't say that I am pessimistic, because I am not," Anthony Fauci told me when I went to visit him at the National Institutes of Health (NIH), where, as the director of the National Institute of Allergy and Infectious Diseases, he is responsible for funding much of the AIDS research in the United States. "A fully effective vaccine against HIV is by no means impossible. It will eventually happen. But there are many problems we need to solve in order to produce one. The best ways to vaccinate don't work with HIV. We need to come up with something new."

"Let's be realistic for five minutes," Larry Corey, who is responsible for organizing the NIH-supported network of vaccine trials, told me. "To create a vaccine that works maybe forty per cent of the time, that costs a thousand dollars, and that has side effects such that you have to go to a lab and get a blood test every six weeks," which is the case with drug regimens, "is crap. What we need is a ninety-per-cent biologically active product that has no side effects, and that, at the most, costs around a hundred and fifty to two hundred dollars."

Almost no one who does AIDS research thinks that a genuine cure will be discovered soon. "I would have to say the virus is winning, not us," Anthony Fauci told me. Fauci is among the most forthcoming members of the American AIDS establishment. When I asked him whether we will have anything significant 10 years from now, he winced. "My God, I hope so," he said. "I really do."

●

Bouncing along on one of Uganda's few good roads, you can easily spend 3 hours on the 95-mile journey from Kampala to the Masaka district. The drive takes you straight across the equator, around the western edge of Lake Victoria, and toward the border with Tanzania.

It is in regions like Masaka that the debate about the standard of medical treatment for volunteers turns into a question of how long and how well someone will live. At the same time, volunteers face basic uncertainties about whether the AIDS-vaccine trials will benefit them at all. "We are asking the Third World to take risks that we have actually never taken ourselves," Larry Corey told me. "Every other time that we have gone in with a vaccine—whether polio, measles, mumps—we have been able to say, 'It works on our people.' With AIDS, we can't say that. Now I have to build a global HIV network, and I have to go to my colleagues in Botswana, Kenya, or Malawi and say, 'I have no idea if I have schlock or I have gold. But you need it and we need it, so we will have to test it on you.' There are really no other choices."

I never met a healthcare professional in Africa who didn't understand this. African doctors live every day with uncertainty and inequity. More clearly than any disease before, AIDS has demonstrated the vast and unbridgeable gulf between the affluent north and the impoverished south. How can one compare the health care available in the United States or Europe with that of the Third World? Curable illnesses such as diarrhea still kill more people every year than AIDS does. Even in Uganda, the rate of childhood vaccination—perhaps the best way to judge the overall health of a nation—has declined recently, from 47% in 1995 to 37% last year.

In Masaka, I toured the village of Kalungu with a census-taker named Irene. Her goal was simply to identify all the people who lived in the pale-yellow huts of the village and then to ask basic questions about their age and marital status.

We walked over to the local clinic, where a young medical student was on duty. I asked whether he thought it would be fair for the people in this village to enter a trial for a new AIDS vaccine if those who became infected did not receive antiretroviral drugs. He snorted and made a dismissive wave at the shelves on the wall. There were about two dozen neatly lettered red labels for a variety of pharmaceuticals. Half the labels—including those for aspirin and Paracetamol—had empty spaces above them. The selection was spotty; there was Fansidar (a highly effective malaria drug), but no ordinary, inexpensive antibiotic. Eight women sat on a bench in the waiting room; they all had children with them. A couple of the babies were crying, but most just stared blankly into space. "We are not getting the care you get," the medical student told me without a shred of bitterness in his voice. "We never will. But I would line up tomorrow to test anything that might help us in any way. And I am sure the rest of the village would, too."

Anyone who offers himself as a test subject for a vaccine that could end a plague surely deserves the best possible medical care. Perhaps that care should be better than the care that other people would receive in the same community; or perhaps entire villages should be entitled to the first access to new treatments. But medicine in Uganda will never be as good as it is at the Mayo Clinic or even at a typical hospital in Moscow. Most people in Africa can't even afford to take a bus to get care at a free clinic. "Where does it start, and where does it end?" Seth Berkley asked me when we spoke one day. "Is it the best treatment for people in the trial? Is there an obligation to pay for current therapies? What about better therapies in the future? Are we supposed to pay for the state of the art for eternity? Nobody could afford it." There is a malady called Chagas' disease, or American trypanosomiasis. It can destroy the esophagus, the bowel, and the heart. End-stage Chagas' disease often results in heart failure. The only treatment is a heart transplant. Does this mean that in order to try to cure this disease in places like Mexico and Brazil, where it is endemic, everyone should receive a transplant? "We have always had this idea, which is simplistic, that justice requires treating everyone, everywhere exactly the same way," Ezekiel Emanuel, who is the chief of the bioethics branch at the NIH, told me. "Justice requires no such thing. Justice simply requires us to treat people fairly." If the rules of clinical trials required participants to receive the best care on earth, there would be no clinical trials.

Some activists in the West talk as if this were a price worth paying to avoid the risk of exploitation. In a speech that Marcia Angell gave at Princeton, she said, "People are not guinea pigs. Research must hold human welfare above the interest of society and science. If you breach this principle, you're on a slippery slope where first humans are exploited for worthwhile purposes, then for not so worthwhile purposes." This position suggests that one cannot hold the interests of society above the interests of an individual, that individual well-being is paramount. Yet in countries that have been devastated by AIDS, balancing the needs of society against those of the individual has never seemed more essential.

Five years ago, Angell led a highly public attack on Western scientists who were conducting trials in Africa, attempting to find a cheap, effective way to prevent a mother from passing the AIDS virus to her child at birth. The research was based on one of the more exciting discoveries of the past decade: women who took the drug AZT during pregnancy could cut the risk of transmission by as much as two-thirds. But the drug regimen was too expensive and complicated for the women who needed it most, and public-health officials began looking for cheaper alternatives. They decided to follow more than 14,000 women in Thailand and Africa and gave AZT to a third of them in various doses. The rest received placebos. At the time, Angell wrote that allowing the women to go without AZT—when doctors knew it worked and Western women would have received it—was "a retreat from ethical principles," and she invoked that most incendiary of comparisons, the Tuskegee experiment. Peter Lurie, who is South African and no stranger to the clinics of the Third World, said that the tests proved there was a two-tiered standard for health care in the world—one set of rules for rich people and another for those who are poor. The recriminations were harsh, and their effects have lingered.

African scientists saw it differently, however. "The women were not going to get any treatment anyway," Pontiano Kaleebu told me. "Instead, thousands received AZT, and that saved their babies. And we found out that it works in much smaller doses—and it has been one of the great discoveries for us in the entire epidemic. If Marcia Angell had her way, though, we still wouldn't know what works, because we would never have been able to do the studies."

The day I left Uganda, I went to see Edward Mbidde, who is the director of the Uganda Cancer Institute and among Africa's most internationally prominent vaccine advocates. Mbidde is a powerfully built, imposing man. He wore a dark-green dashiki and spoke in the rich, deliberate tones of the English-educated African elite. His office is at the Old Mulago Hospital, which for years was at the center of the AIDS epidemic; it sits on a hill overlooking the streets of Kampala. Despite ample reason for despair, Mbidde has always remained determined and optimistic.

"In many ways, these last fifteen years have been the best Uganda has ever seen," he told me. I must have gasped because he laughed and then said, "What I mean by that is simple enough. We have leadership, we have support, and we are united. Who else in Africa can say that? Can you imagine what would have happened to Uganda if AIDS had come along during the time of Idi Amin?" Mbidde travels widely, and he long ago decided that without an AIDS vaccine, Africa is in peril, and the only way to find one that works is to experiment on people—his people.

"If you are living in New York or Florida, you can sit on the beach or work in a skyscraper. You have a different view of what the world is like than we do," he said. "Perhaps it is a better world. Yet if we need to go to work, and we cannot afford a Mercedes-Benz, should we refuse to ride on a motorcycle? Or should we get there by the best route we have? You do what you can in this life, and in Kampala, we cannot do everything. Principles matter as much to us as they do to Americans. But we have been dying for a long time, and you cannot respond to death with principles."

11   Ethical Considerations in Biomedical HIV Prevention Trials (*Excerpt*)

UNAIDS*

Well into the third decade of the HIV pandemic, there remains no effective HIV preventive vaccine, microbicide, product, or drug to reduce the risk of HIV acquisition. As the numbers of those infected by HIV and dying from AIDS continue to increase, the need for such biomedical HIV preventive interventions becomes ever more urgent. Several such products are at various stages of development, including some currently in phase III efficacy trials. The successful development of effective HIV preventive interventions requires that many different candidates be studied simultaneously in different populations around the world. This in turn will require a large international cooperative effort drawing on partners from various health sectors, intergovernmental organizations, government, research institutions, industry, and affected populations. It will also require that these partners be able and willing to address the difficult ethical concerns that arise during the development of biomedical HIV prevention products.

Following deliberations during 1997–1999 involving lawyers, activists, social scientists, ethicists, vaccine scientists, epidemiologists, nongovernmental organization (NGO) representatives, people living with HIV, and people working in health policy from a total of 33 countries, UNAIDS published a guidance document on ethical considerations in HIV preventive vaccine research in 2000. Since then, there have been numerous developments related to the conduct of biomedical HIV prevention trials, including vaccine trials. Consultations have been held to explore key issues such as:

• Creating effective partnerships, collaboration, and community participation in HIV prevention trials;
• The inclusion of adolescents in HIV vaccine trials;
• Gender considerations related to enrollment and informed consent; provision of support, care, and treatment to participants and the community engaged in HIV prevention trials; and
• Post-trial responsibilities of sponsors, researchers, and local providers;

* Originally published by UNAIDS/ONUSIDA, 2012. Reprinted with permission.

In light of these consultations and evolution in the level of prevention, treatment, and care available in the era of "Toward Universal Access," the 2000 guidance document was revised and updated. The revision incorporates developments that have taken place since the original publication, including lessons learned in the field of biomedical HIV prevention research. Many different strategies for HIV prevention are now being explored, including microbicides, vaccines, female-initiated barrier methods, herpes simplex virus-2 (HSV-2) treatment/suppression, index partner treatment, antiretroviral pre-exposure prophylaxis, prevention of mother-to-child transmission, and drug substitution/maintenance for injecting drug users.

This document does not purport to capture the extensive discussion, debate, consensus, and disagreement that have taken place among stakeholders in HIV prevention research. Rather it highlights, from the perspective of UNAIDS and WHO, some of the critical ethical elements that must be considered during the development of safe and effective biomedical HIV prevention interventions.

It is hoped that this document will be of use to potential research volunteers and trial participants, investigators, research staff, community members, government representatives, pharmaceutical companies and other industry partners and trial sponsors, and ethical and scientific review committees involved in the development of biomedical HIV prevention products and interventions. It suggests standards as well as processes for arriving at standards that can be used as a frame of reference from which to conduct further discussion at the local, national, and international levels and can inform the development of national guidelines for the conduct of biomedical HIV prevention trials.

•

Guidance Point 14: Care and Treatment

Participants who acquire HIV infection during the conduct of a biomedical HIV prevention trial should be provided access to treatment regimens from among those internationally recognized as optimal. Prior to initiation of a trial, all research stakeholders should come to agreement through participatory processes on mechanisms to provide and sustain such HIV-related care and treatment.

The obligation on the part of sponsors and investigators to ensure access to HIV care and treatment, including antiretroviral treatment, for participants who become infected derives from some or all of three ethical principles. The principle of beneficence requires that the welfare of participants be actively promoted. The principle of justice as reciprocity calls for providing something in return to participants who have volunteered their time, been inconvenienced, or experienced discomfort by enrolling in the trial. The principle of justice, meaning treating like cases alike, requires that trial participants in high-income and low- and middle-income countries be treated equally regarding access to treatment and care.

A consensus on the level of care and treatment that should be provided to trial participants has emerged in recent years with increasing accessibility of antiretroviral treatment in low- and middle-income countries based on strong commitments from countries, development partners, and multilateral organizations; dramatic decreases in drug prices; and evidence that treatment programs in resource-poor settings are feasible and sustainable. There is consensus that sponsors need to ensure access to internationally recognized optimal care and treatment regimens, including antiretroviral therapy, for participants who become HIV infected during the course of the trial. There is also agreement that prevention trials should contribute constructively to the development of HIV service provision in countries participating in biomedical HIV prevention research, for the sustainable provision of care and treatment after the completion of a trial.

The provision of antiretroviral treatment to trial participants who acquire HIV infection during the trial requires planning for logistics and implementation. Most such participants will not need antiretroviral treatment until years after sero-conversion. However, they may benefit from a comprehensive care and prevention package including cotrimoxazole prophylaxis, isoniazid, nutritional advice, and positive prevention counseling. Biomedical HIV prevention trials should undertake to support such therapy until individuals become eligible for the national program of care and treatment in their country. Countries should include participants in biomedical HIV prevention trials in their priority list for access to antiretroviral treatment under the "Towards Universal Access" program.

Trial sponsors and researchers should collaborate with governments in low- and middle-income countries to explore, develop, and strengthen national and local capacity to deliver the highest possible level of HIV prevention, care, and treatment services through strategic investment and development of trial-related resources. In most situations, no one stakeholder should bear the entire burden of providing resources for such services, and the central responsibility for delivery should lie with local health systems.

Decisions on how these obligations are to be met are best made for each specific trial through a transparent and participatory process that should involve all research stakeholders before a trial starts to recruit participants (see Guidance Point 2). This process should explore options and determine the core obligations applicable to the given situation, in terms of the level, scope, and duration of the care and treatment package, equity in eligibility to access services, and responsibility for provision and delivery. Agreements on who will finance, deliver, and monitor care and treatment should be documented. All stakeholders should recognize that this is a critically important and highly uncertain area that requires all partners to commit themselves to experimentation and the careful documentation of approaches, successes, and failures.

Clinical trials should be integrated into national prevention, treatment, and care plans so that services provided through clinical trials or arrangements brokered for trial participants serve to improve the health conditions of both the trial participants and the community from which they are drawn, and to support and strengthen a country's comprehensive response to the epidemic. Strengthening mechanisms to provide care, treatment, and support for people who acquire HIV infection during the course of a trial will assist in ensuring referral and care provision for people who are deemed ineligible at recruitment to a biomedical HIV prevention trial because they already have HIV infection.

A care and treatment package should include, but not be limited to, some or all of the following items, depending on the type of research, the setting, and the consensus reached by all interested parties before the trial begins:

- counseling
- preventive methods and means
- treatment for other sexually transmitted infections
- prevention of mother to child transmission
- prevention/treatment of tuberculosis
- prevention/treatment of opportunistic infections
- nutrition
- palliative care, including pain control and spiritual care
- referral to social and community support
- family planning
- reproductive health care for pregnancy and childbirth
- home-based care
- antiretroviral therapy

III Vaccine Regulation, Risk-Benefit Assessments, and Safety

In the United States, approval of a new vaccine by the U.S. Food and Drug Administration (FDA) following a successful research and development program is only one of many regulatory, policy, and implementation activities that, together, will determine whether the vaccine is capable of achieving the public health goals envisioned by its proponents. The introduction of new vaccines and ongoing stewardship of vaccination programs are responsibilities shared by a broad partnership of federal, state, and local policymakers and regulators; medical professional societies; individual health-care providers; vaccine manufacturers; and interested citizen, patient, and consumer organizations.

Foremost among the concerns of these stakeholders throughout their work is monitoring the safety of individual vaccines and the overall recommended vaccination schedule. Whether confirmed or simply alleged, vaccine safety concerns pose a grave threat to vaccination programs, particularly to public confidence in vaccination as an important and valuable intervention for themselves or, more commonly, for their children. No vaccine, indeed nothing in medicine, is entirely without risk, and a variety of mechanisms, policies, and programs are in place to rapidly identify and respond to the rare, usually minor adverse events associated with vaccines.

But far more attention and anxiety has been raised not by these rare, minor, known vaccine-associated risks, but by allegations of far more widespread and serious risks that go unacknowledged or unaddressed by health officials. Atop this category of vaccine safety concerns are claims that childhood vaccines are responsible for large observed increases in rates of autism and other developmental conditions, allegations that have been rejected by the mainstream medical and public health communities but remain among some parents of affected children and other critics of contemporary vaccination policy.

This section looks at the design of vaccine policymaking in the United States, from the development of policies and recommendations for the use of vaccines to the efforts to identify, study, and respond to potential vaccine safety concerns. Lance Rodewald, Walter Orenstein, and colleagues begin with an overview of the U.S. vaccination system, highlighting in particular the role of financing programs to ensure broad access to recommended vaccines. Heidi Larson, Louis Cooper, and colleagues next discuss the challenges policymakers worldwide encounter in building and sustaining public confidence in vaccines as part of their work promoting vaccines. Jason Schwartz and Adel Mahmoud then discuss the Advisory Committee on Immunization Practices, the expert advisors to the U.S. Centers for Disease Control and Prevention who shape the design of vaccination programs in the United States and indirectly around their world. Their mission is to combine a rigorous evaluation of evidence in developing policy recommendations with comparable attention to using scarce public health resources wisely, all while sustaining public trust in the U.S. vaccination enterprise.

When safety concerns related to vaccines emerge, a program in the United States has been in place since the 1980s to compensate those who were harmed. Katherine Cook and Geoffrey Evans discuss the National Vaccine Injury Compensation Program, and Michelle Mello then explores the potential rationales—legal, ethical, and policy—for creating this unique program in medicine and public health to deal with vaccine-related injuries.

This section concludes with three chapters that examine the emotional debate alleging an association between childhood vaccines and autism. Jeffrey Baker traces the history of concerns over the health risks of mercury, an ingredient that until the late 1990s could be found in small amounts in many childhood vaccines. Jeffrey Gerber and Paul Offit map the different theories that attempt to connect vaccines with autism, and they summarize many of the studies that have rejected such links. Finally, Fiona Godlee and colleagues look back on the conduct of Andrew Wakefield, the British physician whose 1998 paper—since retracted—on the measles-mumps-rubella vaccine is widely viewed as having spurred a surge of concern about a theorized relationship between vaccines and autism.

Further Reading

Louis Z. Cooper, Heidi J. Larson, Samuel L. Katz. 2008. Protecting Public Trust in Immunization. *Pediatrics* 122 (1):149–153.

Institute of Medicine. 2013. *The Childhood Immunization Schedule and Safety: Stakeholder Concerns, Scientific Evidence, and Future Studies.* Washington, DC: National Academies Press.

Seth Mnookin. 2011. *The Panic Virus: A True Story of Science, Medicine, and Fear.* New York: Simon & Schuster.

Jason L. Schwartz. 2012. The First Rotavirus Vaccine and the Politics of Acceptable Risk. *The Milbank Quarterly* 90 (2):278–310.

U.S. Centers for Disease Control and Prevention. 2015. Vaccine Safety. Available at: http://www.cdc.gov/vaccinesafety/index.html.

12 Immunization in the United States (*Excerpt*)

Lance E. Rodewald, Walter A. Orenstein, Alan R. Hinman, and Anne Schuchat[*]

The immunization system in the United States is a public- and private-sector partnership that works toward common immunization goals and objectives, has a formal process of establishing national immunization recommendations, and uses a set of systems to monitor the health impact, coverage levels, and safety of recommended vaccines. As of 2012, routine immunization protected the U.S. public against 17 vaccine-preventable diseases. Access to vaccines is provided through private and public health insurance for all ages, and financially vulnerable children have a federal government entitlement to vaccines through the Vaccines for Children (VFC) program.

Immunization of young children in the United States has been highly effective. Most vaccine-preventable diseases of children are at record or near record lows in the United States, with small or no disparities by race and ethnicity. Measles, rubella, and polio have been, and remain, eliminated in the United States, and the number of young children not immunized at all remains less than 1%. Immunization of adolescents has become more robust and challenging in the last 5 years as four vaccines have been newly recommended for routine administration (Tdap, meningococcal conjugate vaccine [MCV4], human papillomavirus [HPV], and influenza vaccines). The full benefits of these vaccines are yet to be realized as vaccination coverage levels among U.S. teens have been increasing only moderately and vary substantially across states. Immunization of adults continues to be a growing challenge in the United States as longstanding vaccination coverage objectives have not been fully met, while new vaccines such as zoster, Tdap, and HPV vaccines are being introduced.

Roles of the U.S. Immunization Program

The U.S. Institute of Medicine (IOM) provided a useful conceptual framework for understanding the complex array of roles of the federal, state, and local immunization programs in collaboration with the nation's healthcare delivery system.[1] The IOM identified five key roles: (1) ensure purchase of vaccine, (2) ensure service delivery, (3) control and prevent infectious diseases, (4) conduct surveillance of vaccine coverage and safety, and (5) sustain and improve immunization coverage levels. These roles are used to ensure the ultimate immunization program goal of controlling and preventing infectious diseases. The impact of immunization policies and practices is assessed through careful disease surveillance, vaccine effectiveness studies, and safety monitoring—an evidence base that is used to adjust immunization recommendations as new evidence emerges. All of these activities are supported by a base of immunization finance policies and practices.

Although vaccines are given in private and public sectors, other important components of immunization programs are coordinated by health departments and other public-sector agencies, including surveillance and investigation of disease, outbreak control, promotion of immunization, adverse-events monitoring, assessment of immunization levels, and implementation of regulations and laws regarding immunization.

Ensuring Vaccine Purchase, Supply, and Distribution

Manufacturers sell their vaccines in the private sector directly to immunization providers or indirectly through private-sector pharmaceutical distributors. Private immunization providers purchase vaccines up front for vaccination of their private-sector patients and are reimbursed for the vaccine by private and public health insurance on a fee-for-service basis. In general, private immunization providers receive slightly more in insurance reimbursement than they pay for the vaccines, but private-sector providers are ultimately responsible for the financial risk incurred by the up-front purchase of vaccine.[2]

Approximately half of the childhood vaccine supply is purchased with federal and state government funding using the CDC's vaccine contracts. These contracts allow state and local immunization programs to obtain vaccines at reduced prices and without having to negotiate separate contracts with the vaccine manufacturers. Current CDC contract prices and comparative private-sector catalog prices are available at www.cdc.gov/vaccines/programs/vfc. Discounts from the catalog price vary substantially by vaccine and are in the range of 17% to 63%, with higher discounts for the few formulations of older vaccines still in use. The CDC's vaccine contracts are negotiated annually.

Funding for the purchase of public-sector vaccines is provided by federal, state, and local government resources. Approximately 90% of vaccine funding is provided by the federal VFC entitlement program, with the federal Section 317 program and state/local funding making up the remainder in roughly equal proportions. In fiscal year 2011, $4 billion was used to purchase vaccines using the CDC contracts. State and local immunization programs are provided a credit line of vaccine purchase funding that is awarded through population-based formulas for VFC and Section 317 vaccine.

The CDC operates stockpiles of childhood vaccine that serve as a buffer against short- and medium-term vaccine supply disruptions and to fight outbreaks of vaccine-preventable disease.[3] The stockpiles are operated as storage and rotation inventories of vaccine so that the vaccine that enters the stockpile is used before its expiration. All of the vaccines that are routinely recommended for children and included in the VFC program are included in the stockpiles. The sizes of the stockpiles are equal to a 6-month supply of each of the CDC-contracted pediatric vaccines (i.e., 6 months of vaccine needs purchased through the public sector). Because shortages of vaccine and outbreaks of vaccine-preventable diseases span private and public sectors, the stockpile is able to be used to support the private-sector vaccine supply system by allowing vaccine manufacturers to borrow vaccine from the stockpile to sell to their private customers. Borrowed vaccine must be replaced to the stockpile by the manufacturer after the shortage is resolved. Because the public sector purchases half of the childhood vaccines, CDC's stockpiles can manage a complete vaccine supply disruption of 3 month's duration or longer disruptions that are incomplete (e.g., a vaccine with more than one manufacturer).

Ensuring Access to Vaccines

A critically important step in the assurance of service delivery is to make vaccines available with as few barriers to immunization as possible and with a minimum of missed opportunities to vaccinate. Cost of vaccines is a widely studied and recognized barrier. It is also a barrier that is amenable to government programs that support the purchase of vaccine for financially vulnerable persons and government laws and regulations that require private insurance coverage for immunization—two solutions to the cost barrier that are cornerstones of the U.S. immunization system.

The VFC program rounds out access to vaccine for children by ensuring that financially vulnerable children have access to government-purchased vaccine. The VFC program is an entitlement to eligible children that has mandatory federal funding of CDC/ACIP-recommended vaccines. These vaccines are purchased using CDC's vaccine contracts. Four groups of children are entitled to VFC vaccine: children who are 18 years of age or younger who (1) are eligible for Medicaid health insurance (a federal/ state means-tested health insurance program), (2) have no health insurance, (3) are American Indian or Alaska Native children, or (4) are underinsured and are vaccinated at a Federally Qualified Health Center (FQHC) or Rural Health Clinic (RHC). The combination of VFC and the Affordable Care Act's (ACA) requirement that private health insurance cover ACIP-recommended vaccines ensures that all U.S. children have access to vaccine without out-of-pocket costs for the vaccine.

The CDC also administers the Section 317 program to state and local immunization programs. Although smaller than VFC in terms of resources for vaccine purchase, immunization program grantees can use Section 317 vaccine to vaccinate populations of their choosing, regardless of age or insurance status. The ACA authorized Section 317 permanently and also provided Section 317 with the authority to allow states to purchase vaccine for adults using CDC's vaccine contracts, something that was not authorized previously.

State and local immunization programs are responsible for enrolling providers into VFC. States also enroll non-VFC providers who can receive state or locally purchased vaccine or Section 317–purchased vaccine for the state/local priority populations. These networks of providers are vital to the success of government vaccine programs. The majority of VFC providers are private providers who use a combination of VFC vaccine and privately purchased vaccine to immunize children in their practices. VFC has approximately 45,000 providers enrolled, and three quarters of these providers are private providers. VFC providers may also see insured children. In total, VFC providers take care of approximately 90% of American children.[4]

The governmental program role in ensuring access to vaccines for adults has been more limited than the governmental role for ensuring access to vaccines for children. Medicare Part B covers pneumococcal and influenza vaccination services for all persons 65 years or older enrolled in Medicare Part B (>95% of the older-than-65 population) and hepatitis B vaccine for people undergoing dialysis of any age. State Medicaid programs, supported by federal contributions, may cover recommended vaccines for younger adults enrolled in Medicaid, but there is not a requirement that Medicaid cover vaccines for adults. In 2005, Medicare Part D was enacted to cover prescription drugs, including vaccines other than those included in Part B. Thus, all vaccines recommended for the Medicare population will be covered by Medicare Part B or Medicare Part D for persons who pay to participate.

Control and Prevent Infectious Diseases

The desired outcome of immunization is reduction, elimination, or eradication of disease or disability and prevention or control of outbreaks and their associated disruption. The goals of an immunization program determine how intensively a vaccine-preventable disease is monitored. When programs aim to achieve or sustain disease elimination, intensive efforts are needed surrounding each suspected case. Control programs may also require rapid identification and reporting of cases so that interventions can be offered promptly to reduce complications or limit transmission. Recognition of disease outbreaks is important to limit their scope. Outbreaks may also serve as sentinel events because they may provide the first indication of important program deficiencies or unanticipated limitation in vaccine performance.

Reports of the occurrence of vaccine-preventable diseases have been the means of evaluating the impact of most of the vaccine-preventable disease programs.[5,6] Information is obtained through state health departments, which have authority for mandating reporting of selected diseases to the state level by physicians and other healthcare providers.[7] The Council of State and Territorial Epidemiologists, in consultation with the CDC, establishes the list of nationally notifiable diseases. In the United States, most vaccine-preventable diseases of childhood are reported to the National Notifiable Diseases Surveillance System.

Surveillance data are analyzed to determine whether reductions of disease occur with increasing vaccine coverage; greater than expected reductions and changes in incidence beyond the target age groups may signal important herd effects.[8,9] Surveillance can also determine whether cases are a result of failure of vaccine or failure to vaccinate.[10,11]

Barriers to Vaccination

Since the 1989 to 1991 measles resurgence, a great deal of research has been conducted to understand barriers that prevent timely immunization of U.S. preschool children, and, with increasing recommendations for vaccination of adolescents and adults, barriers in older age groups have also been studied. Key barriers are lack of affordable access to vaccines, lack of a provider recommendation to be vaccinated, lack of knowledge that a vaccine is due, lack of perceived need for a vaccine, and concern about vaccine side effects (e.g., parental hesitancy to vaccinate and perception that influenza vaccine causes influenza).

Conclusion

Development and use of vaccines in the United States has had a profound effect on the occurrence of vaccine-preventable diseases. The success represents a blend of public–private and federal, state, and local partnerships. Measles, rubella, and polio remain eliminated as indigenous diseases in the United States. Childhood vaccination coverage levels have remained high for many years, with small or no disparities by race and ethnicity. The number of children receiving no vaccines has remained less than 1% in the last 4 years.

There are numerous challenges. During the past 20 years, the number of vaccine-preventable diseases of childhood has doubled, from 8 to 16. Since 2004, vaccines against influenza, hepatitis A, meningococcal disease, rotavirus, and HPV have been routinely recommended for children and/or adolescents. In addition, an adolescent booster has become available for pertussis, a second dose of varicella vaccine has been recommended, and a new vaccine for zoster is recommended for all adults older than 60 years. Ensuring financial barriers to access are removed, sustaining high coverage among children, and attaining high levels of coverage among adolescents and adults will be major challenges for the next several years as the U.S. immunization system works to achieve the Healthy People 2020 immunization objectives.

References

1. Hinman, A. R., W. A. Orenstein, and A. Schuchat. 2011. Vaccine-preventable diseases, immunizations, and MMWR, 1961–2011. *MMWR Surveill Summ* 60 (Suppl 4):49–57.

2. Freed, G. L., A. E. Cowan, S. Gregory, and S. J. Clark. 2008. Variation in provider vaccine purchase prices and payer reimbursement. *Pediatrics* 122:1325–1331.

3. Lane, K. S., S. Y. Chu, and J. M. Santoli. 2006. The United States pediatric vaccine stockpile program. *Clin Infect Dis* 42 (Suppl. 3):S125–S129.

4. Santoli, J. M., L. E. Rodewald, E. F. Maes, M. P. Battaglia, and V. G. Coronado. 1999. Vaccines for Children program, United States, 1997. *Pediatrics* 104:e15.

5. Orenstein, W. A., and R. H. Bernier. 1990. Surveillance: Information for action. *Pediatr Clin North Am* 37:709–734.

6. Wharton, M., and P. M. Strebel. 1994. Vaccine preventable diseases. In: *From Data to Action: CDC's Public Health Surveillance for Women, Infants, and Children*, eds. L. S. Wilcox and J. S. Marks, 281–290. Atlanta, GA: Centers for Disease Control and Prevention.

7. Chorba, T. L., R. L. Berkelman, S. K. Safford, N. P. Gibbs, and H. F. Hull. 1989. Mandatory reporting of infectious diseases by clinicians. *JAMA* 262:3018–3026.

8. Whitney, C. G., M. M. Farley, J. Hadler, L. H. Harrison, N. M. Bennett, R. Lynfield, et al. 2003. Decline in invasive pneumococcal disease after the introduction of protein-polysaccharide conjugate vaccine. *N Engl J Med* 348:1737–1746.

9. Adams, W. G., K. A. Deaver, S. L. Cochi, B. D. Plikaytis, E. R. Zell, C. V. Broome, and J. D. Wenger. 1993. Decline of childhood *Haemophilus influenzae* type b (Hib) disease in the Hib vaccine era. *JAMA* 269:221–226.

10. Orenstein, W. A., W. Atkinson, D. Mason, and R. H. Bernier. 1990. Barriers to vaccinating preschool children. *J Health Care Poor Underserved* 1:315–330.

11. Schuchat, A., and B. Bell. 2008. Monitoring the impact of vaccines postlicensure: New challenges, new opportunities. *Expert Rev Vaccines* 7:437–456.

13 Addressing the Vaccine Confidence Gap (*Excerpt*)

Heidi J. Larson, Louis Z. Cooper, Juhani Eskola, Samuel Katz, and Scott Ratzan[*]

Tremendous progress has been made in the development of new vaccines, along with increasing access to new and underused vaccines in the lowest income countries. But vaccines—often lauded as one of the greatest public health interventions—are losing public confidence. Some vaccine experts describe the problem as a "crisis of public confidence" and a "vaccination backlash."[1,2]

Several factors drive public questions and concerns: perceptions of business and financial motives of the vaccine industry and their perceived pressures on public institutions—such as during the H1N1 influenza response; coincidental rather than causal adverse events that are perceived as vaccine related; challenges in management and communication of uncertainty about risks (including serious, albeit rare, ones); less risk tolerance for vaccines given to those who are healthy than for drugs given to treat an illness; skepticism of scientific truths, which later become untruths or amended truths as new research becomes available;[3] elitism of a group of people that believe they should not risk vaccination of their child if enough other children are being vaccinated; and, in some cases, outright nonacceptance of scientific evidence, such as in the case of antivaccine movements that persist in the belief that autism can be caused by thimerosal or the measles-mumps- rubella (MMR) vaccine, despite an abundance of scientific evidence that shows no causal effect.[4,5]

Although communication of candid, evidence-based information to the public about the safety of specific vaccines and their benefit–risk ratios is crucial, this information alone will not stop public distrust and dissent against vaccines. Public decision making related to vaccine acceptance is not driven by scientific or economic evidence alone; it is also driven by a mix of scientific, economic, psychological, sociocultural, and political factors, all of which need to be understood and taken into account by policy and other decision makers.

We discuss factors in the changing global environment that have precipitated what some in the specialty of climate change call "an erosion of trust,"[6] caused by a small minority of climate change skeptics. The vaccine community faces similar challenges. We examine key determinants of trust, with specific examples in which public distrust undermined vaccine acceptance and interrupted immunization programs and then what was done to restore trust. Finally, we outline ways to improve public trust, including future research and actions that can be taken now.

The Changing Global Environment

Many proposed explanations exist as to why vaccines are questioned by the public, what exactly is being questioned, and what can be done to restore public confidence. One common perception is that waning public trust in vaccines is because vaccines have become a victim of their own success—whereby they have been so effective for the prevention of disease that more attention has now been focused on the potential risks of vaccines than on the risks of the now less prevalent diseases they prevent. In high-income countries, lack of familiarity with vaccine-preventable diseases is present in the healthcare community (e.g., nurses, physicians, and others who administer vaccines), many of whom are too young to have seen these illnesses.

Increased public questioning of vaccines in low-income countries, where vaccine-preventable diseases are still prevalent, point to other underlying reasons for public distrust or dissent besides the absence of vaccine-preventable disease. These reasons can be cultural, religious, or sometimes economic or political, as in the case of the polio vaccination boycott in northern Nigeria, where marginalized communities asserted their voice by refusing or challenging government-driven initiatives.[7]

New Media and Horizontal Communication

Democratization movements and the advent of the Internet have changed the environment around vaccines from top-down, expert-to-consumer (vertical) communication toward nonhierarchical, dialogue-based (horizontal) communication, through which the public increasingly questions recommendations of experts and public institutions on the basis of their own, often web-based, research. Such public questioning is not unique to vaccines but is part of a broader environment of increasing public questioning and the emergence of dissent groups, particularly in areas that include risks such as climate change.

The Internet, social media—which allows interactive exchange between many users—and mobile phone networks have shifted the methods and speed of communication substantially, allowing information about vaccines and immunization to be gathered, analyzed, and used—especially through blogs—differently compared with even a decade ago. The amount of information available has increased greatly, including scientifically valid data and evidence-based recommendations alongside poor quality data, personal opinions, and misinformation.

Media attempts to balance coverage by provision of equal opportunity to all viewpoints exacerbates the challenges to public confidence in vaccines by allowing outlier views and small extremist opinions the same media space as views validated through a rigorous process of peer review by the scientific community. This disproportionate share of outlier views has been further amplified by celebrities—such as Jim Carrey or Jenny McCarthy—who encourage parents to question vaccines, often telling highly emotional stories of children who were perceived to have been harmed by vaccines.[8]

The new mix of highly varied and often conflicting information contributes to the skepticism of some vaccine consumers. These views need to be far better understood as they are developing, rather than when vaccination rates start to decline because of distrust.

Effects of Public Distrust

Evidence about the effects of misinformation, rumors, and antivaccine groups on vaccine coverage and consequent disease outbreaks in many countries is well documented. In addition to the polio, tetanus, and MMR vaccine examples, increases in pertussis outbreaks have occurred in Russia,[9] Japan, the United States, Sweden, and England and Wales after antivaccine activity.[10] In France, the political decision to suspend hepatitis B vaccines in schools exacerbated public concerns associating hepatitis B vaccines with autism, multiple sclerosis, and leukemia and led to low levels of hepatitis B vaccination.[11] In Ukraine, scares and negative public reaction to a measles and rubella vaccination campaign led to quarantining of the vaccine and suspension of the campaign, which was targeting 7.5 million people but only reached 116,000.[12]

In all of these situations, management of the effects of declines in vaccine uptake, consequent disease outbreaks, and loss of public trust in the vaccines have taken a toll on human and financial resources in addition to long-term reputational costs to individual vaccines and immunization programs.

New methods of communication, dialogue, and engagement are urgently needed across all vaccine stakeholders—vaccine experts, scientists, industry, national and international health organizations, policymakers, politicians, health professionals, the media, and the public. No single player can reverse the vaccine confidence gap.

The Way Forward: Who Needs to Do What?

The foregoing examples show that the process of building, rebuilding, and sustaining public trust in vaccines is highly variable and depends on a thorough understanding of the community and its socioeconomic status, previous experience, views of those they trust (and distrust) including religious or political leaders, and understanding the risks and benefits of vaccines versus the diseases they prevent.

Traditional principles and practices of vaccine communication remain valid,[13] especially those that ensure timely and accurate communication of information about where, when, and why vaccines are given, and those that ensure mutual respect in health provider–patient interaction. However, additional emphasis should be placed on listening to the concerns and understanding the perceptions of the public to inform risk communication, and to incorporate public perspectives in planning vaccine policies and programs.

To build public confidence, it is key to understand what drives public trust in each community[14–16] and what are the local perceptions of vaccines and their risks.[1,17–22] According to a U.S. National Research Council report, risk communication "emphasizes the process of exchanging information and opinion with the public."[23] Building public trust is not about telling them what they need to understand better, and it is not merely about being clearer or teaching parents about risk–benefit decision making. Trust is built through dialogue and exchange of information and opinion. Valuable models can be drawn from environmental-risk research, which emphasize the importance of listening to public concerns and can protect against simplistic solutions to complex problems.[24]

Research is needed to understand who the public trusts. The UK Department of Health, for example, continues to monitor not only public perceptions of different vaccines but also who the public trusts. Similar studies are in progress in academic institutions[25] and in the CDC.[1] Such efforts should be encouraged and funded.

The immunization enterprise is a complex matrix involving academia, government, industry, private clinicians and other health providers, and public-health systems. Every one of these entities is vulnerable to public mistrust. Improved communication, dialogue, and trust building across these entities are essential. The private sector is conscious of consumer confidence levels as a metric of success and acceptance of their products. The public health community needs similar attentiveness to ensure consumer confidence if we are to achieve the potential benefits of new and existing vaccines.

Conclusion

Vaccination is a complex social act that affects both direct, perceived self-interest, the interest of one's children, and the broader community. The decision leading to immunization remains a personal summation of each individual's perception of the complexity of information they receive and their trust in the institutions that produce, legislate, and deliver vaccines. For vaccines to realize their full potential in protection of health, public and private health practices need to take into account the range of social and political factors that affect the public's willingness to accept vaccines.

The immunization community, including scientists, policymakers, and health providers, needs to come to terms with the reality that individuals and groups will continue to question and refuse vaccines. Extremist antivaccination groups whose minds will not change will exist. Many people—the majority—who accept vaccines could change their mind. The focus should be on building and sustaining trust with those who accept and support vaccines while working to understand and address the growing confidence gap.

References

1. Black, S., and R. Rappuoli. 2010. A crisis of public confidence in vaccines. *Science* 61:61.

2. Shetty, P. 2010. Experts concerned about vaccination backlash. *Lancet* 375:970–971.

3. Clements, C. J., and S. Ratzan. 2003. Misled and confused? Telling the public about MMR vaccine safety. *J Med Ethics* 29:22–26.

4. Institute of Medicine. 2004. *Immunization Safety Review: Vaccines and Autism*. Washington, DC: National Academies Press.

5. Honda, H., Y. Shimizu, and M. Rutter. 2005. No effect of MMR withdrawal on the incidence of autism. *J Child Psychol Psychiatry* 46:572–579.

6. Tollefson, J. 2010. An erosion of trust. *Nature* 466:24–26.

7. Yahya, M. 2006. Polio vaccines—difficult to swallow. The story of a controversy in northern Nigeria. Working paper 261. Institute of Development Studies. Available at: http://www.eldis.org/vfile/upload/1/document/0708/DOC21227.pdf. Accessed January 6, 2011.

8. Jenny McCarthy joins the defense of Andrew Wakefield. Available at: http://www.liquida.com/article/15670682/andrew-wakefield-autism-jenny-mccarthy/. Accessed March 30, 2011.

9. Galazka, A. M., S. E. Robertson,, and P. Oblapenko. 1995. Resurgence of diphtheria. *Eur J Epidemiol* 11:95–105.

10. Gangarosa, E. J., A. M. Galazka, C. R. Wolfe, L. M. Phillips, R. E. Gangarosa, E. Miller, and R. T. Chen. 1998. Impact of anti-vaccine movements on pertussis control: The untold story. *Lancet* 351:356–361.

11. Parry, J. 2008. No vaccine for the scaremongers. *Bull World Health Organ* 86:425–426.

12. Martin, R. 2009, February 19. *Lessons learned from SIAs: Magnification of the opportunities and risks to routine immunization programmes.* Paper presented at the 4th Annual Global Immunization Meeting, New York, NY.

13. McAlister, A., P. Puska, J. Salonen, H. Tuomilehto, and K. Koskela. 1982. Theory and action for health promotion: Illustrations from the North Karelia project. *Am J Public Health* 72:1.

14. Flynn, J., W. Burns, and C. K. Mertz. 1992. Trust as a determinant of opposition to a high-level radioactive waste repository: Analysis of a structural model. *Risk Anal* 12:417–429.

15. Alesina, A. 2002. Who trusts others? *J Public Econ* 85:207.

16. Das, J., and Das, S. 2003. Trust, learning, and vaccination: A case study of a north Indian village. *Soc Sci Med* 57:97–112.

17. Savage, I. 1993. Demographic influences on risk perceptions. *Risk Anal* 13:413.

18. Fowler, G. L., A. Kennedy, L. Leidel, K. S. Kohl, A. Khromava, G. Bizhanova, et al. 2007. Vaccine safety perceptions and experience with adverse events following immunization in Kazakhstan and Uzbekistan: A summary of key informant interviews and focus groups. *Vaccine* 25:3536–3543.

19. Bedford, H, and D. Elliman. 2000. Concerns about immunization. *BMJ* 320:240.

20. Streefland, P. H. 2001. Public doubts about vaccination safety and resistance against vaccination. *Health Policy* 55:159–172.

21. Wroe, A. L., A. Bhan, P. Salkovskis, and H. Bedford. 2005. Feeling bad about immunising our children. *Vaccine* 23:1428–1433.

22. Streefland, P, A. M. R. Chowdhury, and P. Ramos-Jimenez. 1999. Patterns of vaccination acceptance. *Soc Sci Med* 49:1705–1716.

23. Stern, P. C., and H. V. Feinberg, eds. 1996. *Understanding Risk: Informing Decisions in a Democratic Society.* Washington, DC: National Research Council, National Academy Press.

24. Pidgeon, N., and B. Fischhoff. 2011. The role of social and decision sciences in communication uncertain climate risks. *Nat Clim Chang* 1:35–41.

25. Freed, G. L., S. J. Clark, A. T. Butchart, D. C. Singer, and M. M. Davis. 2010. Parental vaccine safety concerns in 2009. *Pediatrics* 125:654–659.

14   A Half-Century of Prevention—The Advisory Committee on Immunization Practices

Jason L. Schwartz and Adel Mahmoud[*]

Shortly after the Salk and Sabin polio vaccines had demonstrated the transformative benefits of childhood vaccination but long before the ill-informed controversy over the measles-mumps-rubella (MMR) vaccine became fodder for refusal movements and television talk shows, the Vaccination Assistance Act of 1962 established a U.S. vaccination program against polio, diphtheria, tetanus, and pertussis. With that effort launched and growing attention directed toward imminent vaccination campaigns against influenza, measles, and rubella, Secretary of Health, Education, and Welfare Anthony Celebrezze approved the establishment of a committee of outside experts to advise the federal government on vaccination activities. That group, the Advisory Committee on Immunization Practices (ACIP), marked its 50th anniversary in 2014.

A panel providing guidance to the Centers for Disease Control and Prevention (CDC), the ACIP is a globally respected voice in vaccination policy and profoundly influences the design, scope, and funding of U.S. vaccination efforts. Its recommendations inform the use of vaccines in every U.S. child, adolescent, and adult. The committee has been an arbiter of controversies in vaccine science and policy, a model for similar advisory bodies around the world, and ahead of its time in demonstrating how U.S. health agencies can promote the use of medical interventions beyond matters related to licensure and regulatory oversight.

The first ACIP meeting in May 1964 was chaired by CDC Director James Goddard; he and his agency successors would hold this position for the ACIP's first 15 years. Its nine other founding members included D. A. Henderson, a CDC physician who also served as secretary to the committee, along with state health officials, academic physicians, and representatives of other Public Health Service divisions. At the committee's first few meetings, members considered how ACIP recommendations could comple-ment, rather than duplicate, those of other existing vaccine advisory bodies, such as those at the American Academy of Pediatrics and the U.S. Department of Defense. Members agreed to focus on public health practice, to make state health departments—which bore primary responsibility for vaccination efforts—their primary audience, and to rapidly update guidance as new evidence emerged.[1] Possessing no legal or regulatory authority, the committee could rely only on the strength of its evidence and analysis to influence public health practice.

In the late 1960s, when the Nixon administration called for a government-wide moratorium on appointing new members to outside advisory committees, the CDC sought an exemption for the ACIP, arguing that it filled "a vitally important role for the United States in regularly evaluating the full range of vaccines and other immuniz-ing agents available for prevention and control of important diseases in this country and elsewhere." The committee's judgments, the CDC authors wrote, "are based on an intensive evaluation of the risks and benefits of available vaccines, of their applicability in contemporary health practice, and of the relationships which must exist in promot-ing uniform immunization activities supported by various medical, public health, and voluntary health groups."[2]

This description remains apt today. The ACIP has been actively involved in essen-tially every significant development in U.S. vaccination policy since its creation. The committee has substantially shaped the addition of many new vaccines (such as hepa-titis B, varicella, and meningococcus) to the recommended schedules, the vaccination programs against swine influenza in 1976 and H1N1 influenza in 2009, the removal of thimerosal from most vaccines beginning in 1999, and the evaluation of innumerable other alleged and confirmed vaccine-safety concerns (such as those involving whole-cell pertussis vaccines and the timing of the childhood vaccination schedule). Its adop-tion of the Grading of Recommendations, Assessment, Development, and Evaluation (GRADE) approach in 2010 systematized its methods for evaluating evidence, an activ-ity central to its development of recommendations.

Because the ACIP advises the CDC, its assessments and recommendations formally apply only to the U.S. population, but they have been closely watched by international public health authorities, even as other countries have developed their own immuniza-tion advisory groups.[3] At times, ACIP evaluations of the risks and benefits of specific vaccines in the U.S. context have served as de facto global judgments, as was the case with the first rotavirus vaccine in 1999.[4]

Yet the ACIP faces multiple challenges moving forward, the most important of which relates to the policymaking responsibilities it holds along with its scientific advisory role. The committee has had this dual identity since the 1994 establishment of the Vaccines for Children Program, which provides ACIP-recommended vaccines free to uninsured and underinsured children. Vaccines newly recommended by the ACIP are added to this entitlement program, whose annual budget now exceeds $4 billion. The Affordable Care Act (ACA) has expanded the ACIP's policymaking role because the vaccinations it recommends are automatically included among the preventive services that new insurance policies are required to cover. A strong ACIP recommendation has long been viewed as an essential determinant of the success or failure of a U.S. vaccination program, and these delegated policy-setting responsibilities add to the committee's importance in this regard.

In developing its recommendations, the ACIP routinely considers cost-effectiveness.[5] Unfavorable results of economic modeling are a common justification for narrow recommendations that ultimately limit access to and affordability of the vaccines in question. Cost issues have influenced ACIP recommendations on vaccines against human papillomavirus, varicella, pneumococcus, and Lyme disease, for example. This aspect of the ACIP's work long predates the ACA, which largely prohibits using cost-effectiveness analyses in government evaluations of medical interventions. Economic costs are not considered by the U.S. Preventive Services Task Force (USPSTF), which evaluates evidence regarding nonvaccine-based preventive care strategies. Favorable USPSTF assessments also result in coverage requirements under the ACA.

Although it is increasingly essential to spend limited healthcare resources wisely, it is less clear that vaccination programs should be held to a higher standard in this regard than other preventive or therapeutic interventions, as is currently the case in the United States. Even if evaluating economic analyses is viewed as an appropriate and desirable activity for the federal government, a public health advisory body largely composed of state and local health officials, infectious-disease specialists, and pediatric and family medicine clinicians may not be the best group to undertake such work. We believe that the formation of a separate group for examination of economic issues could have significant value.

A more general challenge for the ACIP has been defending the independence of its findings and recommendations. In its early years, independence from its CDC sponsors was a principal concern of critics, who questioned whether the committee's structure allowed for truly independent advice. The Federal Advisory Committee Act of 1972 led to significant reforms of the ACIP's membership and operations: voting members were no longer permitted to be government employees, the CDC director stopped chairing the committee, and the public was given far greater access to committee meetings and materials.

Recently, more attention has been paid to financial relationships between committee members and vaccine manufacturers. The adequacy of the procedures for monitoring and addressing conflicts of interest for federal advisory groups has been questioned frequently by Congress, consumer groups, and even the Office of Inspector General of the Department of Health and Human Services, and the ACIP has been a specific focus of several inquiries. Ongoing efforts to identify and eliminate meaningful threats to the committee's independence, whatever their source, remain essential to preserving the value of the ACIP's recommendations and public confidence in government vaccination activities.

For a half-century, U.S. vaccination efforts have benefited greatly from the ACIP's expertise. Outside advisors frequently contribute to the government's regulatory work in health and medicine—for example, by evaluating products' safety and efficacy for the U.S. Food and Drug Administration. Groups providing evidence-based guidance on using such products are far less common. As the ACIP continues to play its influential role, its foremost challenge will be preserving its reputation as an inclusive and credible voice on vaccination. Success requires not simply continued attention to rigorous analyses and high-quality recommendations but also a similar focus on dissemination of its guidance and its reception by clinicians, parents, and patients. With hesitancy regarding vaccines posing a growing threat to vaccination efforts, insights from the fields of health communication, decision making, and related social and behavioral sciences will be increasingly important to the ACIP's work and the continued success of U.S. vaccination activities.

References

1. Minutes. 1964. From the meeting of Surgeon General's Advisory Committee on Immunization Practice, May 25–26, 1964, June 8, 1964. CDC Papers RG 442, 75A69. Morrow, GA: National Archives and Records Administration.

2. Policy guidelines and procedures for public advisory committees. 1969, May 7. CDC Papers RG 442, 10–003. Morrow, GA: National Archives and Records Administration.

3. Duclos, P., L. Dumolard, N. Abeysinghe, A. Adjagba, C. B. Janusz, R. Mihigo, et al. 2013. Progress in the establishment and strengthening of national immunization technical advisory groups: Analysis from the 2013 WHO/UNICEF joint reporting form, data for 2012. *Vaccine* 31:5314–5320.

4. Schwartz, J. L. 2012. The first rotavirus vaccine and the politics of acceptable risk. *Milbank Q* 90:278–310.

5. Smith, J. C. 2010. The structure, role, and procedures of the U.S. Advisory Committee on Immunization Practices (ACIP). *Vaccine* 28 (Suppl 1):A68–A75.

15 The National Vaccine Injury Compensation Program

Katherine M. Cook and Geoffrey Evans[*]

In response to a vaccine-liability crisis in the 1980s, the National Childhood Vaccine Injury Act of 1986 established the National Vaccine Injury Compensation Program (VICP) as a streamlined and less adversarial alternative to the traditional civil law system for resolving claims that arise from vaccine injury.[1]

The act's public-policy goals are to ensure an adequate supply of vaccines, stabilize vaccine costs, and establish and maintain an accessible and efficient setting for providing generous compensation to people found to have been injured by certain childhood vaccines. In addition, the legislation called for the reporting of adverse events after vaccination, the creation of vaccine-information materials that detail vaccine benefits and risks, and Institute of Medicine studies of possible vaccine-related injuries and encouraged research and development of new and safer vaccines.[2]

Operational since October 1988, the VICP has been a key component in stabilizing the U.S. vaccine market through liability protection to both vaccine companies and healthcare providers. As a no-fault alternative to the traditional tort system, petitioners (claimants) must first file with the VICP before pursuing legal remedies in state or federal civil courts. In contrast to civil courts, compensation is not determined on the basis of negligence on the part of the vaccine manufacturer or administering physician (thus, the "no-fault" designation). Funding for the program is provided through an excise tax placed on covered vaccines.

The VICP covers all vaccines recommended by the Centers for Disease Control and Prevention for routine administration to children. As of January 2011, 16 vaccines were covered, including diphtheria, tetanus, pertussis (DTP, DTaP, TdaP, DT, TT, or Td), measles-mumps-rubella (MMR or any components), polio (oral polio vaccine [OPV] or inactivated polio vaccine [IPV]), hepatitis A, hepatitis B, *Haemophilus influenza* type b

(Hib), varicella (chickenpox), rotavirus, pneumococcal conjugate, trivalent influenza (given annually), meningococcus, and human papillomavirus (HPV), whether administered individually or in combination. Although only vaccines recommended for routine use in children are covered by the VICP, there are no age restrictions on filing. In fact, more than half of the claims received annually are filed on behalf of adults.

The VICP comprises three government entities: the U.S. Department of Health and Human Services (HHS), the U.S. Department of Justice, and the U.S. Court of Federal Claims (CFC). Within the HHS, the program is administered by the Health Resources and Services Administration. Petitioners, either through their attorney or on their own, may file a petition with the HHS and the CFC, which begins the review-and-adjudication process.

The National Childhood Vaccine Injury Act provides compensation to people who can demonstrate that a serious injury was related to a vaccine covered under the VICP and who file within the statute of limitations (information on filing deadlines for claims that allege an injury or death is available on the VICP website at http://www.hrsa.gov/vaccinecompensation/howtofile/index.html).

There are three means to qualify for compensation: a petitioner must (1) show that an injury found on the vaccine injury table occurred in the prescribed time interval, (2) prove that the vaccine caused the condition, or (3) prove that the vaccine significantly aggravated a preexisting condition. The table,[3] which lists specific injuries or conditions and the time frames of onset after a vaccine is administered, allows a legal "presumption of causation." If a petitioner cannot establish a table injury, or no table injuries are listed for a particular vaccine, a petitioner has the option of proving causation.

In addition to satisfying one of the three compensation qualifications, the petitioner must also demonstrate that the effects of the injury (1) lasted >6 months after the vaccine was administered, (2) resulted in a hospital stay and surgery, or (3) resulted in a death. Petitioners are not eligible for compensation if the court determines that there is greater evidence of a nonvaccine cause for the injury.

An HHS physician reviews medical records for each petition to determine whether medical criteria for compensation are met. On the basis of these findings, a U.S. Department of Justice attorney will present the HHS's position to one of eight special masters, who are attorneys appointed by the CFC and have expertise in the legal and medical issues associated with adverse reactions to vaccines. The special master makes the final decision on whether to award compensation under the VICP. The special master can also approve settlements negotiated between the parties.

If a petition is found eligible for compensation, either by the HHS conceding the case or a special master's decision, the amount of the award is usually negotiated between the U.S. Department of Justice and the petitioner or petitioner's attorney. If the parties cannot agree, the special master must determine the amount of compensation. Successful petitioners may receive compensation for unreimbursed past and unreimbursable future medical expenses, lost wages, and pain and suffering. Attorneys' fees and costs are also reimbursed by the program, even if the petitioner is not found eligible for compensation, provided the claim was filed in good faith and on a reasonable basis. For this reason, although a petitioner does not need an attorney to file a claim, most petitioners are represented by counsel.

Appeal of a special master's decision, by either party, goes first to a judge of the CFC and then to the U.S. Court of Appeals for the Federal Circuit and may be further appealed to the U.S. Supreme Court.

Although a claim must first be filed with the VICP, petitioners retain their right to file a lawsuit in the civil court system if petitioners reject a decision, regardless of whether there was an award of compensation or a decision or judgment has not been rendered within the time period provided by law. The program is aware of only a small number of VICP claims that go on to the civil (tort) system.

Generally speaking, VICP claims are processed in a timely manner; the average time for adjudication of a compensable claim from filing to payment averages between 2 and 3 years. However, sometimes the court groups claims together, uses a small number of test cases, and applies the evidence from the test cases to a larger number of claims with similar facts. Such is the case with the Omnibus Autism Proceeding.

Beginning in 2001, petitioners began filing claims under the VICP alleging autism (or autism spectrum disorder) from MMR vaccine, thimerosal-containing vaccines, or both.[4] In 2002, the Chief Special Master of the Court created the Omnibus Autism Proceeding to adjudicate the thousands of claims expected. As of January 2011, more than 5,600 autism cases have been filed.[5] Of these 5,600 cases, more than 4,800 cases are pending, and more than 800 claims have been dismissed at the request of petitioners or dismissed by the court because they were filed outside the VICP statute of limitations for injury claims. Some families have gone on to the tort system to pursue legal remedies. Several hundred suits alleging vaccine-related autism were pending adjudication at the beginning of 2010.

Entitlement hearings on general causation and three test cases for each theory under consideration were held in 2007 and 2008. In February 2009, three special masters ruled in favor of the HHS on the first theory (a combined theory that both MMR vaccines and thimerosal-containing vaccines cause autism or autism spectrum disorder). Appeals in each case were made to judges of the CFC, who all ruled in favor of the HHS.

Appeals in two of the three cases to U.S. Court of Appeals for the Federal Circuit also resulted in decisions in favor of HHS.[6]

Special master's decisions for general causation and three test cases for the second theory (thimerosal-containing vaccines cause autism or autism spectrum disorder) were handed down in favor of HHS in March 2010. None of the test cases was appealed by petitioners.[6] A general causation hearing for the third theory (MMR vaccine alone causes autism or autism spectrum disorder) was canceled after petitioners indicated that they did not plan to introduce new evidence and would rely on the evidence presented for the first theory.

As of January 2011, the VICP has awarded compensation to more than 2,500 families and individual people totaling more than $2.1 billion.[5] The vaccine marketplace remains healthy; liability-related vaccine shortages are a distant memory, new vaccines are being licensed, and many are in various stages of development. A number of lawsuits alleging autism from either MMR vaccine or the thimerosal in vaccines are pending in more than 20 states. In contrast, non-autism-related vaccine litigation remains quite low and averaged approximately one dozen lawsuits per year from 2000 to 2005 for all VICP-covered vaccines. Therefore, the VICP continues to fulfill the intent of Congress by providing an accessible and efficient alternative for people found to be injured by certain childhood vaccines and ensuring viability of the vaccine marketplace.

References

1. Pub L No. 100–203 §§4301 et seq 101 Stat. 1330–221, codified at 42 USCA §§300aa-1 et seq (1989).

2. Smith, M. H. 1988. National Childhood Vaccine Injury Compensation Act. *Pediatrics* 82 (2):264–269.

3. U.S. Department of Health and Human Services, Health Resource and Services Administration. Vaccine injury table. Available at: http://www.hrsa.gov/vaccinecompensation/vaccineinjurytable .pdf. Accessed January 25, 2011.

4. U.S. Department of Health and Human Services, Health Resources and Services Administration. About the Omnibus Autism Proceeding. Available at: http://www.hrsa.gov/nvicp/ omnibusautism.html. Accessed January 25, 2011.

5. U.S. Department of Health and Human Services, Health Resource and Services Administration. 2011, January 3. Monthly Statistics Report. Available at: http://www.hrsa.gov/ vaccinecompensation/data/index.html. Accessed January 25, 2011.

6. U.S. Court of Federal Claims. Autism decisions and background information. Available at: http://www.uscfc.uscourts.gov/autism-decisions-and-background-information. Accessed January 25, 2011.

16 Rationalizing Vaccine Injury Compensation

Michelle M. Mello[*]

In November 2005, President Bush outlined a national preparedness strategy for a pandemic influenza outbreak.[1] The plan called on Congress to pass liability protection for vaccine manufacturers to "remove one of the greatest obstacles to domestic vaccine production."[2] Subsequently adopted legislation has given producers of pandemic vaccines near-total immunity from civil lawsuits for vaccine-related injuries.[3] Providing such immunity has ample historical precedent, but an extraordinary feature of the recent legislation is that it contains no alternative provision for compensating individuals injured by covered vaccines.

This omission—which sets pandemic countermeasure vaccinees apart from all other persons with vaccine-related injuries—has ignited objections in the United States[4] and highlighted broader questions about the rationality and consistency of the American approach to vaccine-injury compensation. Policies in this area reflect political pressures and economic considerations more than any cognizable set of principles. Because the issue is likely to recur as new disease threats emerge, it is timely to consider what a less ad hoc policy for vaccine injury compensation grounded in principles of public health ethics might look like.

This chapter identifies a set of morally relevant principles that could guide decisions about the circumstances in which vaccine injuries should be compensated, both inside and outside public health emergencies. The concept of what constitutes adequate compensation for a given injury is not straightforward,[5] but that issue is distinct from the question of the circumstances under which compensation should be offered and is beyond the scope of this chapter. For the purposes of this discussion, "compensation" can be defined as restitution in the amount of past and expected future economic losses (such as lost income and medical expenses), perhaps supplemented by an amount given in consideration of the injured person's pain and suffering.

* Originally published in *Bioethics*, 2008, 22 (1):32–42. Republished with permission of John Wiley and Sons.

Current Provisions for Vaccine Injury Compensation

For many vaccines, persons who believe they have a vaccine-related injury may file a tort lawsuit against the manufacturer. Such claims are usually heard by state courts and based on state-law doctrines of product liability. Plaintiffs may allege that the vaccine was defectively manufactured or defectively designed (unreasonably unsafe), or that the manufacturer failed adequately to warn of the risks. Claims that reach trial are generally decided by a jury.

This process is problematic for both claimants and vaccine makers. From the claimant's perspective, litigation is adversarial, protracted, and uncertain, and it requires that an attorney agree to take the case, which may pose a considerable obstacle for claimants with low earnings or fairly minor injuries. Tort doctrine in most states sets the liability standard for vaccines and other drugs relatively high, making it difficult for plaintiffs to prevail on design-defect claims. Vaccine manufacturers dislike tort because of the uncertainty involved in allowing juries to determine injury causation and damages awards. Even if catastrophically large awards rarely occur, the threat of them weighs heavily on manufacturers and their insurers.[6]

Historically, when vaccine makers have objected that tort liability makes vaccines too risky to manufacture, the government has responded by creating an alternative legal remedy.[7] In 1976, the federal government banned lawsuits against swine flu vaccine manufacturers and assumed liability for vaccine-related injuries. In 1986, Congress created the Vaccine Injury Compensation Program (VICP), which provides no-fault, administrative compensation for adverse effects that have been scientifically established as linked to covered vaccines. Vaccinees can file a lawsuit only after going through the VICP, and special rules make those suits difficult to win. Originally limited to vaccines recommended by the Centers for Disease Control and Prevention for routine administration to children, the VICP has recently been expanded to cover smallpox vaccine and trivalent influenza vaccine, including injuries to adults.

Although the addition of influenza reflected concerns that manufacturers might be unwilling to make the vaccine, the addition of smallpox stemmed from the need to encourage vaccination. In December 2002, the Bush Administration announced a plan for voluntary smallpox vaccination of 500,000 healthcare workers as part of bioterrorism preparedness. Physicians and nurses, who were aware of the vaccine's risks,[8] balked; after 6 months, only 7% of the targeted group had volunteered.[9] Among their concerns was that the plan made inadequate provision for compensating vaccinees who experienced adverse effects.

The Homeland Security Act had, in fact, created a legal remedy: although vaccinees could not sue a smallpox vaccine manufacturer, they could sue the federal government.[10] In some states, workers' compensation programs would also provide limited compensation. This "incomplete and confusing patchwork" of remedies failed to lead to widespread uptake of vaccination,[11] however, so the government added smallpox vaccine to the VICP in 2003.[12]

The history of vaccine injury compensation has been that when the government closes a door, it opens a window. Legal protection for vaccine manufacturers is coupled with an administrative remedy for vaccinees. The alternative remedy is not always provided in a timely fashion, however. For smallpox vaccine, it was not created until it became clear that the voluntary vaccination strategy was failing without it.

The smallpox story raises the question of whether an approach to pandemic preparedness that begins with the presumption of no compensation could risk delay in achieving needed rates of vaccination. Because this presumption was present in the recent legislation, it is timely to consider its defensibility. To be sure, smallpox and pandemic flu present different challenges because of differences in the perceived imminence of the threat and the known risks of vaccination. But both should lead us to ask: On what basis, and in what circumstances, should compensation be available for vaccine-related injuries? In particular, when is the government ethically obliged to assume responsibility for providing compensation?

Rationales for Government Compensation

At first, pandemics and other public health emergencies may seem to present a weaker case for government compensation of injuries than routine vaccinations. It might be argued that emergencies are special; ordinary presuppositions about fairness and compensation find little applicability in a context in which urgency and necessity govern the choice of policy interventions. Moreover, providing compensation for all of the inevitable adverse effects of emergencies could severely encumber public budgets at a time when they are already straining under the burden of responding to vast social needs.

This is not, however, a view the United States has consistently taken toward the victims of emergencies. Families affected by September 11, Hurricane Katrina, and other disasters have had access to large government compensation funds. A pandemic infectious disease could present disaster on a much larger and more costly scale, but the point stands that our approach to emergencies is not generally to ask those who are injured to bear the full costs.

If it is justifiable to think about vaccinations inside and outside the context of emergencies similarly, then there are a number of arguments in favor of providing government compensation for vaccine-related injuries under various other conditions. Some arguments are utilitarian, pointing to social benefits that outweigh the costs of compensation. Others are nonconsequentialist, grounded in notions of fairness and other deontological principles.

Vaccination as a Collective-Action Problem

Underpinning many of the arguments for compensation is the concept that under some circumstances, vaccination presents a collective-action problem. Collective-action problems arise where there is an outcome that makes all members of a group better off, but which they cannot achieve because they cannot agree on how to share the costs or cannot enforce that all members share the cost. The canonical collective-action problem is the "free-rider problem," wherein the group would be better off if all cooperated toward production of a social good, but many members do not cooperate because they believe they can get away with enjoying the benefits of the good without contributing toward its cost. In the context of vaccination programs, the relevant public good is herd immunity against the disease.

Individuals benefit from vaccination both by gaining disease immunity themselves and through herd immunity. The optimal situation for an individual is generally that enough people participate in a vaccination scheme to achieve a sufficient level of herd immunity that the individual's risk of catching the disease will be very low, but the individual opts out of vaccination, avoiding the risk of a vaccine injury. If enough people decline vaccination, however, herd immunity will be insufficient. In this "volunteer dilemma," the individually rational decision, if chosen by enough individuals, leads to the worst outcome for all. The volunteer dilemma is a special kind of free-rider problem in which free-riding is encouraged only when most people are not free-riding.

The payoff matrix associated with getting preemptively vaccinated for a potentially pandemic disease varies with the risk of contracting the disease, as well as the risk associated with vaccination.[13] When the risk of disease is high, either because there is a high risk of an outbreak or because the disease is highly transmissible, the collective-action problem dissipates. When the risk is low (especially relative to the risk of vaccine injury), there will be little incentive for people to volunteer for vaccination if they believe most other people will volunteer. This insight has implications for vaccine injury compensation. It should also be noted that pandemic vaccines present special difficulties in calculating a payoff matrix because the risks of new vaccines are not initially clear.

Utilitarian Arguments for Vaccine Injury Compensation

Encouraging Voluntary Vaccination

The primary motivation for offering compensation for smallpox-vaccine-related injuries was to encourage first responders to submit to voluntary vaccination. Encouraging parents to seek early childhood vaccinations was also one of the motivations for creating the VICP (vaccinations are not required until children enter school). The operating assumption here is that some individuals will be willing to undergo vaccination if they know that compensation for resulting injuries is easily obtainable through an administrative program but not if the only remedy is to file a lawsuit or if there is no remedy at all.

If compensation programs really are effective in boosting vaccination rates, they could conceivably preclude the need for mandatory vaccination laws. They would constitute a less restrictive alternative to coercive laws, which is desirable according to principles of public health ethics and law. This will only be the case, however, if voluntary programs with compensation are as effective as coercion (or nearly so).

At present, there is little evidence to support the assumption that easy availability of compensation increases willingness to undergo vaccination. News reports[14] and commentaries[15] have emphasized the possible role that compensation concerns played in decisions regarding smallpox vaccination, and the advocacy of several healthcare worker unions and professional organizations was influential in putting such concerns on the policy agenda.[16] The issue, however, has never been comprehensively studied. Small survey studies[17] have concluded that compensation concerns were not a significant predictor of physicians' willingness to receive smallpox vaccination. Rather, unwillingness to receive the vaccine appears to hinge largely on the perception that the risk of disease outbreak was extremely low.[18]

If these findings are generalizable, then an offer of compensation alone is unlikely to be effective in substantially boosting voluntary vaccination rates. It is possible, however, that these findings may not generalize to a scenario in which the risk of an outbreak is perceived to be appreciable. It may be that a perception of near-zero risk is sufficient to turn people against vaccination, but when the perceived risk is higher, people may weigh a range of factors in making their decision. However, it is also possible that public mention of the availability of compensation could discourage vaccination by highlighting the safety risks associated with it.

Encouraging Vaccine Production

An alternative rationale for vaccine injury compensation programs—the one that most strongly drove the creation of the VICP—is to respond to vaccine manufacturers' objections that tort liability costs make vaccines too expensive to produce. There is a strong social need to maintain an adequate number of vaccine suppliers. Companies may be especially reluctant to produce new vaccines against a threatening pandemic because time pressure may mean less opportunity to test the vaccine fully and, therefore, greater risk of injury.[19] Alternatively, companies may produce vaccines but price them high to cover their expected liability costs (a socially undesirable outcome).

Such concerns may argue for eliminating manufacturer liability, but they do not squarely address the question of whether injured vaccinees should have access to compensation. Manufacturers could be relieved of liability with or without the creation of an alternative compensation mechanism. As long as they are not subject to liability, there is no reason to think that their willingness to make vaccines is increased by the presence of a government compensation fund. In fact, manufacturers might prefer it if the VICP did not exist because the scheme is funded through a vaccine tax, which raises the price of their products.

Overall, utilitarian arguments provide a weaker foundation for government compensation of vaccine injuries than is frequently assumed. More persuasive are several nonconsequentialist principles.

Nonconsequentialist Arguments for Compensation

Fairness to Persons Subject to Coercion

It is a well-accepted principle of public health law and ethics that the government may exercise its coercive powers to restrict individual liberty in ways that are reasonably calculated to achieve public health goals. Accompanying the exercise of coercive power, however, should be measures to promote fairness to individuals who are burdened by it. One such measure is to provide due process before a person is deprived of liberty or property; another is to require that the government select the least restrictive intervention that will achieve its public health objective.

Arguably, a third measure should be to require that individuals who are harmed by the exercise of coercive power (such as through mandatory vaccination) be offered restitution, to the extent that the government can reasonably provide it. Such a policy would follow from the same impulse that leads us to prefer the least restrictive alternative: the notion that we should take whatever steps are practically available to minimize the intrusion on the individual. If it is not possible to lighten the burden of the intervention (e.g., by making vaccination voluntary rather than mandatory or developing a vaccine that presents little or no risk of injury), we can at least mitigate the collateral harm that results from the intervention for an unlucky few. This harm consists of the physical suffering of a vaccine-related adverse event and the economic loss (lost income, medical expenses, and other costs) that result from it. The physical suffering cannot be prevented, but the secondary losses that flow from it can be recompensed.

Although fairness to persons subject to mandatory vaccination did not drive the creation of the VICP, it is frequently cited as an ex post justification for the program. Commentators describe the VICP as a means of caring for children who are injured as a result of mandatory school entry vaccinations.[20] The coercion argument also has considerable moral force and resonates strongly with American political ideology, with its emphasis on individual autonomy.

Nevertheless, it might be pointed out that the government generally does not, in fact, offer compensation to individuals who have been deprived of liberty due to an exercise of public health powers; it usually offers only procedural protections against wrongful deprivations. But arguably, the burdens associated with vaccination requirements are special: they go beyond dignitary harms and economic losses to actual physical injury; severe consequences will occur with statistical certainty; and the victims are often children, the elderly, or other vulnerable persons. Consequently, this form of coercion should be viewed as particularly ethically problematic, triggering fairness concerns. This would suggest that vaccine injuries—at least severe injuries—should be compensated whenever the vaccination was mandatory.

Fairness to Persons with Professional Obligations

Another strand of fairness argument for vaccine injury compensation relates to the professional obligations of health workers. Longstanding principles of medical ethics emphasize physicians' and nurses' duty to treat patients in need, even if it endangers their own health. Although some ethicists have argued that the duty to treat diminishes as risk increases,[21] others argue that in the context of a threatening epidemic, a sliding scale of professional obligation cannot be entertained; the risk is a biological given, and excusing some providers from it would mean unfairly shifting the risk to others.[22] Physicians appear sympathetic to this view: in one survey, 80% reported that they would be willing to care for patients in the event of an outbreak of an unknown but potentially deadly disease.[23]

If doctors and other emergency responders have a professional ethical obligation to care for patients during infectious-disease outbreaks, arguably this entails an obligation to take the necessary measures to minimize the likelihood that they will fall ill and cannot work. Therefore, where vaccination is available, it becomes, by extension, obligatory. When individuals encounter the risk of a vaccine injury out of professional duty, it is reasonable to argue that they should not be left to bear the financial burdens associated with that injury.

Some may argue that health and safety professionals assume these obligations out of a sense of altruism and duty, not in the expectation of a quid pro quo. But their motivation for service is not necessarily relevant. Regardless of their reasons for choosing their profession, we do routinely compensate those who protect public safety and suffer injury as a result. For example, injured soldiers, police officers, and firefighters and their families receive a range of benefits for injuries sustained in the line of duty. These policies arise from a sense that even if compensation is not expected by these public servants, it is still fair, virtuous, and perhaps morally obligatory to offer it because they have entered into a "special relationship of service" to society,[24] from which all benefit. Compensation is a way of providing some reciprocity in this relationship or at least of showing gratitude.

The principle that those who undertake these professional obligations deserve a basic safety net arguably extends to healthcare workers who must be vaccinated to be able to care for patients in a disease outbreak. In the aforementioned survey, 88% of physicians felt that society should ensure that health professionals were optimally protected against health threats in the course of their work.[25] Although this line of thinking does not justify compensation of all vaccine injuries, it does support compensation of injuries sustained by health professionals and others who are on the front lines of a (potential) disease outbreak. Notably, this argument has both deontological and utilitarian strands: compensation is merited by fairness concerns but also because it is socially important to maintain an adequate supply of emergency responders who are willing and able to care for victims of disease outbreaks.

Fairness to Those Who Act against Self-Interest

Part of the appeal of the argument from professional obligation is the notion that health workers and emergency responders operate out of a sense of duty, which verges on altruism. If other-regarding behavior is a legitimate ethical reason to compensate vaccine injuries, then perhaps the compensation policy should also extend to other private citizens who get vaccinated in circumstances in which they likely have more to lose than to gain by vaccination. That is, perhaps fairness demands that vaccine injuries be compensated where vaccination was voluntary and contrary to the individual's self-interest.

The collective-action problem described earlier is helpful in analyzing such a claim. For many vaccinations, the public-health benefits of herd immunity are greater than the benefit that vaccination confers on any individual vaccinee; indeed, the risk/benefit calculus for the individual may weigh against preemptive vaccination (vaccination before an actual outbreak occurs). This is likely to be the case when the individual's risk of contracting the disease without vaccination is low because the risk of a disease outbreak is low and/or the disease is not highly transmissible. Some individuals will accept preemptive vaccination in these circumstances even in the absence of a mandate, out of a sense of obligation to contribute to herd immunity. Conversely, there may be a vaccine with an injury risk so low that as long as there is any risk at all of disease outbreak, it would be individually irrational not to be vaccinated.

One possible compensation policy would be to offer compensation where the circumstances of the injured person's vaccination fit the description of a collective-action problem. That is, compensation should be available when the person accepted vaccination notwithstanding a personal risk/benefit calculation suggesting that he should refuse it but not where vaccination was clearly in the person's self-interest. Even if we accept that it seems unlikely that the offer of compensation will encourage more individuals to get vaccinated, such a policy would be justified on the basis of fairness to those who voluntarily risk personal harm for the benefit of the community or by a social desire to reward behavior that is perceived as virtuous. A strong version of this argument would posit that a community which benefits from an individual's altruistic act has a moral obligation to provide restitution to the individual; a weaker version would simply assert that although compensation is not morally required, it is morally desirable as a charitable act.[26]

Such a rule has moral appeal but might be difficult to operationalize. It is clear that some types of vaccinations are sought primarily out of self-interest and confer substantial benefit on the vaccinee. Vaccinations obtained in advance of travel to regions where infectious diseases are endemic are one example; vaccines against human papillomavirus are another (with parents acting on behalf of their children's best interests).[27] Other vaccinations maintain herd immunity against a disease that individuals are unlikely to be exposed to in the United States, such as polio. Those vaccinations are not generally sought out of self-interest; they are generally mandatory.

For a third group of vaccinations, however, the risk/benefit calculus for individuals is much less clear. Vaccines developed in anticipation of potential new pandemics or bioterrorist attacks fit this description because the likelihood of a disease outbreak is not known with reasonable certainty. Nor, in the case of new infectious agents such as mutated strains of influenza, is the transmissibility of the agent known with precision.[28]

Also, the risk of vaccine-associated adverse effects will be murky for new vaccines. In such circumstances, the principle of fairness to those who act against self-interest does not point to a clear answer about compensating vaccine injuries. Because this group of vaccinations is likely large, such a principle does not create a workable compensation rule.

A second objection to the self-interest principle relates to the definition of a benefit to the vaccinee. Even if a disease outbreak never in fact occurs, individuals arguably receive a benefit from vaccination in the form of protection against a possible risk. The argument is best explained by analogy to purchasing insurance: even if the risk of loss is uncertain at the time of purchase and, in retrospect, extremely low, it still does not seem right to say that the insured received no benefit from having bought insurance. The benefit could be described as peace of mind or complete security from risk. Thus, an expansive concept of individual benefit would hold that there are no circumstances in which vaccination is contrary to self-interest. If this is the case, then the self-interest principle is not useful for identifying vaccine injuries that merit compensation. (A counterargument might be that although individuals may receive a security benefit, it may not outweigh the risks of vaccination in some circumstances; therefore, the self-interest principle could distinguish circumstances under which compensation is and is not warranted.)

Solidarity

Many countries around the world have implemented compensation schemes for vaccine injuries, not primarily out of a utilitarian desire to keep vaccine markets well supplied or encourage vaccination but as an expression of solidarity.[29] In some countries, the schemes are an outgrowth of other types of social insurance schemes, reflecting a broader social judgment that medical risks should be shared. In others, vaccine injuries were viewed as special due to their severity, complexity, and propensity to befall children and others who would not qualify for extensive benefits under existing accident insurance programs.[30]

Solidarity tends to wax and wane in American ideology; it has blossomed during times of war, economic depression, and civil rights movements and tends to recede during calmer, more prosperous periods. The ethos may again shift toward an embrace of solidarity, and solidarity is an important part of thinking about vaccine injury compensation elsewhere in the world.[31] Although not explicitly identified as such, solidarity arguments have been influential in deliberations in the United States over whether society has a moral obligation to compensate injured research subjects.[32]

Intrinsic to the concept of solidarity is the notion that every member of the community should share risks and the burdens associated with those risks. This is particularly important where the risks are associated with the production of a public good, such as herd immunity. Solidarity means that members of the community should not have to bear terrible risks alone, and that the community should stand by those who are harmed by the measures we take to protect ourselves.

Versions of the solidarity argument that refer to the injured person's participation in the production of a social benefit resemble general fairness arguments. Both types of argument respond to the fact that among vaccinees, the injured and the uninjured pay unequal shares of the social cost of producing the shared good of herd immunity. In other words, the uninjured are (unintentionally) free-riding on the injured.[33] It is true that all vaccinees have borne the same share of risk of injury, but the burden of injury itself is unequally distributed. Fairness and solidarity both militate in favor of a safety net for those whose sacrifice is especially large. Other versions of the solidarity argument, which refer not to individual sacrifices in the course of producing a social good but to the general virtue of not allowing members of the community to bear catastrophic losses alone, apply even when fairness concerns do not.

The principle of solidarity supports a policy of compensating those vaccine injuries that, in the judgment of the community, individuals and families cannot reasonably be expected to bear alone. Compensation might be limited to rare and severe adverse reactions, for example. There would be no distinctions drawn based on the reasons for which the individual obtained the vaccination, including whether it was voluntary. Distinctions might be made on the basis of the individual's ability to bear the financial loss associated with his injury (e.g., compensation might not be offered to millionaires).

The notion of solidarity is out of step with strongly held American values such as self-reliance, voluntary assumption of risk, and individual decision making about whether and how much insurance to buy. The principle seems to find greater traction during emergencies, however, and in other circumstances in which the risk in question is neither voluntarily encountered nor easily insured against. Solidarity could perhaps be used to justify compensation of severe effects of vaccines during public health emergencies, but it is a fragile buttress for a more general policy of compensation of vaccine injuries in the United States.

Failure of Informed Consent

An alternative basis for compensation would be to compensate when the conditions for individuals to give informed consent to vaccination are not present. Ruth Faden has proposed such a policy for smallpox vaccine injuries.[34] In the smallpox vaccination effort, she argued, meaningful informed consent was not possible because the risk of a bioterrorist attack was not known or reasonably knowable; thus, individuals could not accurately weigh the risks and benefits of vaccination.

Similar circumstances apply to other preemptive pandemic vaccinations. They also inhere in the use of all new vaccines because insufficient experience has accumulated to understand the range and risk of adverse reactions. Pandemics and bioterrorist attacks pose additional challenges for informed consent once an outbreak has occurred: during the ensuing emergency, immediate vaccination would be critical, and the chaos in public health systems may make it infeasible to put vaccinees through a detailed informed consent process.[35]

Faden argues that during emergencies, justice requires a social compact in which the usual requirement of informed consent for medical interventions is suspended but, in return, the government offers compensation for serious vaccine injuries. The resonance of this proposition with important provisions of American law is clear—for example, the constitutional provision that the government may not deprive citizens of property without offering just compensation.[36] Some ethicists, however, might object that many ordinary medical treatments involve the kinds of conditions Faden cites as precluding informed consent—yet there is no suggestion that resulting adverse outcomes merit compensation (in the absence of negligence).[37] In a range of medical situations, we accept a patient's informed consent as valid, although it is given under conditions of uncertainty about risk. Also, when medical needs are emergent or pressing, the patient may be ill situated to offer meaningful informed consent or indeed any affirmative consent at all. It is not clear why vaccination should be treated differently from other medical interventions (many of which are equally or more burdensome and disabling), at least when vaccination is voluntary.

The Argument from Reasonableness

A final argument for vaccine injury compensation, which mixes utilitarian and non-consequentialist considerations, is that rational vaccinees would prefer a world in which such an insurance scheme existed, if it could be provided efficiently. Vaccination is a high-stakes scenario in which some individuals will suffer catastrophic losses and in which no one can know who will be injured. Vaccinees are, in this sense, behind a Rawlsian veil of ignorance.

A utilitarian strand of this argument, drawing on principles of rational-choice economics and Harsanyi's theory of average utilitarianism,[38] is that a rational utility maximizer who has decided (or is required) to be vaccinated would support a scheme like the VICP because it improves the expected outcome of vaccination at a very low price (the VICP is funded by a $0.75-per-dose excise tax on covered vaccines[39]). One way of thinking about this is to consider that if each individual who presented for vaccination was offered the option to purchase an insurance policy against vaccine injuries for 75 cents, it is likely that few would turn it down. Another is that it produces greater total disutility for a small number of people to face a catastrophic injury alone than for everyone to pay a small tax on vaccines in order to fund a compensation program.

The nonconsequentialist strand of the reasonableness argument springs from Rawls's theory of justice as fairness.[40] His maximin principle suggests that under the circumstances, individuals would agree to form an insurance plan to protect those who turn out to be big losers in the pursuit of a general social gain. The scheme would likely apply only to severe injuries because the motivation is to minimize terrible outcomes. Thus, reasonableness suggests that severe vaccine injuries should routinely be compensated, regardless of the reasons vaccination was sought.

Conclusions

A number of conclusions emerge from the foregoing. First, although the primary rationales for creation and expansion of the VICP have been utilitarian ones—encouraging vaccination and vaccine production—close analysis reveals these to be relatively weak justifications for compensation. Vaccination decisions do not appear to be strongly linked to the availability of a compensation fund, and the need to maintain vaccine supplies implies a need for liability protections for vaccine makers, not necessarily a compensation fund for vaccinees. Moreover, there are probably better ways to ensure an adequate vaccine supply, such as ensuring a stable market for vaccines.[41]

Second, some nonconsequentialist considerations do form a strong foundation for vaccine injury compensation. Arguments articulating a moral obligation to provide compensation for persons subject to de jure or de facto coercion are especially strong. Where vaccinations are legally mandatory or effectively required for health workers or emergency responders to fulfill their professional duties in the event of a disease outbreak, the government should provide ready access to compensation for injuries that result.

Such circumstances raise profound fairness concerns because the individual's choice set has been limited. Clearly, unfairness does not occur whenever choices are limited; it is not meaningful to speak of unfairness arising because a mere state of the world, such as a pandemic outbreak, limits the range of available choices. In the above circumstances, however, it is not the fact of the disease outbreak that results in limited liberty but, rather, the social decisions to require vaccination and to impose duties on certain individuals to care for others during emergencies. Such decisions are entirely justifiable, but justice requires that redress is made to those who are so burdened, insofar as we can provide it. The obligation seems especially strong when these decisions are implemented in advance of an actual outbreak.

Third, the reasonableness argument is also a compelling justification for a compensation scheme. It supports the extension of compensation beyond those who are required to be vaccinated to those who sustain severe injuries from voluntary vaccinations. In summary, an ethically defensible vaccine compensation policy would make a compensation fund available to all individuals with severe injuries and to individuals with less severe injuries if the vaccination was required by law or professional duty.

Lawrence Gostin has written that "infectious diseases tend to bring out the best and worst in societies."[42] When it comes to vaccine injury compensation policy, the need for a rapid response to each emerging threat has sometimes led to disease exceptionalism in policymaking,[43] rather than consistency in our treatment of those who are harmed by our collective self-defense efforts. The threat of pandemic influenza—particularly now, when it is still theoretical—presents an opportunity to reconsider and rationalize these policies. Reflection suggests the desirability of reaching agreement on a set of ethical principles to govern vaccine compensation and applying them in a consistent fashion, rather than allowing policy to flow from political expediency.

References

1. U.S. Homeland Security Council. 2005. National Strategy for Pandemic Influenza. Available at: http://www.whitehouse.gov/homeland/pandemic-influenza.html. Accessed February 16, 2006.

2. White House. 2005. Fact Sheet: Safeguarding America Against Pandemic Influenza. Available at: http://www.whitehouse.gov/news/releases/2005/11/20051101.html. Accessed November 10, 2005.

3. Public Readiness and Emergency Preparedness Act, P.L. 109–148, 119 Stat. 2680. 109th Congress, 1st Session, 2005.

4. Pelosi, N., S. R Hoyer, R. Menendez, et al. 2005. Letter from Nancy Pelosi and House Democrats to President George W. Bush. Available at: http://www.housedemocrats.gov/news/librarydetail.cfm?library_content_id=553. Accessed February 16, 2006; D. Henderson. 2005, November 8. Bush flu plan eases firms' liability. *Boston Globe*, D1.

5. Boxhill, B. R. 1982. Consent and compensation. In: *Compensating for Research Injuries, Volume Two*. President's Commission for the Study of Ethical Problems in Medicine and Biomedical and Behavioural Research, 41–55. Washington, DC: President's Commission.

6. Mello, M. M., and T. A. Brennan. 2005. Legal concerns and the influenza vaccine shortage. *JAMA* 294 (14):1817–1820.

7. Ibid.

8. Casey, C. G., et al. 2005. Adverse events associated with smallpox vaccination in the United States, January-October 2003. *JAMA* 294 (21):2734–2743.

9. Yih, W. K., et al. 2003. Attitudes of healthcare workers in US hospitals regarding smallpox vaccination. *BMC Public Health* 3:20.

10. Centers for Disease Control and Prevention. 2006. Smallpox Program Implementation: Liability Issues. Available at: http://www.bt.cdc.gov/agent/smallpox/vaccination/vaccination -program-qa.asp?type=cat&cat=Smallpox+Program+Implementation&subCat1=Liability+Issues. Accessed February 16, 2006.

11. Baciu, A., et al., eds. 2005. *The Smallpox Vaccination Program: Public Health in an Age of Terrorism*. Washington, DC: National Academies Press.

12. Smallpox Emergency Personnel Protection Act of 2003, P.L. 108–20, 117 Stat. 638 (April 30, 2003), codified at 42 USC 239.

13. Bauch, C. T., A. P. Galvani, and D. J. Earn 2003. Group interest versus self-interest in smallpox vaccination policy. *Proc Natl Acad Sci USA* 100 (18):10564–10567.

14. Kemper, V. 2003, February 6. Smallpox vaccinations falter over compensation. *Chicago Tribune*: N16.

15. Kuhles, D. J., and D. M. Ackman. 2003. The federal smallpox vaccination program: Where do we go from here? *Health Aff* (Suppl. Web Exclusives):W3–503–10.

16. Baciu et al., op. cit. note 11.

17. Benin, A. L., et al. 2004. Reasons physicians accepted or declined smallpox vaccine, February Through April, 2003. *J Gen Intern Med* 19 (1):85–89; Yih et al., op. cit. note 9.

18. Benin et al., op. cit. note 17; Kwon, N., et al. 2003. Emergency physicians' perspectives on smallpox vaccination. *Acad Emerg Med* 10 (6):599–605.

19. Testimony of Michael O. Leavitt before the Energy and Commerce Committee of the U.S. House of Representatives, Hearing on Pandemic Flu Preparedness, November 8, 2005.

20. Association of American Physicians and Surgeons. 2003, March 27. Doctors: Vaccine Compensation Bill Only Half a Solution. Press Release. Available at: http://www3.scienceblog.com/ community/older/archives/K/2/pub2826.html. Accessed February 16, 2006; National Vaccine Information Center. Homeland Security and Vaccine Compensation. Available at: http://www .nvic.org/vaccine-laws/homeland-security/briefing-paper.aspx. Accessed February 16, 2006.

21. Daniels, N. 1991. Duty to treat or right to refuse? *Hastings Ctr Rep* 21:36–36.

22. Reid, L. 2005. Diminishing returns? Risk and the duty to care in the SARS epidemic. *Bioethics* 19 (4):348–361.

23. Alexander, G. C., and M. K. Wynia. 2003. Ready and willing? Physicians' sense of preparedness for bioterrorism. *Health Aff* 22 (5):189–197.

24. Report of HEW Secretary's Task Force on the Compensation of Injured Research Subjects. 1977. Washington, DC: US Department of Health, Education, and Welfare.

25. Alexander and Wynia., op. cit. note 23.

26. Mariner, W. K. 1987. Compensation programs for vaccine-related injury abroad: A comparative analysis. *St. Louis Univ Law J* 31 (3):599–654; Swazey, J. P., and L. Glantz. 1982. A social perspective on compensation for injured research subjects. In: *Compensating for Research Injuries, Volume Two*. President's Commission for the Study of Ethical Problems in Medicine and Biomedical and Behavioural Research, 3–18. Washington, DC: President's Commission.

27. Bowe, C. 2005, October 21. Viral links spur the search for cancer vaccines. *Financial Times*:13.

28. Mills, C. E., et al. 2006. Pandemic influenza: Risk of multiple introductions and the need to prepare for them. *PLoS Med* 3 (6):e135.

29. Mariner, op. cit. note 26.

30. Ibid. 1999. Evans, G. Vaccine injury compensation programs worldwide. *Vaccine* 17 (Suppl 3):S25–S35.

31. Evans, op. cit. note 30.

32. Mariner, W. K. 1994. Compensation for research injuries. In: *Women and Health Research*, Volume 2, eds. A. C. Mastroianni, R. Faden, and D. Federman, 113–126. Washington, DC: National Academy Press; President's Commission for the Study of Ethical Problems in Medicine and Biomedical and Behavioural Research. 1982. *Compensating for Research Injuries*, Volume One. Washington, DC: President's Commission.

33. Smith, H. M. 1982. Compensating research-related injuries: Ethical considerations. In: *Compensating for Research Injuries*, Volume Two, 19–39. President's Commission for the Study of Ethical Problems in Medicine and Biomedical and Behavioural Research. Washington, DC: President's Commission.

34. Faden, R. R., H. A. Taylor, and N. K. Seiler. 2003. Consent and compensation: A social compact for smallpox vaccine policy in the event of an attack. *Clin Infect Dis* 36 (12):1547–1551.

35. Ibid.

36. U.S. Constitution, Amendment V.

37. I am grateful to Dan Wikler and Dan Brock for this suggestion.

38. Harsanyi, J. C. 1953. Cardinal utility in welfare economics and in the theory of risk-taking. *J Polit Econ* 61:453–455.

39. U.S. Department of Health and Human Services, Health Resources and Services Administration. 2006. *National Vaccine Injury Compensation Program: Funding.* Accessed February 21, 2006.

40. Rawls, J. 1971. *A Theory of Justice.* Cambridge, MA: Belknap Press of Harvard University Press.

41. Mello & Brennan, op. cit. note 6.

42. Gostin, L. O. 2005. Public health preparedness and ethical values in pandemic influenza. In *The Threat of Pandemic Influenza: Are We Ready?*, eds. S. L. Knobler et al., 357–372. Washington, DC: National Academies Press.

43. Lazzarini, Z. 2001. What lessons can we learn from the exceptionalism debate (finally)? *J Law Med Ethics* 29:149–151.

17 Mercury, Vaccines, and Autism: One Controversy, Three Histories

Jeffrey P. Baker[*]

Despite the reassurance of no less than eight safety review panels conducted by the Institute of Medicine (IOM) since 2001, many parents continue to fear that childhood vaccines can cause a host of adverse effects ranging from immune dysfunction to attention deficit disorder and autism.[1] Several trends no doubt contribute to this anxiety: fading memory of vaccine-preventable diseases, adverse media coverage, misinformation on the Internet, and litigation.[2] Yet global explanations of this sort fail to do justice to the fact that controversies over vaccines have often followed quite disparate trajectories in different settings. For example, although the alleged relationship between childhood vaccines and autism has been the dominant controversy over child immunization of recent years, British anxiety has centered on the measles-mumps-rubella (MMR) vaccine, whereas Americans have focused much more on the role of mercury in vaccine preservatives.[3]

I examine the origins of the American debate surrounding vaccines, mercury, and autism to illuminate how historical analysis can contribute to understanding public attitudes toward vaccine safety. It is not my intent to answer whether mercury in vaccines explains the increasing prevalence of autism; the IOM has already determined over the course of two reviews that available evidence fails to support such a conclusion.[4] Instead, I examine the historical questions that have been raised in the debate but only superficially addressed by the IOM. Why was the mercury-containing preservative thimerosal introduced in infant vaccines in the first place? Why was its use not questioned until the late 1990s, long after the toxic effects of mercury had been recognized? Why was autism perceived to be "epidemic" in the 1990s, and how did it become linked to vaccines in the public's mind?

* Reprinted from Baker, J. P., 2008. Mercury, vaccines, and autism: One controversy, three histories. *American Journal of Public Health* 98 (2):244–253. Republished with permission of American Public Health Association.

I argue that the thimerosal story is best envisioned in terms of three historical "streams" dating back to the early twentieth century that converged unexpectedly and momentously in the summer of 1999. These three tributaries, corresponding to the histories of vaccine preservatives, mercury poisoning, and autism, are examined successively to illuminate why various groups responded so differently to the debates beginning in that year.

Thimerosal and Vaccines

Understanding why mercury was first incorporated into childhood vaccines leads back to the preantibiotic era, a time when physicians employed a variety of compounds known as "germicides" to combat bacteria. Perhaps the best known was Joseph Lister's carbolic acid, developed in the 1860s for surgical antisepsis and later employed as a germicide and preservative known as phenol.[5] Yet a variety of mercury compounds were also used for the same purpose. No less an authority than Robert Koch championed the use of mercury chloride as an antiseptic, although the product's propensity to cause tissue irritation limited its use. In the early twentieth century, investigators synthesized a new class of compounds they claimed to be both more effective and less toxic, the organomercurials. Often brilliantly colored, these products soon found widespread usage, from operating suites to home medicine cabinets.[6]

Thimerosal was one of the most promising new organomercurials that excited the pharmaceutical industry after World War I. It was a white, crystalline powder, approximately 50% mercury by weight, in the form of ethylmercury bound to thiosalicylate. The emerging pharmaceutical giant Eli Lilly and Company provided grant support for its synthesis at the University of Chicago and in 1928 patented it under the trade name Merthiolate.[7] Over the next several years, Lilly's investigators H. M. Powell and W. A. Jamieson conducted extensive in vitro testing, showing that thimerosal was 40 to 50 times as effective as phenol against Staphylococcus aureus. The two men evaluated toxicity by injecting the compound into more than 300 rabbits and a variety of other animals observed for a week's time. The animals appeared to tolerate significant doses—up to 20 mg per kg body weight in rabbits and still higher in rats—without apparent injury.[8]

These encouraging results prompted the Lilly team in 1929 to offer their product to the Indiana General Hospital during an epidemic of meningococcal meningitis. Hospital physicians gave 22 patients as much as 180 mL of a 1% solution of thimerosal intravenously divided over five doses. From a therapeutic standpoint, the trial was a failure, but investigators were struck by how well the patients seemed to tolerate such high doses.[9] Combined with the animal studies, the data further reinforced the impression that thimerosal was far more benign than earlier mercurials, preparing the way for its incorporation at low concentrations into a wide range of biological products as a preservative. Vaccines would become an especially important niche.

One of the most troublesome safety issues afflicting early twentieth-century child immunization was that of bacterial contamination. This could easily occur on a sporadic basis, when general practitioners might have to draw vaccines from multidose vials under poor hygienic conditions. Contamination of entire lots could be much more spectacular. In Columbia, South Carolina, in 1916, a tainted batch of typhoid vaccine stored at room temperature caused 68 severe reactions, 26 abscesses, and 4 deaths. A still more disturbing incident took place in 1928 in Queensland, Australia, where 12 of 21 children inoculated with contaminated diphtheria vaccine died of multiple staphylococcal abscesses and toxemia. The need for effective preservatives was readily apparent and represented one of the most important safety issues for the promoters of new vaccines.[10]

In this context, Powell and Jamieson's studies suggested that Merthiolate had an unexpected advantage. The problem with existing preservatives such as phenol and cresol was that they often reduced the potency of the biological products they were intended to protect. By contrast, thimerosal not only inhibited bacterial growth in vaccines and antisera at concentrations as low as 1:10000 but also had no such deleterious effects.[11] A series of other investigators confirmed these findings over the next several years, and by 1940, thimerosal was incorporated into diphtheria toxoid, meningococcal serum, pertussis vaccine, and a host of other biological products.[12] Indeed, in 1938, Lilly's assistant director of research listed Merthiolate along with insulin as one of the five most important drugs ever developed by the company.[13]

Thimerosal's efficacy was sometimes challenged during the first 50 years following its synthesis but rarely its safety. In 1948, the American Medical Association's (AMA's) Council on Pharmacy and Chemistry issued a report calling attention to a series of investigations asking whether organomercurials were any more effective as germicides than inorganic mercury compounds had previously been.[14] The AMA's council, it should be noted, played an important role before 1950 in providing independent assessments and approvals of drugs; the U.S. Food and Drug Administration (FDA) did not require manufacturers to submit prelicensure safety testing until 1938 or efficacy testing until the 1960s.[15] Despite these voices of dissent, thimerosal remained popular in practice. Its defenders pointed to their own studies and the simple fact that contamination incidents had become exceedingly uncommon following its introduction.[16] Although Jonas Salk's experience with inactivated polio vaccine in field trials from

1954 to 1955 suggested that in some cases thimerosal, contrary to expectation, did in fact harm vaccine immunogenicity, this case was regarded as an exception to the rule.[17]

The first real questions regarding thimerosal's safety were raised in the 1970s, provoked (as will be described in the next section) by rising awareness of the dangers of organic mercury poisoning. Although the latter debate centered on the organomercurial methylmercury found in fish and industrial pollution, ethylmercury did not escape scrutiny. A series of case reports demonstrated the compound's potential for neurotoxicity when given in large volumes, such as when used as a topical antiseptic to "paint" large omphaloceles.[18,19] These exposures exceeded those in vaccines, however, by many orders of magnitude. Only one routine infant vaccine in the 1970s, the diphtheria-tetanus-pertussis combination, contained thimerosal. A formal review of thimerosal by the FDA concluded in 1976 that no dangerous quantity of mercury was likely to be received from vaccines and other biological products over a lifetime.[20]

Concerns over neurotoxicity in infants receiving thimerosal from vaccines were never raised by medical or governmental authorities before the late 1990s. To be sure, some bacteriologists continued to question its efficacy in the laboratory. As noted by dermatologists (and eventually the FDA), skin testing revealed that contact with thimerosal caused hypersensitivity in many people. There was no evidence, however, that this phenomenon had any medical significance.[21] Thimerosal's toxicity at high doses was clearly established by the 1970s, but the comparatively miniscule exposures involved in vaccines were well within all published guidelines for mercury exposure. The overwhelming consensus was that ethylmercury in low concentrations was safe and effective in practice.

What broke this consensus was the convergence of the history of ethylmercury with the parallel history of methylmercury in the mid-1990s. This story, known better to environmental scientists than vaccinologists, evolved in a direction that eventually suggested that even relatively low exposures to organic mercury could be dangerous to the fetus and young infant.

Methylmercury and the Developing Brain

Methylmercury, the form of mercury linked most closely in the public mind with environmental pollution, has a history as public and infamous as the history of ethylmercury has been quiet and inconspicuous. Much in the thimerosal debate hinges on the alleged similarity, or dissimilarity, of ethylmercury to methylmercury. The two compounds sound alike, differ by only one methylated side chain in their structure, and tend to be mentioned interchangeably in the popular press. Yet the chemical distinction is not trivial; it may be compared with that between ethanol (the form of alcohol in wine) and its highly lethal counterpart methanol. Methylmercury was once used widely in developing countries as a fungicide as part of the "Green Revolution" that transformed agriculture after 1945. It is also synthesized by bacteria living in mercury-polluted waters, where it is passed up the food chain and concentrated in fish. The dangers of methylmercury in both contexts have been vividly demonstrated in a series of environmental disasters.

The first and best remembered of these took place in the fishing community of Minamata Bay, Japan. In the early 1950s, the Chisso chemical company constructed a factory that began expelling large quantities of effluent into the bay. The area's inhabitants soon began witnessing a variety of disturbing events. Seagulls fell from the sky, dead fish washed ashore, and frenzied cats were seen whirling in a mad dance ending in death. Soon thereafter, doctors began seeing patients with a staggering gait, numbness in the hands and feet, and more profound neurological impairments. A new form of viral encephalitis was initially suspected. An investigation by Kumamoto University, however, pointed instead to the similarity of the symptoms to those described in an obscure 1940 case report of four workers in a manufacturing plant producing methylmercury as a seed disinfectant. Bacteria in the bay, the researchers concluded, had converted inorganic mercury discharged from the plant into methylmercury.[22]

The Minamata Bay disaster became one of the defining events in the rise of environmental awareness of the toxic effects of mercury. The Chisso company long resisted pressure to improve its discharge system, and victims continued to appear in the 1960s in both Minamata and Niigata, Japan, the site of a second outbreak. Only in 1968 did the Japanese government release a formal statement implicating methylmercury in the outbreaks. A series of lawsuits began shortly thereafter that would last until the end of the century. The magnitude of the disaster remains hard to determine, but as of 2003, more than 2,265 patients had been certified to have had Minamata disease.[23] The spectacle was brought to American eyes in the 1960s on the pages of *Life* magazine through the poignant work of documentary photographer and activist W. Eugene Smith.[24]

Some of Smith's most enduring images depicted children with mercury poisoning, some of whom, born to asymptomatic mothers, had been exposed in utero. Here was the first indication that the fetus was more vulnerable than the adult. Infants with "congenital Minamata disease" manifested the hallmarks of profound neurological injury: spasticity, seizures, deafness, and severe mental deficiency. The shame associated with the syndrome was so great, however, that investigators had a great deal of difficulty enrolling patients for formal studies.[25]

Tragically, a still greater disaster soon provided researchers another opportunity. In Iraq in 1971 and 1972, an estimated 6,530 farmers and family members were hospitalized for methylmercury poisoning, of whom 459 died. The source was homemade bread derived from seed wheat that had been contaminated by fungicide.[26] Extensive study of the Iraqi victims provided the basis for the first standards defining safe organic mercury exposure for adults. Specifically, the FDA drew on these data, as well as a variety of animal studies and reports from other mercury poisoning incidents, when it proposed in the 1970s an acceptable daily intake of 0.4 μg per kg of body weight per day, based on the threshold at which paresthesia occurs in adults.[27]

Determining safe exposure for the fetus and newborn proved much more challenging.[28] At an early point, investigators in Iraq identified cases of severe congenital mercury poisoning characterized by profound retardation and spasticity similar to those that had been described in Japan.[29] Only gradually did it become apparent that these infants represented the extreme of a continuum of toxicity. The first published studies of apparently asymptomatic Iraqi infants exposed to intrauterine or postnatal (through breastmilk) methylmercury were reassuring, with tests revealing normal development at age 1 year. As surveillance of these children continued into the 1980s, however, a disproportionate number began to show signs of delays in language acquisition.[30] The probability that mercury might be analogous to lead, which was also shown to have more subtle yet real cognitive effects by researchers in the same time period, was becoming more compelling.[31]

Two major longitudinal studies were launched during the 1980s in the hope of answering whether relatively low maternal methylmercury exposures could result in any degree of neurological injury to the fetus. Both were conducted in isolated island populations consuming large quantities of fish. The first, based in the Seychelles in the Indian Ocean, used global measures such as overall IQ and the Denver Developmental Screening test, whereas the second, based in the Faroe Islands in the North Atlantic, employed more-specialized, domain-related tests of function.

The two studies produced different results. The Seychelles children did not appear to suffer any adverse outcomes. By contrast, the Faroe children demonstrated deficits in language, attention, and memory at age 7 years. It is unclear whether these differences reflect testing strategies, different genetic vulnerabilities, or the source of mercury. The Faroe Islanders consumed mercury in more of a "bolus" fashion in the form of meals, including pilot whale blubber, which is heavily contaminated with fat-soluble pollutants such as polychlorinated biphenyl (PCB) and pesticides. Still, the more-specific types of testing in the Faroes led many environmental experts to give the results there precedence.[32,33]

The stage was now set for the confusing array of advisory recommendations on methylmercury that emerged in the 1990s. Agencies differed with respect to directing recommendations at adults or pregnant women, balancing the conflicting data for the Seychelles and Faroes, and determining how much of an uncertainty factor to take into account the extent to which individuals may metabolize mercury differently. As of 1999, the FDA continued to set its acceptable daily intake at 0.4 μg per kg of body weight per day, the standard proposed for adults in the 1970s. It noted that this figure should probably be set lower for pregnant women. By contrast, in 1994, the U.S Environmental Protection Agency (EPA) lowered its reference dose for methylmercury exposure to 0.1 μg per kg of body weight per day on the basis of the Iraqi data on women and children. To make the situation still more confusing, the Agency for Toxic Substances and Disease Registry lowered its minimal risk level to 0.1 μg per kg of body weight per day in 1994, only to raise it back to 0.3 μg per kg of body weight per day in 1999, prioritizing the Seychelles over the Faroes studies.[34]

Beyond the discrepancy between official recommendations, two other points deserve emphasis. First, there was an emerging consensus among environmental scientists that the fetus was indeed more sensitive to methylmercury than the adult and that this toxicity was better expressed as a continuum than a clear-cut syndrome. The second point is that this concern had to do with relatively subtle cognitive and language delays, detectable in older children through domain-specific testing. Autism was not even discussed. It was not described among either the profoundly injured children in disasters such as Minamata Bay and Iraq or the milder delays described in the Faroes. Autism only entered the discourse in 1999, represented by a third set of communities with their own historical memories.

Autism and Its Histories

The hypothesis that thimerosal-containing vaccines could explain the remarkable rise in the prevalence of autism arose not among environmental scientists but among the communities that have emerged over the past 20 years of parents and professionals caring for autistic children.[35] Specifically, parents and clinicians who have framed autism in biomedical terms (such as immune or gastrointestinal dysfunction) have been critical agents in promoting both the concept of the "autism epidemic" and the primacy of vaccines as its cause. The passion behind their arguments stems from a long history of advocacy on behalf of their children, often in the face of psychiatric theories perceived as "parent blaming" and inadequately funded developmental and educational resources in many communities.

The psychoanalyst Leo Kanner first coined the term "autistic" in a classic 1948 case report of 11 children exhibiting what he characterized as "an extreme autistic aloneness" shutting out all social contact, as well as an "obsessive desire for the maintenance of sameness" in their play and daily routines. The typical autistic child in his series eventually acquired language but used it in a mechanical way devoid of emotion, sometimes combined with striking rote memory. One preschool child could recite 25 questions of the Presbyterian Catechism, another could distinguish 18 symphonies from one another. Kanner (along with his contemporary Hans Asperger, who described a similar syndrome in 1944) was especially struck that all the children were born to highly intelligent parents.[36] Over the next two decades, autism researchers such as Bruno Bettelheim developed an explicitly Freudian explanation to account for the association: autism arose in infancy in response to rejection by an emotionally distant (although typically well-educated) parent—a so-called "refrigerator mother."[37]

In 1965, psychologist Bernard Rimland (himself the father of an autistic child) rejected the psychogenic model of autism in his ground-breaking *Infantile Autism*, proposing that the condition was instead rooted in biology.[38] The collapse of the psychoanalytic model gave rise, however, to two rather different explanatory frameworks in its place. The ways in which these have diverged and have been embraced by different communities of parents and professionals is of critical importance to understanding the current debate over the existence of an autism epidemic.

What might be characterized as the "mainline" community of autism researchers has reconceptualized autism as a neurodevelopmental condition.[39] Four tenets have characterized most approaches by these researchers. First, the cause of autism is fundamentally biological and no more attributable to parental behavior than is cerebral palsy or Down syndrome. Although the nature of the cause remains unknown, a variety of studies (ranging from radiographic imaging to genetic twin studies and family pedigree analysis) have increasingly highlighted the importance of genetics.[40] Second, autism is conceptualized as a spectrum of disorders. In the 1970s, investigators modified Kanner's original restrictive diagnosis to encompass children with greater intellectual and language impairment and then expanded it in the opposite direction to encompass higher functioning children with labels such as "pervasive developmental disorders" and "autistic spectrum disorders."[41]

Third, if autism represents a spectrum disorder rooted in biology as proffered in the first two tenets, its treatment must be largely rehabilitative rather than curative. For example, Eric Schopler of the University of North Carolina developed the influential Teaching and Education of Autistic and related Communication-handicapped Children (TEACCH) program as a model combining parental education and therapy to assist parents in understanding their children prior to setting realistic management approaches.[42] Fourth, as with other developmental disorders, early referral and intervention offer the greatest hope for a positive outcome. Many autism researchers and parent allies have worked tirelessly to promote screening tools and special education programs in the schools. In 1991, autism was officially added to the list of covered disabilities in the Individuals with Disabilities Education Act passed the preceding year, providing a major boost to its diagnosis and early treatment.[43]

The essential point to understand is that the rise of autism diagnoses in the 1990s was exactly what the mainline researchers expected.[44] It represented the logical consequence of their ongoing efforts to expand its definition and promote its recognition in developmental evaluation centers and the schools. What perhaps was not expected, and certainly not welcome, was the gap that frequently appeared between the supply of and rising demand for autistic services. All too often, parents confronted with their child's diagnosis in the 1990s were met with long waiting lists and primary care doctors who seemed barely familiar with the condition. Placed in this predicament, parents not surprisingly turned to one another and the Internet.

Parents frustrated by the mainline approach to autism were likely to meet what might be characterized as the "alternative" community of autism research. This approach viewed autism in biomedical terms. Rather than viewing autism as a continuum of disability, it characterized the condition as a heterogenous collection of discrete entities with different etiologies sharing a common presentation. Most important, this viewpoint offered hope that at least some forms of autism are not simply treatable but curable. Many such cures have been proposed. Among the most popular were those focusing on special diets, based on studies suggesting that an abnormality in intestinal permeability (a so-called "leaky gut") may admit intestinal toxins or opioids affecting the nervous system at an early age. Although promoted by researchers who viewed themselves as "dissident" with respect to mainline thinking, these theories recast autism as biomedical in origin and potentially curable in ways that profoundly reflected late twentieth-century American hopes in the power of medical technology.[45]

The most notable organization promoting this framework is the Autism Research Institute in San Diego, California, which through its Defeat Autism Now! conferences and educational materials seeks to provide parents with the tools to understand and treat their own child. Parents provide much of the leadership and energy in this and related organizations. A smaller cadre of professionals participate as well, some of whom are prominent in their own right. The Autism Research Institute was organized with the full support of psychologist Bernard Rimland, who had earlier played such a pivotal role in dethroning the psychogenic approach.[46]

It was among these parental advocacy groups, not the medical or educational professions, that the notion of an autism "epidemic" first took root. These organizations provided a context to bring parents out of isolation and into a realization that others—many others—shared their hopes and frustrations. Against this background, an alarming possibility became more plausible: the cause of autism was not only biological but environmental, the consequence of some new exposure faced by young children. Indeed, it seemed fair to speak of an autism epidemic as a means of summoning the sense of urgency the situation required.

In 1998, British gastroenterologist Andrew Wakefield proposed a hypothesis linking the "leaky gut" etiologic framework of autism to a new environmental factor explaining its rise. In that year, he published a report describing a small number of patients who developed autistic regression and diarrhea following their MMR immunization.[47] Wakefield's study launched a major controversy in Britain, despite the failure of large epidemiological studies to confirm its results.[48] Aided by the Internet, the controversy soon crossed the Atlantic and was viewed with concern by many parents of autistic children as well as the parallel network of parent groups opposing compulsory immunization. Both groups gained a powerful ally when Congressman Dan Burton (R, Ind) began a series of congressional hearings on autism and vaccine safety after his own grandchild was diagnosed with autism following the 12-month vaccinations.[49]

By 1999, a growing body of articulate and well-organized parents of autistic children was set on a trajectory destined to collide with that of the vaccine community. Their collective experience had taught them the importance of challenging conventional wisdom and expertise. Many were highly capable individuals, such as Rick Rollens, an associate of California Governor Gray Davis (and, again, the father of an autistic child), who persuaded the legislature to fund millions of dollars for autism research at the University of California at Davis, as well as a study examining the historical trend in children receiving services for autism in the state's public school system.[50] Released on March 1, 1999, the report indicated that the rate of autism had increased 273% over the past 10 years. Reported widely in the press, the California Department of Developmental Services study gave new urgency to calls for investigation of an autism "epidemic" as the summer approached.[51]

Confluence

The events that would bring these three histories together began in 1997, when New Jersey Representative Frank Pallone, representing a district concerned about environmental mercury poisoning, appended a rider to the FDA Modernization Act of that year to assess all of the agency's products for mercury content.[52] In response, the Center for Biologics Evaluation and Research (CBER) at the FDA initiated a formal risk assessment of thimerosal in vaccines beginning in April 1998. By this point, the vaccine schedule had expanded, and three of the vaccines routinely given to infants (diphtheria-tetanus-acellular pertussis, *Haemophilus influenzae* type b conjugate, and hepatitis B) potentially contained thimerosal. The analysis was completed in the spring of 1999. The actual cumulative exposure varied considerably, given that not all manufacturers used the preservative, but the CBER scientists calculated that a minority of infants could receive as much as 187.5 µg of ethylmercury during the first 6 months of life. Lacking any standard for ethylmercury, the CBER team compared this exposure to standards for methylmercury and discovered that it exceeded that set by the EPA. Although acknowledging the many uncertainties involved, the FDA responded by inviting vaccine advisory bodies for consultation in June 1999.[53]

There followed a rapid series of meetings and conference calls involving representatives of the American Academy of Pediatrics and the Centers for Disease Control and Prevention (CDC), culminating in a joint statement released on July 9, 1999. Although noting that there was no evidence that the use of thimerosal as a vaccine preservative had caused any true harm, the groups agreed that "thimerosal-containing vaccines should be removed as soon as possible" given the concerns raised by the Environmental Protection Agency's guidelines.[54] The controversy was now out in the open.

Many have criticized the process leading to the release of the joint statement, charging that it took place too rapidly and without proper consultation from important parties.[55] Its call to suspend the use of hepatitis B virus vaccine in infants younger than 6 months until thimerosal-free vaccine became widely available was particularly contentious. Although the ban only lasted for several months, it resulted in considerable confusion and inconsistency in hepatitis B virus vaccine delivery in some hospital nurseries.[56] One study later found that the proportion of hospitals failing to vaccinate infants born to seropositive mothers rose by more than six times (from 1% to 7%) during the suspension.[57] The consequences of this were harder to calculate but clearly worrisome given the high (up to 90%) chance that infants who acquire hepatitis B infection at birth will develop the infection in a chronic form, with a significant (25%) risk of liver cancer.[58] By contrast, the statement's defenders asserted the prime importance of preserving the public's trust in the vaccine system, particularly given the rising influence of populist "vaccine safety" groups since the 1970s. Manufacturers, moreover, did successfully mobilize to remove thimerosal from their routine infant vaccines in a remarkably short time; the effort was largely complete by the summer of 2001.[59,60]

Meanwhile, the third of the historical streams, represented by parents within the "alternative" autism community, rapidly entered the debate. As detailed by journalist David Kirby, it was in fact a group of parents of autistic children (rather than parental organizations critical of vaccination, such as the National Vaccine Information Center) that first seized on thimerosal as an explanation for the autism epidemic. In keeping with their identity as participants in shaping research, some spent long hours on the computer or in libraries researching studies on mercury. Eventually, their efforts led to a published study in *Medical Hypotheses* that compared the features of autism to various signs reported in past studies and case reports of mercury exposure.[61] The publication of this study in turn helped to legitimize the hypothesis and thereby reinforce a growing body of individual testimonies across the Internet and in conferences.

Parents organized effectively in the political realm as well. The self-designated "Mercury Moms" created an advocacy organization, Safe Minds. They were instrumental in persuading Congressman Burton to shift his focus from MMR to thimerosal in his congressional hearings. They organized successfully to oppose a rider to the Homeland Security Bill in 2003 that would protect thimerosal's manufacturer from legal action.[62]

These events are chosen among many that have taken place since 1999 to illustrate the polarization that soon characterized the entire debate. Although a full analysis cannot be provided here, two themes deserve emphasis. One is the issue of trust. Physicians and public health leaders have generally turned to the scientific process to sort out the controversy and have been reassured by the negative conclusions of the IOM reports. Vaccine opponents have repeatedly rejected these studies, charging that the data have been manipulated for political reasons.[63] The second factor has been the entry of personal injury lawyers into the debate, accompanied by full-page advertisements in prominent newspapers and an infusion of financial support. Although hardly the primary agent in the story, litigation has without doubt fueled the polarization of the debate and further obscured scientific testimony through the promotion of expert witnesses dissenting from the IOM position.[64] Today, the mercury–autism hypothesis continues to be widely accepted among parents of autistic children.

Conclusion

At this point, it is fair to ask whether this narrative should more properly have focused on the story of the thimerosal controversy since 1999. Has not a new group of actors, including members of Congress, professional groups, antivaccine organizations, and personal injury lawyers, assumed central relevance since that time? Is it really necessary to understand the long-term historical trends that converged just prior to the 1999 joint statement?

There are three answers, each corresponding to one of the historical streams already examined. The first is directed at the insinuation prevalent on the Internet that thimerosal was a dubious product smuggled into vaccines by avaricious drug companies bent on profits rather than the welfare of children. A more sober assessment would suggest that thimerosal was the result of ethical scientific and corporate research in the 1920s and 1930s, specifically to improve vaccine safety. Despite questions regarding its efficacy, it has performed well in practice and posed toxicity so low as to be considered negligible until recent years.

The second point concerns the history of mercury poisoning. Central to the public story of thimerosal has been a battle over the meaning of "mercury." Those in the scientific community take it as axiomatic that all forms of mercury are not created equal; in particular, there are good reasons to believe that the ethylmercury used in vaccines is different from the methylmercury studied in environmental science. In public discourse, however, such distinctions are subsumed under a single entity, mercury, with a long and public history. Perhaps unfairly, history has endowed mercury in all of its forms with a notoriety that is not easy to erase, as will quickly be discovered by any pediatrician trying to convince an anxious mother that a "trace" of mercury in a vaccine is safe. One cannot simply brush aside this perception in constructing policy.

Finally, however important personal injury lawyers, vaccine skeptics, and their allies in Congress may have been in shaping the thimerosal controversy since 1999, they did not create it. Parents within the "alternative" wing of the autism community were the primary agents in popularizing the concepts that autism had become epidemic and vaccines were its cause. Jumping from the first to the second proposition may have been highly conjectural, but the question of whether the rise in autism is real or defined (or both) remains open to reasonable debate. There is genuine anger in the autism community that has fueled the polarization of the thimerosal debate, but this anger is best understood in terms of frustration with the medical and educational systems, not the cynical manipulation of lawyers.

Although historical understanding may not readily translate into policy guidelines, it is essential for those responsible for conducting and implementing such policy. A polarized debate both draws on and contributes to polarized understandings of history. Participants within each of this story's three streams judged the same data using different sets of assumptions, each shaped by history. Articulating and sharing these narratives represent a first step toward transcending the powerful boundaries shaping today's vaccine controversies.

References

1. The eight reports are available at: www.iom.edu/?ID=4705/. Accessed October 9, 2007.

2. Colgrove, J., and R. Bayer. 2005. "Could it happen here? Vaccine risk controversies and the specter of derailment. *Health Affairs* 24:729–739; Wilson, C. B., and E. K. Marcuse. 2001. Vaccine safety—vaccine benefits: Science and the public's perception. *Nature Reviews Immunology* 1:160–165.

3. Michael, F. 2005. *MMR and Autism: What Parents Need to Know*. London: Routledge; Kirby, D. 2005. *Evidence of Harm: Mercury in Vaccines and the Autism Epidemic: A Medical Controversy*. New York: St. Martin's Press.

4. Institute of Medicine. 2001. *Immunization Safety Review: Thimerosal-Containing Vaccines and Neurodevelopmental Disorders*. Washington, DC: National Academies Press; Institute of Medicine. 2004. *Immunization Safety Review: Vaccines and Autism*. Washington, DC: National Academies Press.

5. Porter, R. 1997. *The Greatest Benefit to Mankind: A Medical History of Humanity*. New York: W.W. Norton.

6. Brewer, J. H. 1950. Mercurials as antiseptics. *Annals of the New York Academy of Sciences* 53:211–219; Goldwater, L. J. 1972. *Mercury: A History of Quicksilver*. Baltimore: York Press.

7. AMA Council on Pharmacy and Chemistry. 1929. New and nonofficial remedies. *Journal of the American Medical Association* 93:1809.

8. Powell, H. M., and W. A. Jamieson. 1931. Merthiolate as a germicide. *American Journal of Hygiene* 13:296–310.

9. Smithburn, K. C., G. E. Kempf, L. G. Zerfas, and L. H. Gilman. 1930. Meningococcic meningitis: A clinical study of one hundred and forty-four cases. *Journal of the American Medical Association* 95:776–780; Powell and Jamieson, Merthiolate as a Germicide, 306–307.

10. Wilson, G. S. 1967. *The Hazards of Immunization*. London: Athalone Press.

11. Jamieson, W. A., and H. M. Powell. 1931. Merthiolate as a preservative for biological products. *American Journal of Hygiene* 14:218–224.

12. Powell, H. M., and W. A. Jamieson. 1937. On the efficacy of "merthiolate" as a biological preservative after ten years' use. *Proceedings of the Indiana Academy of Science* 47:65–70; Povitsky, O. R., and Eisner, M. 1935. Merthiolate versus phenol as a preservative for diphtheria toxoids. *Journal of Immunology* 28:209–213.

13. Madison, J. H. 1989. *Eli Lilly: A Life, 1885–1977*. Indianapolis: Indiana Historical Society.

14. AMA Council on Pharmacy and Chemistry. 1948. Report to the council: Organomercurial compounds. *Journal of the American Medical Association* 136:36–41.

15. Swann, J. P. 1998. Food and Drug Administration. In: *A Historical Guide to the US Government*, ed. G. T. Kurian, 248–254. New York: Oxford University Press.

16. Powell, H. M. 1948. Antibacterial action of "merthiolate" against hemolytic streptococci. *JAMA* 137:862–864; Brewer, Mercurials as antiseptics, 211–219. Robert Martenson's analysis of the literature concluded that later investigators' confidence in thimerosal's safety by the 1950s was grounded in their own experience, not earlier publications from the Eli Lilly team; Martenson, R. L. 1948. Analysis Report in the Matter of Easter vs Eli Lilly and Company. Unpublished.

17. Oshinsky, D. 2005. *Polio: An American Story*. Oxford: Oxford University Press.

18. Axton, J. H. M. 1972. Six cases of poisoning after a parental organic mercurial compound (merthiolate). *Postgraduate Medicine* 48:417–421.

19. Fagan, D. G., J. S. Pritchard, T. W. Clarkson, and M. R. Greenwood. 1977. Organ mercury levels in infants with omphaloceles treated with organic mercurial antiseptic. *Archives of Disease in Children* 52:962–964.

20. Gibson, S. 1976, February 27. Memorandum from assistant director, Bureau of Biologics, FDA to director, Bureau of Biologics, "Use of Thimerosal in Biologics Production. Quoted in Ball, L. K., R Ball, and R. D. Pratt. 2001. An assessment of thimerosal use in childhood vaccines. *Pediatrics* 107:1147–1154.

21. Cox, N. H., and Forsyth, A. 1988. Thimerosal allergy and vaccination reactions. *Contact Dermatitis* 18:229–233; Moller, H. 1994. All these positive tests to thimerosal. *Contact Dermatitis* 31:209–213. Hypersensitivity concerns prompted the FDA to propose rules on the use of thimerosal as a preservative on two occasions; see Department of Health, Education, and Welfare, Food and Drug Administration. 1977, September 30. Skin test antigens: Proposed implementation of efficacy review. *Federal Register* 42:52719–52721; Department of Health, Education, and Welfare, Food and Drug Administration. 1982, January 5. Mercury-containing drug products for topical antimicrobial over-the-counter human use: Establishment of a monograph. *Federal Register* 47:436–442.

22. Masazumi, H. 1995. Minamata disease: Methylmercury poisoning in Japan caused by environmental pollution. *Critical Reviews in Toxicology* 25:1–24. For the original description of the symptoms of methylmercury poisoning, see Hunter, D., R. Bromford, and D. Russell. 1940. Poisoning by methyl mercury compounds. *Quarterly Journal of Medicine* 9:193–214.

23. Masazumi, H. 2004. *Minamata Disease* (T. Sachie and T. S. George, Trans.). Tokyo: Iwanami Shoten.

24. Eugene, S. W., and A. M. Smith. 1975. *Minamata*. New York: Holt, Rinehart, and Winston.

25. Masazumi, H. 1978. Congenital Minamata disease: Intrauterine methylmercury poisoning. *Teratology* 18:285–288.

26. Bakir, F., S. F. Damluji, L. Amin-Zaki, et al. 1973. Methylmercury poisoning in Iraq. *Science* 181:230–241.

27. Mahaffey, K. R. 1999. Methylmercury: A new look at the risks. *Public Health Reports* 114: 403, 407.

28. For a review of the state of knowledge in the 1970s, see Koos, B. J., and L. D. Longo. 1976. Mercury toxicity in the pregnant woman, fetus, and newborn infant. *American Journal of Obstetrics and Gynecology* 126:390–409.

29. Laman, A.-Z., S. Elhassani, M. A. Majeed, et al. 1974. Intra-uterine methylmercury poisoning in Iraq. *Pediatrics* 54:587–595.

30. Laman, A.-Z., S. Elhassani, M. A. Majeed, et al. 1974. Studies of infants postnatally exposed to methylmercury. *Journal of Pediatrics* 85:81–84; Laman, A.-Z., S. B. Elhassani, M. A. Majeed, et al. 1980. Methylmercury poisoning in mothers and their suckling infants. *Developments in Toxicology and Environmental Science* 8:75–78; Marsh, D. O. 1987. Clarkson, T. W., C. Cox, et al. 1987. Fetal methylmercury poisoning: Relationship between concentration in single strands of hairs and child effects. *Archives of Neurology* 44:1017–1022.

31. Fowler, A., D. C. Bellinger, R. L. Bornschein, et al. 1993. *Measuring Lead Exposure in Infants, Children, and Other Sensitive Populations*. Washington, DC: National Academy of Sciences Press.

32. Grandjean, P., P. Weihe, R. F. White, et al. 1997. Cognitive deficit in 7-year-old children with prenatal exposure to methylmercury. *Neurotoxicology and Teratology* 19:417–428.

33. Davidson, P. W., Myers, G. J., C. Cox, et al. 1998. Effects of prenatal and postnatal methylmercury exposure from fish consumption on neurodevelopment: Outcomes at 66 months of age in the Seychelles Child Development Study. *Journal of the American Medical Association* 280: 701–707.

34. Mahaffey, Methylmercury, 403, 407–411.

35. On the role of parental communities in shaping the diagnosis and treatment of autism, see Silverman, C. 2004. *A Disorder of Affect: Love, Tragedy, Biomedicine, and Citizenship in American Autism Research, 1943–2003* [PhD dissertation]. Philadelphia: University of Pennsylvania.

36. Kanner, L. 1943. Autistic disturbances of affective contact. *Nervous Child* 2:217–250. Asperger's paper was published in German during wartime and "re-discovered" later by Anglo-American autism researchers; see Frith, U. 1991. Asperger and his syndrome. In: *Autism and Asperger Syndrome*, ed. U. Frith, 1–36. Cambridge: Cambridge University Press.

37. Bettelheim, B. 1967. *The Empty Fortress: Infantile Autism and the Birth of the Self*. New York: Free Press, 1967.

38. Rimland, B. 1965. *Infantile Autism: The Syndrome and Its Implications for a Neural Theory of Behavior*. London: Methuen.

39. Prominent exponents of this approach have included Eric Schopler in the United States and Michael Rutter and Lorna and John Wing in Britain. See Wing, J. K., ed., 1966. *Early Childhood Autism: Clinical, Educational, and Social Aspects*. Oxford: Pergamon Press; Schopler, E., S. S. Brehm,

M. Kinsbourne, and R. J. Reichler. 1971. Effect of treatment structure on development in autistic children. *Archives of General Psychiatry* 24:415–421.

40. Folstein, S., and M. Rutter. 1977. Infantile autism: A genetic study of 21 twin pairs. *Journal of Child Psychology and Psychiatry* 18:297–321; Szatami, P. 2003. The causes of autism spectrum disorders. *British Medical Journal* 326:173–174.

41. Michael Rutter added impaired language to Kanner's two criteria of impaired social relationships and preoccupation with sameness, developing the autistic triad underlying most definitions ever since; Rutter, M. 1978. Diagnosis and definition of childhood autism. *Journal of Autism and Childhood Schizophrenia* 8:139–161. On the concept of an autistic spectrum, see Wing, L. 1996. *The Autistic Spectrum*. London: Constable. In the United States, both developments are reflected in successive revisions of *Diagnostic and Statistical Manual of Mental Disorders*, Revised Third Edition. 1987. Washington, DC: American Psychiatric Association; and *Diagnostic and Statistical Manual of Mental Disorders*, Fourth Edition. 1994. Washington, DC: American Psychiatric Association.

42. Schopler, E., and R. J. Reichler. 1971. Parents as cotherapists in the treatment of psychotic children. *Journal of Autism and Childhood Schizophrenia* 1:87–102. Behavioral therapy ranges from the primarily rehabilitative approach exemplified by Schopler to the more optimistic claims of applied behavioral analysis and similar methodologies; see Lovass, O. I. 1987. Behavioral treatment and normal rducational and intellectual functioning in young autistic children. *Journal of Consulting and Clinical Psychology* 55:3–9; Aman, M. G. 2005. Treatment planning for parents with autism spectrum disorders. *Journal of Clinical Psychiatry* 66 (suppl 10):38–45.

43. Palfrey, J. S., and J. S. Rodman. 1999. Legislation for the education of children with disabilities. In: *Developmental-Behavioral Pediatrics*, 3rd edition, ed. M. D. Levine, W. B. Carey, and A. C. Crocker, 869–872. Philadelphia: W.B. Saunders.

44. Wing, L. 1996. Autistic spectrum disorders: No evidence for or against an increase in prevalence. *British Medical Journal* 312:327–328; Fombonne, E. 2001. Is there an epidemic of autism? *Pediatrics* 107:411–413.

45. Silverman, A Disorder of Affect, 360–451.

46. Pangorn, J., and S. Baker. 2005. *Autism: Effective Biomedical Treatments (Have We Done Everything We Can for This Child?): Individuality in an Epidemic*. San Diego: Autism Research Institute.

47. Wakefield, A. J., S. H. Murch, A. Anthony, et al. 1998. Ileal–lymphoid–nodular hyperplasia, non-specific colitis, and pervasive developmental disorder in children. *Lancet* 351:637–641.

48. Fitzpatrick, *MMR and Autism*.

49. Autism: Present Challenges, Future Needs—Why the Increased Rates? Hearing Before the Committee on Government Reform, House of Representatives, 106th Cong, 2nd Sess (April 6, 2000); Vastag, B. 2001. Congressional autism hearings continue: No evidence MMR vaccine causes disorder. *Journal of the American Medical Association* 285:2567–2568.

50. Kirby, *Evidence of Harm*, 89–90.

51. *Changes in the Population of Persons with Autism and Pervasive Developmental Disorders in California's Developmental Services System: 1987 Through 1998: A Report to the Legislature.* 1999, March 1. Sacramento: California Department of Developmental Services.

52. Allen, A. 2002, November 10. The not-so-crackpot autism theory. *New York Times Magazine.*

53. Ball, L. K., R. Ball, and R. D. Pratt. 2001. An assessment of thimerosal use in childhood vaccines. *Pediatrics* 107:1147–1154.

54. Joint Statement of the American Academy of Pediatrics (AAP) and the United States Public Health Service (USPHS). 1999. *Pediatrics* 104:568–569.

55. For details on the negotiations leading to the joint statement, see Freed, G. L., M. C. Andrae, A. E. Cowan, and S. L. Katz. 2002. The process of public policy formation: The case of thimerosal in vaccines. *Pediatrics* 109:1153–1159; Uproar over a little-known preservative, thimerosal, jostles US Hepatitis B vaccination policy. 1999. *Hepatitis Control Reports* 4 (Summer 1999):1–10.

56. Seal, J. B., and R. S. Daum. 2001. What happened to primum non nocere? *Pediatrics* 201: 1177–1179.

57. Clark, S. J., M. D. Cabana, T. Malik, H. Yusuf, and G. L. Freed. 2001. Hepatitis B vaccination pactices in hospital nurseries before and after changes in vaccine recommendations. *Archives of Pediatrics and Adolescent Medicine* 135:915–920; Impact of the 1999 AAP/USPHS Joint Statement on Thimerosal in Vaccine on Infant Hepatitis B Vaccination Practices. 2001. *MMWR Morbidity and Mortality Weekly Report* 50:94–97.

58. Mahoney, F. J., and M. Kane. 1999. Hepatitis B vaccine. In: *Vaccines*, 3rd edition, ed. S. A. Plotkin and W. A. Orenstein, 159–160. Philadelphia: W.B. Saunders.

59. Halsey, N. 1999. Limiting infant exposure to thimerosal and other sources of mercury. *JAMA* 282:1763–1765; American Academy of Pediatrics Committee on Infectious Diseases and Committee on Environmental Health.1999. Thimerosal in vaccines—An interim report to clinicians. *Pediatrics* 104:570–574; Halsey, N., and L. Goldman. 2001. Balancing risks and benefits: Primum non nocere is too simplistic. *Pediatrics* 108:466–467.

60. On the modern revival of vaccine resistance, see Colgrove, J. 2006. *State of Immunity: The Politics of Vaccination in Twentieth-Century America.* Berkeley: University of California Press; Baker, J. P., The pertussis vaccine controversy in Great Britain, 1974–1986. *Vaccine* 21:4003–4010; Johnston, R. D. 2004. Contemporary anti-vaccination movements in historical perspective. In: *The Politics of Healing: Histories of Alternative Medicine in Twentieth-Century North America,* ed. Robert D. Johnston, 259–286. New York: Routledge.

61. Bernard, S., A. Enyati, L. Redwood, H. Roger, and T. Binstock, 2001. Autism: A novel form of mercury poisoning. *Medical Hypotheses* 56:462–471; Kirby, *Evidence of Harm*, 46–78.

62. Kirby, *Evidence of Harm*, 1–7.

63. One reason that many parents have not accepted the IOM Report's conclusion is their belief that the CDC deliberately manipulated data in early analyses of the Vaccine Safety Datalink, a charge that the primary researchers have patently denied. See Kirby, *Evidence of Harm*, 270–299; Verstraeten, T., R. L. Davis, F. deStefano, et al. 2003. Safety of thimerosal-containing vaccines: A two-phased study of computerized health maintenance organization databases. *Pediatrics* 112:1039–1048.

64. Among many examples, see Geier, D. A., and M. R. Geier. 2003. An assessment of the impact of thimerosal on childhood neurodevelopmental disorders. *Pediatric Rehabilitation* 6:97–102.

18   Vaccines and Autism: A Tale of Shifting Hypotheses

Jeffrey S. Gerber and Paul A. Offit[*]

A worldwide increase in the rate of autism diagnoses—likely driven by broadened diagnostic criteria and increased awareness—has fueled concerns that an environmental exposure like vaccines might cause autism. Theories for this putative association have centered on the measles-mumps-rubella (MMR) vaccine, thimerosal, and the large number of vaccines currently administered. However, both epidemiological and biological studies fail to support these claims.

MMR

On February 28, 1998, Andrew Wakefield, a British gastroenterologist, and colleagues[1] published an article in *The Lancet* that described eight children whose first symptoms of autism appeared within 1 month after receiving an MMR vaccine. All eight of these children had gastrointestinal symptoms and signs and lymphoid nodular hyperplasia revealed on endoscopy. From these observations, Wakefield postulated that MMR vaccine caused intestinal inflammation that led to translocation of usually nonpermeable peptides to the bloodstream and, subsequently, to the brain, where they affected development.

Several issues undermine the Wakefield et al. interpretation of this case series. First, the self-referred cohort did not include control subjects, which precluded the authors from determining whether the occurrence of autism following receipt of the MMR vaccine was causal or coincidental. Because ~50,000 British children per month received MMR vaccine between ages 1 and 2 years—at a time when autism typically presents—coincidental associations were inevitable. Indeed, given the prevalence of autism in England in 1998 of 1 in 2,000 children,[2] ~25 children per month would receive a

* Reprinted from Gerber, J. S., and P. A. Offit. Vaccines and autism: A tale of shifting hypotheses. *Clinical Infectious Diseases* 2009 48 (4):456–461, by permission of Oxford University Press.

diagnosis of the disorder soon after receiving the MMR vaccine by chance alone. Second, endoscopic or neuropsychological assessments were not blind, and data were not collected systematically or completely. Third, gastrointestinal symptoms did not predate autism in several children, which is inconsistent with the notion that intestinal inflammation facilitated bloodstream invasion of encephalopathic peptides. Fourth, measles, mumps, or rubella vaccine viruses have not been found to cause chronic intestinal inflammation or loss of intestinal barrier function. Indeed, a recent study by Hornig et al.[3] found that the measles vaccine virus genome was not detected more commonly in children with or without autism. Fifth, putative encephalopathic peptides traveling from the intestine to the brain have never been identified. In contrast, the genes that have been associated with autism spectrum disorder to date have been found to code for endogenous proteins that influence neuronal synapse function, neuronal cell adhesion, neuronal activity regulation, or endosomal trafficking.[4]

Although no data supporting an association between MMR vaccine and autism existed and a plausible biological mechanism was lacking, several epidemiologic studies were performed to address parental fears created by the Wakefield et al. publication. Fortunately, several features of large-scale vaccination programs allowed for excellent descriptive and observational studies—specifically, large numbers of subjects, which generated substantial statistical power; high-quality vaccination records, which provided reliable historical data; multinational use of similar vaccine constituents and schedules; electronic medical records, which facilitated accurate analysis of outcome data; and the relatively recent introduction of the MMR vaccine in some countries, which allowed for before and after comparisons.

Ecological Studies

Researchers in several countries performed ecological studies that addressed the question of whether the MMR vaccine causes autism. Such analyses employ large databases that compare vaccination rates with autism diagnoses at the population level.

• In the United Kingdom, researchers evaluated 498 autistic children born from 1979 through 1992 who were identified by computerized health records from eight health districts.[5] Although a trend toward increasing autism diagnoses by year of birth was confirmed, no change in the rates of autism diagnoses after the 1987 introduction of the MMR vaccine was observed. Further, MMR vaccination rates of autistic children were similar to those of the entire study population. Also, investigators did not observe a clustering of autism diagnoses relative to the time that children received the MMR vaccine, nor did they observe a difference in age at autism diagnosis between those vaccinated and not vaccinated or between those vaccinated before or after 18 months of age. These authors also found no differences in autism rates among vaccinated and unvaccinated children when they extended their analysis to include a longer time after MMR exposure or a second dose of MMR.[6]

• Also in the United Kingdom, researchers performed a time-trend analysis using the General Practice Research Database—a high-quality, extensively validated electronic medical record with virtually complete vaccination data.[7] More than 3 million person-years of observation during 1988–1999 confirmed an increase in autism diagnoses despite stable MMR vaccination rates.

• In California, researchers compared year-specific MMR vaccination rates of kindergarten students with the yearly autism case load of the California Department of Developmental Services during 1980–1994.[8] As was observed in the United Kingdom, the increase in the number of autism diagnoses did not correlate with MMR vaccination rates.

• In Canada, researchers estimated the prevalence of pervasive developmental disorder with respect to MMR vaccination in 27,749 children from 55 schools in Quebec.[9] Autism rates increased coincident with a decrease in MMR vaccination rates. The results were unchanged when both exposure and outcome definitions varied, including a strict diagnosis of autism.

Additional population-based studies considered the relationship between the MMR vaccine and the "new variant" form of autism proposed by Wakefield et al.—specifically, developmental regression with gastrointestinal symptoms. Although it is difficult to analyze such a phenomenon when it is unclear that one exists (which complicates the formulation of a case definition), conclusions may be gleaned from the data with respect to developmental regression alone (i.e., autism irrespective of coincident bowel problems).

• In England, researchers performed a cross-sectional study of 262 autistic children and demonstrated no difference in age of first parental concerns or rate of developmental regression by exposure to MMR vaccine.[10] No association between developmental regression and gastrointestinal symptoms was observed.

• In London, an analysis of 473 autistic children used the 1987 introduction of MMR to compare vaccinated and unvaccinated cohorts.[11] The incidence of developmental regression did not differ between cohorts, and the authors observed no difference in the prevalence of gastrointestinal symptoms between vaccinated and unvaccinated autistic children.

Two conclusions are evident from these data. First, the explicit consideration of developmental regression among autistic children does not alter the consistent independence of the MMR vaccine and autism. Second, these data argue against the existence of a new variant form of autism.

Retrospective, Observational Studies

Four retrospective, observational studies addressed the relationship between the MMR vaccine and autism.

• In the United Kingdom, 71 MMR-vaccinated autistic children were compared with 284 MMR-vaccinated matched control children through use of the Doctor's Independent Network, a general practice database.[12] The authors observed no differences between case and control children in practitioner consultation rates—a surrogate for parental concerns about their child's development—within 6 months after MMR vaccination, which suggests that the diagnosis of autism was not temporally related to MMR vaccination.

• In Finland, using national registers, researchers linked hospitalization records to vaccination records in 535,544 children vaccinated during 1982–1986.[13] Of 309 children hospitalized for autistic disorders, no clustering occurred relative to the time of MMR vaccination.

• In Denmark, again using a national registry, researchers determined vaccination status and autism diagnosis in 537,303 children born during 1991–1998.[14] The authors observed no differences in the relative risk of autism between those who did and did not receive the MMR vaccine. Among autistic children, no relationship between date of vaccination and development of autism was observed.

• In metropolitan Atlanta, using a developmental surveillance program, researchers compared 624 autistic children with 1,824 matched control children.[15] Vaccination records were obtained from state immunization forms. The authors observed no differences in age at vaccination between autistic and nonautistic children, which suggests that early age of MMR vaccine exposure was not a risk factor for autism.

Prospective Observational Studies

Capitalizing on a long-term vaccination project maintained by the National Board of Health, investigators in Finland performed two prospective cohort studies. Researchers prospectively recorded adverse events associated with MMR-vaccinated children during 1982–1996 and identified 31 with gastrointestinal symptoms; none of the children developed autism.[16] A further analysis of this cohort revealed no vaccine-associated cases of autism among 1.8 million children.[17] Although this cohort was analyzed using a passive surveillance system, the complete absence of an association between gastrointestinal disease and autism after MMR vaccination was compelling.

Thimerosal

Thimerosal—50% ethylmercury by weight—is an antibacterial compound that has been used effectively in multidose vaccine preparations for >50 years[18] (thimerosal is not contained in live-virus vaccines, such as MMR). In 1997, the U.S. Food and Drug Administration (FDA) Modernization Act mandated identification and quantification of mercury in all food and drugs; 2 years later, the FDA found that children might be receiving as much as 187.5 µg of mercury within the first 6 months of life. Despite the absence of data suggesting harm from quantities of ethylmercury contained in vaccines, in 1999, the American Academy of Pediatrics and the Public Health Service recommended the immediate removal of mercury from all vaccines given to young infants.[19] Widespread and predictable misinterpretation of this conservative, precautionary directive, coupled with a public already concerned by a proposed but unsubstantiated link between vaccination and autism, understandably provoked concern among parents, which led to the birth of several antimercury advocacy groups. However, because the signs and symptoms of autism are clearly distinct from those of mercury poisoning, concerns about mercury as a cause of autism were—similar to those with the MMR vaccine—biologically implausible;[20] children with mercury poisoning show characteristic motor, speech, sensory, psychiatric, visual, and head circumference changes that are either fundamentally different from those of or absent in children with autism. Consistent with this, a study performed by scientists at the Centers for Disease Control and Prevention years later showed that mercury in vaccines did not cause even subtle signs or symptoms of mercury poisoning.[21]

Despite the biological implausibility of the contention that thimerosal in vaccines caused autism, seven studies—again descriptive or observational—were performed.[22–27] Four other studies have been reviewed in detail elsewhere[28] but are not discussed here because their methodology is incomplete and unclear and thus cause difficulty in drawing meaningful conclusions.

Ecological Studies

Three ecological studies performed in three different countries compared the incidence of autism with thimerosal exposure from vaccines. In each case, the nationwide removal of thimerosal—which occurred in 1992 in Europe and in 2001 in the United States—allowed robust comparisons of vaccination with thimerosal-containing and thimerosal-free products as follows.

In Sweden and Denmark, researchers found a relatively stable incidence of autism when thimerosal-containing vaccines were in use (1980–1990), including years when children were exposed to as much as 200 µg of ethylmercury (concentrations similar to peak U.S. exposures).[22] However, in 1990, a steady increase in the incidence of autism began in both countries and continued through the end of the study period in 2000, despite the removal of thimerosal from vaccines in 1992.

In Denmark, researchers performed a study comparing the incidence of autism in children who had received 200 µg (1961–1970), 125 µg (1970–1992), or 0 µg of thimerosal (1992–2000) and again demonstrated no relationship between thimerosal exposure and autism.[23]

In Quebec, researchers grouped 27,749 children from 55 schools by date of birth and estimated thimerosal exposure on the basis of the corresponding Ministry of Health vaccine schedules. School records were obtained to determine age-specific rates of pervasive developmental disorder.[9] Thimerosal exposure and pervasive developmental disorder diagnosis were found to be independent variables. Similar to previous analyses, the highest rates of pervasive developmental disorder were found in cohorts exposed to thimerosal-free vaccines. The results were unchanged when both exposure and outcome definitions varied.

Cohort Studies

Four cohort studies that examined thimerosal exposure and autism have been performed, as follows:

• In Denmark, researchers examined >1,200 children with autism that was identified during 1990–1996, which comprised ~3 million person-years. They found that the risk of autism did not differ between children vaccinated with thimerosal-containing vaccines and those vaccinated with thimerosal-free vaccines or between children who received greater or lower quantities of thimerosal.[24] They also found that the rates of autism increased after the removal of thimerosal from all vaccines.

• In the United States, using the Vaccine Safety Data Link, researchers at the Centers for Disease Control and Prevention examined 140,887 U.S. children born during 1991–1999, including >200 children with autism.[25] The researchers found no relationship between receipt of thimerosal-containing vaccines and autism.

• In England, researchers prospectively followed 12,810 children for whom they had complete vaccination records who were born during 1991–1992, and they found no relationship between early thimerosal exposure and deleterious neurological or psychological outcomes.[26]

• In the United Kingdom, researchers evaluated the vaccination records of 100,572 children born during 1988–1997, using the General Practice Research Database, 104 of whom were affected with autism.[27] No relationship between thimerosal exposure and autism diagnosis was observed.

Too Many Vaccines

When studies of the MMR vaccine and thimerosal-containing vaccines failed to show an association with autism, alternative theories emerged. The most prominent theory suggests that the simultaneous administration of multiple vaccines overwhelms or weakens the immune system and creates an interaction with the nervous system that triggers autism in a susceptible host. This theory was recently popularized in the wake of a concession by the Vaccine Injury Compensation Program with regard to the case of a 9-year-old girl with a mitochondrial enzyme deficiency whose encephalopathy, which included features of autism spectrum disorder, was judged to have worsened following the receipt of multiple vaccines at age 19 months.[29] Despite reassurances by the Centers for Disease Control and Prevention that the Vaccine Injury Compensation Program's action should not be interpreted as scientific evidence that vaccines cause autism, many in the lay press and the public have not been reassured.

The notion that children might be receiving too many vaccines too soon and that these vaccines either overwhelm an immature immune system or generate a pathologic, autism-inducing autoimmune response is flawed for several reasons.

Vaccines do not overwhelm the immune system. Although the infant immune system is relatively naive, it is immediately capable of generating a vast array of protective responses; even conservative estimates predict the capacity to respond to thousands of vaccines simultaneously.[30] Consistent with this theoretical exercise, combinations of vaccines induce immune responses comparable to those given individually.[31] Also, although the number of recommended childhood vaccines has increased during the past 30 years, with advances in protein chemistry and recombinant DNA technology, the immunologic load has actually decreased. The 14 vaccines given today contain <200 bacterial and viral proteins or polysaccharides, compared with >3,000 of these immunological components in the 7 vaccines administered in 1980.[30] Further, vaccines represent a minute fraction of what a child's immune system routinely navigates; the average child is infected with four to six viruses per year.[32] The immune response elicited from the vast antigen exposure of unattenuated viral replication supersedes that of even multiple, simultaneous vaccines.

Multiple vaccinations do not weaken the immune system. Vaccinated and unvaccinated children do not differ in their susceptibility to infections not prevented by vaccines.[33–35] In other words, vaccination does not suppress the immune system in a clinically relevant manner. However, infections with some vaccine-preventable diseases predispose children to severe, invasive infections with other pathogens.[36,37] Therefore, the available data suggest that vaccines do not weaken the immune system.

Autism is not an immune-mediated disease. Unlike autoimmune diseases such as multiple sclerosis, there is no evidence of immune activation or inflammatory lesions in the central nervous system of people with autism.[38] In fact, current data suggest that genetic variation in neuronal circuitry that affects synaptic development might in part account for autistic behavior.[39] Thus, speculation that an exaggerated or inappropriate immune response to vaccination precipitates autism is at variance with current scientific data that address the pathogenesis of autism.

No studies have compared the incidence of autism in vaccinated, unvaccinated, or alternatively vaccinated children (i.e., schedules that spread out vaccines, avoid combination vaccines, or include only select vaccines). These studies would be difficult to perform because of the likely differences among these three groups in healthcare-seeking behavior and the ethics of experimentally studying children who have not received vaccines.

Conclusions

Twenty epidemiologic studies have shown that neither thimerosal nor the MMR vaccine causes autism. These studies have been performed in several countries by many different investigators who have employed a multitude of epidemiologic and statistical methods. The large size of the studied populations has afforded a level of statistical power sufficient to detect even rare associations. These studies, in concert with the biological implausibility that vaccines overwhelm a child's immune system, have effectively dismissed the notion that vaccines cause autism. Further studies on the cause or causes of autism should focus on more promising leads.

References

1. Wakefield, A. J., S. H. Murch, A. Anthony, J. Linnell, D. M. Casson, M. Malik, et al. 1998. Ileal-lymphoid-nodular hyperplasia, non-specific colitis, and pervasive developmental disorder in children. *Lancet* 351:637–641.

2. Chen, R. T., and F. DeStefano. 1998. Vaccine adverse events: Causal or coincidental? *Lancet* 351: 611–612.

3. Hornig, M., T. Briese, T. Buie, M. L. Bauman, G. Lauwers, U. Siemetzki, et al. 2008. Lack of association between measles virus vaccine and autism with enteropathy: A case-control study. *PLoS One* 3:e3140.

4. Sutcliffe, J. S. 2008. Genetics: Insights into the pathogenesis of autism. *Science* 321:208–209.

5. Taylor, B., E. Miller, C. P. Farrington, M. C. Petropoulos, I. Favot-Mayaud, J. Li, and P. A. Waight. 1999. Autism and measles, mumps, and rubella vaccine: No epidemiological evidence for a causal association. *Lancet* 353:2026–2029.

6. Farrington, C. P., E. Miller, and B. Taylor. 2001. MMR and autism: Further evidence against a causal association. *Vaccine* 19:3632–3635.

7. Kaye, J. A., M. del Mar Melero-Montes, and H. Jick. 2001. Mumps, measles, and rubella vaccine and the incidence of autism recorded by general practitioners: A time trend analysis. *BMJ* 322:460–463.

8. Dales, L., S. J. Hammer, and N. J. Smith. 2001. Time trends in autism and in MMR immunization coverage in California. *JAMA* 285:1183–1185.

9. Fombonne, E., R. Zakarian, A. Bennett, L. Meng, and D. McLean-Heywood. 2006. Pervasive developmental disorders in Montreal, Quebec, Canada: Prevalence and links with immunizations. *Pediatrics* 118:e139–e150.

10. Fombonne, E., and S. Chakrabarti. 2001. No evidence for a new variant of measles-mumps-rubella-induced autism. *Pediatrics* 108:e58.

11. Taylor, B., E. Miller, R. Lingam, N. Andrews, A. Simmons, and J. Stowe. 2002. Measles, mumps, and rubella vaccination and bowel problems or developmental regression in children with autism: Population study. *BMJ* 324:393–396.

12. DeWilde, S., I. M. Carey, N. Richards, S. R. Hilton, and D. G. Cook. 2001. Do children who become autistic consult more often after MMR vaccination? *Br J Gen Pract* 51:226–227.

13. Makela, A., J. P. Nuorti, and H. Peltola. 2002. Neurologic disorders after measles-mumps-rubella vaccination. *Pediatrics* 110:957–963.

14. Madsen, K. M., A. Hviid, M. Vestergaard, D. Schendel, J. Wohlfahrt, P. Thorsen, et al. 2002. A population-based study of measles, mumps, and rubella vaccination and autism. *N Engl J Med* 347:1477–1482.

15. DeStefano, F., T. K. Bhasin, W. W. Thompson, M. Yeargin-Allsopp, and C. Boyle. 2004. Age at first measles-mumps-rubella vaccination in children with autism and school-matched control subjects: A population-based study in metropolitan Atlanta. *Pediatrics* 113:259–266.

16. Peltola, H., A. Patja, P. Leinikki, M. Valle, I. Davidkin, and M. Paunio. 1998. No evidence for measles, mumps, and rubella vaccine-associated inflammatory bowel disease or autism in a 14-year prospective study. *Lancet* 351:1327–1328.

17. Patja, A., I. Davidkin, T. Kurki, M. J. Kallio, M. Valle, and H. Peltola. 2000. Serious adverse events after measles-mumps-rubella vaccination during a fourteen-year prospective follow-up. *Pediatr Infect Dis J* 19:1127–1134.

18. Baker, J. P. 2008. Mercury, vaccines, and autism: One controversy, three histories. *Am J Public Health* 98:244–253.

19. Centers for Disease Control Prevention. 1999. Thimerosal in vaccines: A joint statement of the American Academy of Pediatrics and the Public Health Service. *MMWR Morb Mortal Wkly Rep* 48:563–565.

20. Nelson, K. B., and Bauman, M. L. 2003. Thimerosal and autism? *Pediatrics* 111:674–679.

21. Thompson, W. W., C. Price, B. Goodson, D. K. Shay, P. Benson, V. L. Hinrichsen, et al. 2007. Early thimerosal exposure and neuropsychological outcomes at 7 to 10 years. *N Engl J Med* 357:1281–1292.

22. Stehr-Green, P., P. Tull, M. Stellfeld, P. B. Mortenson, and D. Simpson. 2003. Autism and thimerosal-containing vaccines: Lack of consistent evidence for an association. *Am J Prev Med* 25:101–106.

23. Madsen, K. M., M. B. Lauritsen, C. B. Pedersen, P. Thorsen, A. M. Plesner, P. H. Andersen, and P. B. Mortensen. 2003. Thimerosal and the occurrence of autism: Negative ecological evidence from Danish population-based data. *Pediatrics* 112:604–606.

24. Hviid, A., M. Stellfeld, J. Wohlfahrt, and M. Melbye. 2003. Association between thimerosal-containing vaccine and autism. *JAMA* 290:1763–1766.

25. Verstraeten, T., R. L. Davis, F. DeStefano, T. A. Lieu, P. H. Rhodes, S. B. Black, et al. 2003. Safety of thimerosal-containing vaccines: A two-phased study of computerized health maintenance organization databases. *Pediatrics* 112:1039–1048.

26. Heron, J., and J. Golding. 2004. Thimerosal exposure in infants and developmental disorders: A prospective cohort study in the United Kingdom does not support a causal association. *Pediatrics* 114:577–583.

27. Andrews, N., E. Miller, A. Grant, J. Stowe, V. Osborne, and B. Taylor. 2004. Thimerosal exposure in infants and developmental disorders: A retrospective cohort study in the United Kingdom does not support a causal association. *Pediatrics* 114:584–591.

28. Parker, S. K., B. Schwartz, J. Todd, and L. K. Pickering. 2004. Thimerosal-containing vaccines and autistic spectrum disorder: A critical review of published original data. *Pediatrics* 114:793–804.

29. Offit, P. A. 2008. Vaccines and autism revisited—the Hannah Poling case. *N Engl J Med* 358:2089–2091.

30. Offit, P. A., J. Quarles, M. A Gerber, C. J. Hackett, E. K. Marcuse, T. R. Kollman, et al. 2002. Addressing parents' concerns: Do multiple vaccines overwhelm or weaken the infant's immune system? *Pediatrics* 109:124–129.

31. King, G. E., and S. C. Hadler. 1994. Simultaneous administration of childhood vaccines: An important public health policy that is safe and efficacious. *Pediatr Infect Dis J* 13:394–407.

32. Dingle, J. H., G. F. Badger, and W. S. Jordan, Jr. 1964. *Illness in the Home: A Study of 25,000 Illnesses in a Group of Cleveland Families*. Cleveland, OH: Press of Western Reserve University.

33. Black, S. B., J. D. Cherry, H. R. Shinefield, B. Fireman, P. Christenson, and D. Lampert. 1991. Apparent decreased risk of invasive bacterial disease after heterologous childhood immunization. *Am J Dis Child* 145:746–749.

34. Davidson, M., G. W. Letson, J. I. Ward, A. Ball, L. Bulkow, P. Christenson, and J. D. Cherry. 1991. DTP immunization and susceptibility to infectious diseases: Is there a relationship? *Am J Dis Child* 145:750–754.

35. Storsaeter, J., P. Olin, B. Renemar, T. Lagergård, R. Norberg, V. Romanus, and M. Tiru. 1988. Mortality and morbidity from invasive bacterial infections during a clinical trial of acellular pertussis vaccines in Sweden. *Pediatr Infect Dis J* 7:637–645.

36. O'Brien, K. L., M. I. Walters, J. Sellman, P. Quinlisk, H. Regnery, B. Schwartz, and S. F. Dowell. 2000. Severe pneumococcal pneumonia in previously healthy children: The role of preceding influenza infection. *Clin Infect Dis* 30:784–789.

37. Laupland, K. B., H. D. Davies, D. E. Low, B. Schwartz, K. Green, and A. McGeer. 2000. Invasive group A streptococcal disease in children and association with varicella-zoster virus infection: Ontario Group A Streptococcal Study Group. *Pediatrics* 105: e60.

38. McCormick, M. C. 2004. *Immunization Safety Review: Vaccines and Autism*. Washington, DC: Institute of Medicine.

39. Morrow, E. M., S. Y. Yoo, S. W. Flavell, T. K. Kim, Y. Lin, R. S. Hill, et al. 2008. Identifying autism loci and genes by tracing recent shared ancestry. *Science* 321:218–223.

19   Wakefield's Article Linking MMR Vaccine and Autism Was Fraudulent (*Excerpt*)

Fiona Godlee, Jane Smith, and Harvey Marcovitch[*]

"Science is at once the most questioning and … skeptical of activities and also the most trusting," said Arnold Relman, former editor of the *New England Journal of Medicine*, in 1989. "It is intensely skeptical about the possibility of error, but totally trusting about the possibility of fraud."[1] Never has this been truer than of the 1998 *Lancet* paper that implied a link between the measles-mumps-rubella (MMR) vaccine and a "new syndrome" of autism and bowel disease.

In a series of articles starting this week, and 7 years after first looking into the MMR scare, journalist Brian Deer now shows the extent of Wakefield's fraud and how it was perpetrated. Who perpetrated this fraud? There is no doubt that it was Wakefield. Is it possible that he was wrong but not dishonest—that he was so incompetent that he was unable to fairly describe the project or report even 1 of the 12 children's cases accurately? No. A great deal of thought and effort must have gone into drafting the article to achieve the results he wanted: the discrepancies all led in one direction: misreporting was gross.

Furthermore, Wakefield has been given ample opportunity to either replicate the article's findings, or say he was mistaken. He has declined to do either. He refused to join 10 of his coauthors in retracting the article's interpretation in 2004,[2] and he has repeatedly denied doing anything wrong at all. Instead, although now disgraced and stripped of his clinical and academic credentials, he continues to push his views.[3]

Meanwhile the damage to public health continues, fueled by unbalanced media reporting and an ineffective response from government, researchers, journals, and the medical profession.[4-5] Although vaccination rates in the United Kingdom (UK) have recovered slightly from their 80% low in 2003–2004,[6] they are still below the 95% level recommended by the World Health Organization to ensure herd immunity. In 2008, for the first time in 14 years, measles was declared endemic in England and Wales.[7] Hundreds of thousands of children in the UK are currently unprotected as a result of the scare, and the battle to restore parents' trust in the vaccine is ongoing.

But perhaps as important as the scare's effect on infectious disease is the energy, emotion, and money that have been diverted away from efforts to understand the real causes of autism and how to help children and families who live with it.[8]

There are hard lessons for many in this highly damaging saga. First, for the coauthors. The GMC panel was clear that it was Wakefield alone who wrote the final version of the article. His coauthors seem to have been unaware of what he was doing under the cover of their names and reputations. Although only two (John Walker-Smith and Simon Murch) were charged by the GMC, and only one, the paper's senior author Walker-Smith, was found guilty of misconduct, they all failed in their duties as authors. The satisfaction of adding to one's CV must never detract from the responsibility to ensure that one has been neither party to nor duped by a fraud. This means that coauthors will have to check the source data of studies more thoroughly than many do at present—or alternatively describe in a contributor's statement precisely which bits of the source data they take responsibility for.

What of Wakefield's other publications? In light of this new information, their veracity must be questioned. Past experience tells us that research misconduct is rarely isolated behavior.[9] Over the years, the *BMJ* and its sister journals, *Gut* and *Archives of Disease in Childhood*, have published a number of articles, including letters and abstracts, by Wakefield and colleagues. We have written to the vice provost of UCL, John Tooke, who now has responsibility for Wakefield's former institution, to ask for an investigation into all of his work to decide whether any more articles should be retracted.

The *Lancet* article has of course been retracted but for far narrower misconduct than is now apparent. The retraction statement cites the GMC's findings that the patients were not consecutively referred and the study did not have ethical approval, leaving the door open for those who want to continue to believe that the science, flawed although it always was, still stands. We hope that declaring the article a fraud will close that door for good.

References

1. Schechter, A. N., J. B. Wyngaarden, J. T. Edsall, J. Maddox, A. S. Relman, M. Angell, et al. 1989. Colloquium on scientific authorship: Rights and responsibilities. *FASEB J* 3:209–217.

2. Murch, S. H., A. Anthony, D. H. Casson, M. Malik, M. Berelowitz, A. P. Dhillon, et al. 2004. Retraction of an interpretation. *Lancet* 363:750.

3. Shenoy, R. 2010, December 17. Controversial autism researcher tells local Somalis disease is solvable. Minnesota Public Radio. Available at: http://www.mprnews.org/story/2010/12/17/somali-autism/.

4. Hilton, S., K. Hunt, M. Langan, V. Hamilton, and M. Petticrew. 2009. Reporting of MMR evidence in professional publications: 1988–2007. *Arch Dis Child* 94:831–833.

5. Bedford, H. E., and D. A. C. Elliman. 2010, February 2. MMR vaccine and autism. *BMJ* 340:c655.

6. Health Protection Agency. Completed primary course at two years of age: England and Wales, 1966–1977, England only 1978 onwards. Available at: https://www.gov.uk/government/publications/completed-primary-courses-at-2-years-of-age-england-and-wales/.

7. Health Protection Agency. Confirmed cases of measles, mumps and rubella 1996–2009. Available at: https://www.gov.uk/government/publications/measles-confirmed-cases/.

8. Oakley, G. P., and Johnstone, R. B. 2004. Balancing the benefits and harms in public health prevention programmes mandated by governments. *BMJ* 329:41–43.

9. Rennie, D. Misconduct and journal peer review. 2003. In: *Peer Review in Health Sciences*, 2nd ed., eds. F. Godlee and T. Jefferson, 118–129. London: BMJ Books.

IV Vaccination Requirements and Responses to Vaccine Hesitancy

If public anxiety regarding alleged links between vaccines and autism or other medical conditions is the dominant vaccine *science* concern of our time, then the corresponding vaccine *policy* concern of foremost prevalence is the role, use, and appropriate scope of laws that require vaccination of children or other groups. These requirements, often referred to as "mandates," are viewed by advocates of vaccination as a necessary and appropriate tool to protect the health of children and to promote and sustain high vaccination rates among communities. Critics—particularly those with already heightened concerns about the safety, effectiveness, and value of vaccines—reject these policies as an inappropriate government intrusion on parental decision making.

The 2015 outbreaks of measles in the United States linked to visitors to Disneyland in California brought new attention to mandates and their consequences. Public health advocates noted the disproportionate number of unvaccinated children among those sickened, many of whom were not vaccinated because their parents had received exemptions from state vaccination requirements on the basis of their religious or personal beliefs. An ensuing legislative effort in California was successful in eliminating those exemptions for nonmedical reasons, one policy reform among many that have been considered to strengthen the vital "safety-net" role played by requirements in the opinion of most vaccination advocates.

This section explores vaccination requirements and related topics regarding efforts by policymakers, healthcare providers, and medical organizations to produce high vaccination rates, even when some parents or patients may have reservations regarding the vaccines being promoted. In the first two chapters, Daniel Salmon, Saad Omer, and colleagues provide a wealth of information about the history of government vaccination requirements in the United States and other countries, as well as the availability of exemptions from those requirements and their impact on individual and public health. Next, Paul Offit offers an argument for why states should follow California's recent example (and that of West Virginia and Mississippi) by prohibiting exemptions from state vaccination requirements on the basis of parental personal beliefs. (Advocates of vaccination are not of one mind on this policy, however. For a competing viewpoint that sees the continued value of well-crafted, relatively narrow nonmedical exemption policies, see Edgar Marcuse's article listed below.)

Debates over the propriety of state vaccination requirements were particularly prominent in public attention to human papillomavirus (HPV) vaccines following their introduction in 2006. Efforts to require vaccination of preadolescent girls against this virus responsible for 12,000 cases of cervical cancer and 4,000 deaths in the United States each year were met with considerable opposition, nowhere more so than in Texas, where an Executive Order that would have required the vaccine was overwhelmingly rejected by state legislators. Alta Charo considers the ethics and politics of HPV vaccination requirements, and Jason Schwartz and colleagues review the largely unsuccessful early push for HPV vaccination requirements in Texas and other states. Ten years after their introduction, few states have even considered revisiting potential HPV vaccination requirements for their school-age children.

Although mandates may be among the most highly visible tools to promote vaccination, discussions between parents and healthcare providers are known to be profoundly influential in parental vaccination decisions, particularly when parents have questions or concerns about the safety and necessity of recommended vaccines. Writing for the American Academy of Pediatrics, Douglas Diekema and colleagues offer guidance on how physicians should respond when parents feel so strongly regarding vaccines that they wish to delay some or all recommended vaccines or even omit them entirely. This statement offers an important perspective on the ongoing debate regarding whether it is appropriate for physicians and other healthcare providers to dismiss families with such views from their practices.

Finally, hesitancy about vaccines and attention to vaccination requirements is not confined to the childhood population. Similar questions about the ethics and politics of mandatory vaccination emerge in the military, in immigration policy, and, as Tom Talbot and colleagues discuss, for healthcare workers for whom annual influenza vaccination is strongly recommended. A growing number of healthcare facilities have implemented influenza vaccination requirements for their personnel as a condition of employment, policies intended to protect both medical staff and patients but that have nonetheless been met with vocal resistance in some cases.

Further Reading

Armand H. Antommaria. 2013. "An Ethical Analysis of Mandatory Influenza Vaccination of Health Care Personnel: Implementing Fairly and Balancing Benefits and Burdens." *American Journal of Bioethics,* 13(9): 30–37.

Edgar K. Marcuse. 2012. "Prudent Personal Belief Exemptions." *Archives of Pediatrics and Adolescent Medicine,* 166(12): 1093–1094.

Jennifer A. Reich. 2016. *Calling the Shots: Why Parents Reject Vaccines.* New York: New York University Press.

Jason L. Schwartz and Arthur L. Caplan. 2011. "Vaccination Refusal: Ethics, Individual Rights, and the Common Good." *Primary Care,* 38(4): 717–728.

Eileen Wang, et al. 2014. "Nonmedical Exemptions from School Immunization Requirements: A Systematic Review." *American Journal of Public Health,* 104(11): e62–e84.

20 Compulsory Vaccination and Conscientious or Philosophical Exemptions: Past, Present, and Future

Daniel A. Salmon, Stephen P. Teret, C. Raina MacIntyre, David Salisbury, Margaret Burgess, and Neal A. Halsey[*]

Vaccination is one of the greatest achievements in medicine and public health:[1,2] wild-type poliovirus will soon be eradicated,[3] and each year, about 5 million life-years are saved by control of poliomyelitis, measles, and tetanus.[4] Vaccine-preventable diseases in many developed countries have been reduced by 98%–99%.[2,4]

Compulsory vaccination programs have contributed to the achievement of high rates of immunization.[5] Such programs are based on laws that require a population—or population segment—to be vaccinated to have the right to reside in a jurisdiction or receive an entitlement. But not everyone agrees on the merits of compulsory vaccination; experts and the lay public alike have argued that the benefits are outweighed by ethical drawbacks. Most notably, some argue that compulsory vaccination diminishes autonomy for the vaccinee or for parents making decisions on behalf of their children. Others, however, contend that compulsory vaccination ensures greater equity in society because all members share the risks and benefits of vaccination. Without compulsory vaccination, some people receive the indirect benefits of vaccination (i.e., herd immunity) without the risks, however small, associated with vaccines.

The first regulations requiring smallpox vaccination were passed in 1806 in Piombino and Lucca, former Napoleonic Principalities now part of Italy.[6] Many European countries considered, debated, and passed laws to require their citizens to have smallpox vaccination throughout the nineteenth century. In France, the laws were first applied to specific populations (e.g., university students in 1810). In other countries, the original laws required vaccination of the general population: Sweden passed such a law in 1816, and France passed a law for the entire country in 1902.[6] Enforcement was often lax and varied between localities. In Sweden, fines were increased until vaccination was done, but conscientious exemptions were permitted.[6] In Germany and France, conscientious exemptions were not allowed. Anti-vaccination movements, present in nearly all European countries, tended to be strongest in countries where some vaccinations were compulsory.

History of Compulsory Vaccination in the UK

The UK has a history of struggle with compulsory vaccination. After a report in 1850 by the Epidemiology Society, the Vaccination Act of 1853 required smallpox vaccination in England and Wales.[7] This law galvanized the anti-vaccination movement, which was joined not only by those against vaccination but also by opponents to intrusion by governments on personal autonomy.[7] Political candidates were chosen solely on their position on vaccination.[6] In 1865, 20,000 demonstrators took to the streets of Leicester for an anti-vaccine demonstration.[6]

Local authorities grappled with how best to apply penalties for noncompliance: should a single fine be levied or should fines accrue until vaccination? In some cases, personal property was auctioned to cover payment for accruing fines,[7] and violators were seen as martyrs in the fight against forced vaccination. Local authorities were responsible for implementation of the vaccine law, and rates of enforcement varied between areas. Authorities tended to be influenced by their constituents, especially where opposition to vaccination was strong. In 1889, the Royal Commission on Vaccination was charged with inquiring into and reporting on: the usefulness of vaccination in control of smallpox; what means, other than vaccination, could be used for controlling smallpox; the safety of smallpox vaccination; what could be done to improve the safety of smallpox vaccination; and whether any changes should be made to compulsory vaccination laws.

In 7 years, the Commission met 136 times and questioned 187 witnesses, including vaccine supporters and opponents. A final report, issued in 1896, covered each point in detail.

The Commission recognized that the decrease in smallpox incidence was at least partly attributable to vaccination,[8] but it was careful not to dismiss the contribution of improvements to sanitation. The Commission also acknowledged that, despite earlier reports to the contrary, the use of humanized lymph (serum) could spread diseases such as syphilis. Calf lymph, the Commission recommended, should be within reach of all, in view of the compulsory nature and public funding of vaccination.[8]

With regard to prosecution for noncompliance with the vaccination law, the Commission recommended that repeated penalties should no longer be imposed. The Commission went beyond limiting punishment for noncompliance to a single fine by creating a conscientious exemption to vaccination.

The penalty was not designed to punish a parent who may be considered misguided in his views and unwise in his action, but to secure the vaccination of people. If a law less severe, or administered with less stringency, would better secure this end, that seems to us conclusive in its favour ... it would conduce to increase vaccination if a scheme could be devised which would preclude the attempt (so often a vain one) to compel those who are honestly opposed to the practice to submit their children to vaccination, and, at the same time, leave the law to operate, as at present, to prevent children remaining unvaccinated owing to the neglect or indifference of the parent. When we speak of an honest opposition to the practice, we intend to confine our remarks to cases in which the objection is to the operation itself, and to exclude cases in which the objection arises merely from an indisposition to incur the trouble involved.[8]

The Commission recommended a conscientious exemption for people who were "honestly opposed" to vaccination and distinguished them from those who were too lazy or indifferent to have their children vaccinated. Of thirteen members, two opposed allowance of conscientious exemption, and two described vaccination as "objectionable" and, along with two other members, rejected any form of compulsory vaccination.

The result of allowance of conscientious exemption was that the parents of about 200,000 children opted out of vaccination; however, the overall effect was an increase in the number of vaccinated children.[6] Many in the British medical community supported the allowance of conscientious exemption, a feeling embodied by a supportive editorial in the *British Medical Journal*.[9]

Implementation of the conscientious exemption clause varied by locality. Some jurisdictions made it easy for a parent to claim an exemption: they allowed mothers (not only fathers) to claim an exemption, and hearings were held at late hours to accommodate busy parents. "But where magistrates favored vaccination, parents were cross examined or bullied, their motives questioned and certificates refused when strict standards remained unsatisfied."[6]

In 1907, 100 opponents of compulsory vaccination were elected to the 666-seat Parliament, and an amendment to the 1896 Act removed the administrative hurdles to claiming an exemption.[6] This amendment resulted in a substantial drop in the number of vaccinated children.[6] The UK repealed vaccination requirements altogether in 1946 because nearly half of parents in many areas were claiming conscientious exemptions. Vaccination rates fell, although uptake tended to increase when outbreaks occurred. In 1961, legislation allowed for compulsory examination of individuals suspected to have smallpox,[10] and clinically confirmed patients could be "removed at once to a hospital designated by the Regional Hospital Board for the reception of smallpox."[11] However, no legislation compelled vaccination even for the control of smallpox outbreaks.[12] Smallpox vaccination was abandoned in 1971 because the likelihood of smallpox introduction in the UK was low, and although vaccination was a safe and reliable method to protect against smallpox, the risks of vaccine complications outweighed the risks of disease.[12]

In 2004, the British Medical Association revisited the issue of compulsory vaccination, partly because of decreases in vaccine coverage for measles-mumps- rubella (MMR) that resulted from the widespread concern about associations between MMR and autism.[13–15] The British Medical Association concluded that compulsory vaccination was not appropriate for the UK[16] and supported a 2003 Scottish Executive Report,[17] which concluded that "such a policy [compulsory vaccination] is not consistent with key elements of the frameworks or principles for immunization policy. On a practical level, it is not self-evident that it would lead to higher levels of immunization. More substantively, it runs counter to the ... core principle that vaccines should be administered on a voluntary basis."[17]

Vaccination Legislation in Australia

Australia united as a federation of six British colonies in 1901. The federal government controls diseases that require quarantine, but jurisdictions legislate for other communicable diseases. Australia has never legislated requirements for smallpox vaccination.

Legislation that required children to be vaccinated for MMR, DTP (diphtheria, tetanus, pertussis), and polio before school entry started in 1991 during a period of low vaccination coverage (<85%) in the state of Victoria and currently exists in six of the eight Australian states and territories. This legislation mandates provider-authenticated documentation of immunization status before school entry. Conscientious exemptors who sign a form stating that they object to immunization on personal, philosophical, or religious beliefs may enroll in school, but the children are not allowed to attend during an outbreak of a relevant disease. Medical exemptions are also permitted for vaccine contraindications.

In 1997, a federal initiative to increase immunization coverage in Australia[18] included financial incentives for parents and family doctors and recommendations to develop uniform vaccination requirements for school entry. The payment of incentives to family doctors, the main providers of immunization, started in 1998. The scheme has three components, including a payment for medical practices that achieve more than 90% coverage of children younger than 7 years. The legislation underpinning parental incentives, which were in effect by 1999, is the Family Assistance Act. This federal law provides means-tested maternity allowance and universal child-care benefits, contingent on proof of vaccination. This law specifies that a family is eligible for payment "if a recognized immunization provider has certified in writing that he or she has discussed with the adult the benefits and risks of immunizing the child and the adult has declared in writing that he or she has a conscientious exemption to the child being immunized."[19] An Australian study showed that parental financial incentives improved immunization rates, and that 70% of parents could not afford child care without the payments.[20]

Coverage for vaccines due by 12 months of age was 94% in 2001, compared with 75% in 1997,[21] showing that incentives for parents and providers contribute to high immunization rates, even in the jurisdictions that do not have legislation to link school entry with vaccination. Cultural factors might also contribute to acceptance of this type of legislation because Australia has always had a culture of acceptance of legislation for the public good.

Compulsory Vaccination in the United States

In 1809, Massachusetts passed the first immunization law in the United States requiring smallpox vaccination for the general population.[22] The constitutionality of the Massachusetts law was questioned when Henning Jacobson of Cambridge, Massachusetts, refused to be vaccinated against smallpox and, in accordance with the law, was fined US$5.[23] Jacobson believed that he was at increased risk of an adverse reaction. The law permitted children with medical justification to avoid vaccination but made no such exclusion for adults. Jacobson argued that:

A compulsory vaccination law is unreasonable, arbitrary and oppressive, and therefore, hostile to the inherent right of every freeman to care for his own body and health in such way as to him seems best; and that the execution of such a law against one who objects to vaccination, for whatever reason, is nothing short of an assault upon his person.[23]

Jacobson's case was decided in 1905 by the U.S. Supreme Court, which rejected each of his constitutional arguments. The Court found that:

The liberty secured by the constitution of the United States to every person within its jurisdiction does not import an absolute right in each person to be, at all times and in all circumstances, wholly freed from restraint. There are manifold restraints to which every person is necessarily subject for the common good.[23]

The Court affirmed the right of states to require vaccination as a legitimate use of their police powers and clearly stated that the protection of the health of the public supersedes certain individual interests, within reasonable boundaries. The Jacobson case laid the foundation for public health law in the United States. The U.S. Supreme Court also upheld the constitutionality of school vaccination laws in 1922.[24]

At the time of the Jacobson case, eleven states had compulsory vaccination laws, although three-quarters of them did not enforce the law with legal penalties for non-compliance. By 1963, twenty states required immunization against certain diseases for school entrance; by 1970, this number had increased to twenty-nine states.[22] The main intent of modern immunization requirements was to reduce or prevent school-based outbreaks of vaccine-preventable diseases. Outbreaks of measles were not uncommon during the 1970s; investigations of outbreaks indicated that schools were commonly a site of transmission.[25] States with immunization laws had lower rates of measles than did states without laws, and the incidence was much lower in states that strictly enforced the laws than in other states.[26–29] A push for compulsory laws came in 1966 during the national measles eradication campaign.

Secretary Joseph Califano, Department of Health and Human Services, wrote to the governor of every state in April 1977, urging them to enact and enforce compulsory vaccination laws. The Centers for Disease Control and Prevention (CDC) advocated the establishment and universal enforcement for immunization before school entry. As part of their annual program plans to receive federal funds to purchase vaccines and support vaccine infrastructure, states were asked to review their immunization laws and enforcement policies. By 1980, all fifty states had laws that linked vaccination with school entrance.

Laws originally written to require vaccination for school entrance were in many cases amended to include the entire school population, thereby identifying students who entered school before laws were enacted or who eluded the entrance laws. The Task Force on Community Preventive Services, an independent group assessing the evidence base for public-health interventions, concluded that the evidence showed immunization requirements "are effective in reducing vaccine-preventable disease and/or improving vaccination coverage."[30]

State laws provide a safety net ensuring that nearly all children older than 5 years are fully vaccinated. State laws also demonstrate a public and public-health commitment to vaccination, supporting both the individual and community benefit of vaccination. Laws that require vaccination for school entrance allow immunization programs to benefit from additional school system resources as schools take on the burden of checking each child's immunization status and ensuring every child has met the state immunization requirement. Walter Orenstein, former Director of the National Immunization Program, CDC, has noted, "school laws establish a system for immunization, a system that works year in and year out, regardless of political interest, media coverage, changing budget situations, and the absence of vaccine-preventable disease outbreaks to spur interest."[22]

All states allow medical exemptions to school immunization requirements; to qualify, many states require parents or guardians to provide a letter or other documentation from a doctor. Forty-eight states permit nonmedical exemptions,[31] called "religious" or "philosophical" (twenty states). In 1999, the complexity of obtaining an exemption was inversely associated with the proportion of exemptions filed. The nineteen states with the most formal requirements did not have a high proportion of exemptions, compared with states with less formal requirements.[32] In many states, the process of claiming a nonmedical exemption required less effort than fulfilling the immunization requirements, and in some states, there was no contact between parents and health professionals. Only sixteen states reported that exemption requests were ever denied. The local administrative difficulty for claiming an exemption has been associated with the likelihood of children having exemptions.[33]

Children with exemptions to school immunization requirements have had higher rates of vaccine-preventable diseases and contributed to outbreaks of such diseases. The risks of measles and pertussis in school-age children in the United States with nonmedical exemptions have been reported to be 22–35 times and 5–9 times higher, respectively, than those in vaccinated children.[34,35] The community risk associated with exemptions has been demonstrated through modeling[34] and epidemiologic investigations.[35]

Anti-vaccine groups have made concerted efforts to ease exemption requirements and add philosophical exemptions in states where they do not exist. In 1999, legislation was introduced in at least eight states to eliminate state vaccination laws or add philosophical exemptions. Coordinated efforts by workers in the state health department, physicians' groups, and other public-health advocates have thwarted efforts to remove state mandates. The states of Arizona and Arkansas passed legislation to allow philosophical exemptions in 2003 and 2002, respectively.

Lessons Learned

In 1896, The Royal Commission on Vaccination recognized that vaccination should be compulsory only if there is a reliable supply of safe vaccines. In the United States, availability of vaccines was ensured before school immunization requirements were implemented or strictly enforced.[30,36,37] In 2000–2003, vaccine shortages in the United States resulted in temporary suspension of school immunization requirements in several states.[38,39]

For compulsory vaccination to work as planned, the great majority of the population must be willing to be vaccinated. To force vaccination on children of parents who have strong convictions against vaccination could create a public backlash and serve to galvanize anti-vaccine groups. During the public concerns about the safety of MMR in the UK during the early 2000s, introduction of compulsory vaccination probably would have been unacceptable.

There are remarkable similarities between the arguments of the nineteenth-century European anti-vaccination movement and the present movement in the United States, including the belief that compulsory vaccination is a move toward totalitarianism.[40] The main purpose of compulsory vaccination (i.e., to prevent transmission of disease or increase immunization coverage) might also affect the acceptance of compulsory vaccination. Countries such as Sweden, Norway, Denmark, The Netherlands, and the UK, where there are high rates of vaccination without obligatory laws, would probably not be good settings for compulsory vaccination; they would be viewed as unnecessary given the success of their immunization programs.

The allowance of nonmedical exemptions to compulsory vaccination is one approach that could limit public backlash; however, this compromise might have been the beginning of the failure of compulsory vaccination in the UK. A stronger argument could be that the British problems were the result of easily obtainable exemptions, and compulsory laws would have remained effective had administrative requirements for claiming exemptions not been removed. Likewise, in the United States, high exemption rates are associated with jurisdictions where exemptions are easy to obtain. However, rates of immunization in Australia remain high despite the option of conscientious objection perhaps because of the link between vaccination and financial incentives for parents and providers. High rates of exemptions render compulsory vaccination ineffective. Additionally, exemptions raise problems with social equity: children who claim exemptions will benefit from herd immunity but avoid the risks, however small, associated with vaccination.

The U.S. approach to conscientious objectors to military conscription could be used as a model for implementation of nonmedical exemptions to vaccinations.[41] The military conscientious objectors model was based on the British model for immunization exemptions and was recently used to revise exemption legislation in the state of Arkansas.[42] Application of the military model to immunization exemptions would ensure exemptions granted on the basis of strength of conviction rather than the nature of the belief (religious vs. philosophical). Administrative requirements might also discourage applicants who consider exemption as a path of least resistance to school enrollment.

Compulsory vaccination increases the burden on governments to ensure vaccine safety. The Royal Commission acknowledged this responsibility when it stated that government should be required to make calf-lymph vaccine available to all. In the

United States, the compulsory nature of vaccination has been included in the rationale for federal vaccine-safety efforts and the development of the National Vaccine Injury Compensation Program.[43] Australia, however, has no such compensation scheme.

Allowance of local implementation and enforcement of vaccine laws and requirements recognizes that beliefs and cultures can vary between settings. Nevertheless, if these local variations are allowed and laws are not applied equally across populations, there could be clustering of unvaccinated people, which could increase the risk of disease in individuals and the community and also raise social equity issues. In the United States, some variability is inevitable because the compulsory vaccination laws are made by states and not the federal government. In Australia, the school-entry laws are state-based, but the link between immunization and parent financial assistance is made at a national level.

Health-services research is needed to assess the usefulness of compulsory laws, exemptions, and effects of variations in laws on vaccine acceptance and disease incidence. Exploration of perceptions and beliefs about the ethical issues surrounding compulsory vaccination is also important.

Compulsory vaccination should add to, not replace, other strategies to reach and sustain high rates of immunization. In the UK, substantial resources have been used to elucidate parents' perceptions about vaccination and to develop, implement, and evaluate strategies to communicate information about vaccine risks.[44,45] In the UK, there is a public demand for vaccination, and the system relies on the use of physicians' incentives for immunization[46] rather than trying to compel parents to have their children immunized. However, compulsory vaccination in the United States and Australia has achieved high rates of immunization without the resources the UK has devoted to public education. Neither the United States nor Australia has had any drops in coverage of pertussis immunization, such as those that occurred in the UK during campaigns against the use of whole-cell pertussis vaccine in the 1970s and 1980s. Likewise, in Australia and the United States, there has not been a lowered uptake of MMR vaccination since the concerns about safety were raised. The UK has had a series of unique events in health care such as the vCJD outbreak,[47] the Bristol experience,[48] and the whole-cell pertussis vaccination scare,[49] which may have eroded public confidence in the medical profession to a larger degree than has happened in Australia or the United States. The role of these events in shaping attitudes toward immunization in the UK cannot be underestimated.

Individual freedoms must be weighed against public benefits when exploring the viability of compulsory vaccination. Values vary between cultures and countries and can affect the ability of countries to institute and maintain compulsory vaccination programs. Cultures with a higher regard for individual freedoms and a lower regard for the protection of the common good may not be good candidates for compulsory vaccination. Nevertheless, compulsory vaccination has been successful in the United States, a country built on the principles of individual freedom and autonomy.

References

1. Centers for Disease Control and Prevention. 1999. Impact of vaccines universally recommended for children—United States, 1900–1998. *JAMA* 281:1482–1483.

2. Centers for Disease Control and Prevention. 1999. Ten great public health achievements, 1900–1999: Impact of vaccines universally recommended for children. *MMWR Morb Mortal Wkly Rep* 241:243–248.

3. Ehreth, J. 2003. The global value of vaccination. *Vaccine* 21: 596–600.

4. Task Force on Community Preventive Services. 2000. Recommendations regarding interventions to improve vaccination coverage in children, adolescents, and adults. *Am J Prev Med* 18 (suppl 1):92–96.

5. Baldwin, P. 1999. *Contagion and the State of Europe, 1830–1930.* New York: Cambridge University Press.

6. Thomas, E. G. 1980. The old poor law and medicine. *Med Hist* 24:1–19.

7. Williamson, S. 1984. Anti-vaccination Leagues. *Arch Dis Child* 59:1195–1196.

8. Royal Commission on Vaccination. 1986. *Final Report.* London: HM Stationery Office.

9. 1896. Editorial. The future of legislation on vaccination. *BMJ* 2:1396–1397.

10. Anon. 1961. *Public Health Act. Sec 38. Prevention and Notification of Disease.* London: HM Stationery Office.

11. Anon. 1936. *Public Health Act. Sec 169.* London: HM Stationery Office.

12. Department of Health and Social Security and the Welsh Office. 1975. *Memorandum on the Control of Outbreaks of Smallpox, 1964.* London: HM Stationery Office.

13. WHO. 2003. Global Advisory Committee on Vaccine Safety. MMR and autism. *Wkly Epidemiol Rec* 4:17–20.

14. Stratton, K., A. Gable, P. Shetty, M. McCormick, eds. 2001. *Immunization Safety Review: Measles-Mumps-Rubella Vaccine and Autism.* Washington, DC: Institute of Medicine, National Academy Press.

15. Halsey, N. A., S. L. Hyman, Conference Writing Panel. 2001. Measles-mumps-rubella vaccine and autism spectrum disorder: Report from the new challenges in childhood immunizations conference convened in Oak Brook, Illinois, June 12–13, 2000. *Pediatrics* 107:e84.

16. British Medical Association Board of Science and Education. 2003. *Childhood Immunization: A Guide for Healthcare Professionals.* London: BMA.

17. Report of the MMR Expert Group. Scottish Executive Publications. Available at: http://www.gov.scot/Publications/2002/04/14619/3779/. Accessed January 24, 2006.

18. Australian Department of Health and Ageing. 1997. *The Seven Point Plan.*

19. Department of Family and Community Services. Commonwealth of Australia. Family Assistance Act 1999, Section 6 (3). Available at: https://www.legislation.gov.au/Details/C2013C00028/. Accessed June 23, 2005.

20. Lawrence, G. L., C. R. MacIntyre, B. P. Hull, and P. B. McIntyre. 2004. Effectiveness of the linkage of child care and maternity payments to childhood immunization. *Vaccine* 22: 2345–2350.

21. Hull, B. P., G. L. Lawrence, C. R. MacIntyre, and P. B. McIntyre. 2003. Immunization coverage in Australia corrected for under-reporting to the Australian Childhood Immunization Register. *Aust N Z J Public Health* 27:533–558.

22. Orenstein, W. A., and A. R. Hinman. 1999. The immunization system in the United States—the role of school immunization laws. *Vaccine* 17 (suppl 3):S19–S24.

23. Jacobson v Commonwealth of Massachusetts, 197 US 11 (1905).

24. Zucht v King, 260 US 174 (1922).

25. Centers for Disease Control and Prevention. 1981. Age characteristics of measles cases—United States, 1977–1980. *MMWR Morb Mortal Wkly Rep* 30:502.

26. Orenstein, W. A., A. R. Hinman, and W. W. Williams. 1992. The impact of legislation on immunization in the United States. In: *Immunization: The Old and the New. Proceedings of the 2nd National Immunization Conference, May 27–29, 1991*, ed. R. Hall and J. Richters, 58–62. Canberra: Public Health Association of Australia.

27. Orenstein, W. A., N. A. Halsey, G. F. Hayden, D. L. Eddins, J. L. Conrad, J. J. Witte, et al. 1978. From the Center for Disease Control: Current status of measles in the United States, 1973–1977. *J Infect Dis* 37:847–853.

28. Centers for Disease Control Prevention. 1978. Measles and school immunization requirements—US, 1978. *MMWR Morb Mortal Wkly Rep* 27:303–304.

29. Middaugh, J. P., and L. D. Zyla. 1978. Enforcement of school immunization law in Alaska. *JAMA* 239:2128–2130.

30. Briss, P. A., L. E. Rodewald, A. R. Hinman, A. M. Shefer, R. A. Strikas, R. R. Bernier, et al. 2000. Reviews of evidence regarding interventions to improve vaccination coverage in children, adolescents, and adults. *Am J Prev Med* 18 (suppl 1):97–140.

31. Institute for Vaccine Safety. Vaccine exemptions. Available at: http://www.vaccinesafety.edu/cc-exem.htm. Accessed June 23, 2005.

32. Rota, J. S., D. A. Salmon, L. E. Rodewald, R. T. Chen, B F. Hibbs, and E. J. Gangarosa. 2000. Process for obtaining nonmedical exemptions to state immunization laws. *Am J Public Health* 91:645–648.

33. Salmon, D. A., S. B. Omer, L. Moulton, S. Stokley, M. P. Dehart, S. Lett, et al. 2005. The role of school policies and implementation procedures on school immunization requirements and non-medical exemptions. *AJPH* 95:436–440.

34. Salmon, D. A., M. Haber, E. J. Gangarosa, L. Phillips, N. Smith, and R. T. Chen. 1999. Health consequences of religious and philosophical exemptions from immunization laws: Individual and societal risks of measles. *JAMA* 282:47–53.

35. Feikin, D. R., D. C. Lezotte, R. F. Hamman, D. A. Salmon, R. T. Chen, and R. E. Hoffman. 2000. Individual and community risks of measles and pertussis associated with personal exemptions to immunizations. *JAMA* 284:3145–3150.

36. Centers for Disease Control and Prevention. 1981. Measles—Florida, 1981. *MMWR* 30:593–596.

37. Fowinkle, E. W., S. Barid, and C. M. Bass. 1981. A compulsory school immunization program in Tennessee. *Public Health Rep* 96:61–65.

38. Rowland, R. 2002, February 18. Childhood vaccines in short supply. CNN. Available at: http://edition.cnn.com/2002/HEALTH/parenting/02/18/vaccine.shortages/. Accessed June 23, 2005.

39. Santoli, J. M., G. Peter, M. Arvin, J. P. Davis, M. D. Decker, P. Fast, et al. 2003. Strengthening the supply of routinely recommended vaccines in the United States: Recommendations from the National Vaccine Advisory Committee. *JAMA* 290:3122–3128.

40. Wolfe, R. M., and L. K. Sharp. 2002. Anti-vaccinationists past and present. *BMJ* 325:430–432.

41. Salmon, D. A., and A. W. Siegel. 2001. The administration of religious and philosophical exemptions from vaccination requirements: Legal review and lessons learned from conscientious objectors from conscription. *Public Health Rep* 116:289–295.

42. Salmon, D. A., J. Sapsin, J. Jacobs, J. Thompson, S. Teret, and N. A. Halsey. 2005. Public health and the politics of school immunization requirements. *Am J Public Health* 95:778–783.

43. Department of Health and Human Services. 1999. *Vaccine Safety Action Plan: Minutes of the National Vaccine Advisory Committee: January 13, 1999.* Atlanta, GA: National Vaccine Program Office.

44. Salisbury, D. M. 2004. The consumers' perspective. In: *Vaccines: preventing disease and protecting health. Pan American Health Organization Scientific and Technical Publication No. 596,* ed. C. de Quadros, 310–317.Washington, DC: PAHO.

45. Yarwood, J., K. Noakes, D. Kennedy, H. Campbell, and D. Salisbury. 2005. Tracking mothers' attitudes to childhood immunization, 1991 to 2001. *Vaccine* 23:5670–5687.

46. Salisbury, D.M., and S. Dittmann. 1999. Immunization in Europe. In: *Vaccines* (3rd ed.), ed. S. A. Plotkin and W. A. Orenstein, 1033–1046. Philadelphia: W. B. Saunders.

47. Zeidler, M., G. E. Stewart, C. R. Barraclough, D. E. Bateman, D. Bates, D. J. Burn, et al. 1997. New variant Creutzfeldt-Jakob disease: Neurological features and diagnostic tests. *Lancet* 350: 903–907.

48. Dunn, P. M. 1998. The Wisheart affair: Paediatric cardiological services in Bristol, 1990–95. *BMJ* 317:1144–1145.

49. Miller, D. L., E. M. Ross, R. Alderslade, M. H. Bellman,, and N. S. Rawson. 1981. Pertussis immunization and serious acute neurological illness in children. *BMJ* 282:1595–1599.

21 Vaccine Refusal, Mandatory Immunization, and the Risks of Vaccine-Preventable Diseases

Saad B. Omer, Daniel A. Salmon, Walter A. Orenstein, M. Patricia deHart, and Neal Halsey[*]

Vaccines are among the most effective tools available for preventing infectious diseases and their complications and sequelae. High immunization coverage has resulted in drastic declines in vaccine-preventable diseases, particularly in many high- and middle-income countries. A reduction in the incidence of a vaccine-preventable disease often leads to the public perception that the severity of and susceptibility to the disease have decreased.[1] At the same time, public concern about real or perceived adverse events associated with vaccines has increased. This heightened level of concern often results in an increased number of people refusing vaccines.[1,2]

In the United States, policy interventions, such as immunization requirements for school entry, have contributed to high vaccine coverage and record or near-record lows in the levels of vaccine-preventable diseases. Herd immunity, induced by high vaccination rates, has played an important role in greatly reducing or eliminating continual endemic transmission of a number of diseases, thereby benefiting the community overall in addition to the individual vaccinated person.

Recent parental concerns about perceived vaccine safety issues, such as a purported association between vaccines and autism, although not supported by a credible body of scientific evidence,[3–8] have led increasing numbers of parents to refuse or delay vaccination for their children.[9,10] The primary measure of vaccine refusal in the United States is the proportion of children who are exempted from school immunization requirements for nonmedical reasons. There has been an increase in state-level rates of nonmedical exemptions from immunization requirements.[11] In this chapter, we review the evidentiary basis for school immunization requirements, explore the determinants of vaccine

* From *New England Journal of Medicine*, Omer, S. B., D. A. Salmon, W. A. Orenstein, M. P. deHart, and N. Halsey, Vaccine refusal, mandatory immunization, and the risks of vaccine-preventable diseases, 360:1981–1988. Copyright © 2009 Massachusetts Medical Society. Reprinted with permission from Massachusetts Medical Society.

refusal, and discuss the individual and community risks of vaccine-preventable diseases associated with vaccine refusal.

Evolution of U.S. Immunization Requirements

Vaccination was introduced in the United States at the turn of the nineteenth century. The first U.S. law to require smallpox vaccination was passed soon afterward, in 1809 in Massachusetts, to prevent and control frequent smallpox outbreaks that had substantial health and economic consequences.[12–14] Subsequently, other states enacted similar legislation.[13] Despite the challenges inherent in establishing a reliable and safe vaccine delivery system, vaccination became widely accepted as an effective tool for preventing smallpox through the mid-nineteenth century, and the incidence of smallpox declined between 1802 and 1840.[15] In the 1850s, "irregular physicians, the advocates of unorthodox medical theories,"[16] led challenges to vaccination. Vaccine use decreased, and smallpox made a major reappearance in the 1870s.[15] Many states passed new vaccination laws, whereas other states started enforcing existing laws. Increased enforcement of the laws often resulted in increased opposition to vaccination. Several states, including California, Illinois, Indiana, Minnesota, Utah, West Virginia, and Wisconsin, repealed compulsory vaccination laws.[15] Many other states retained them.

In a 1905 landmark case, *Jacobson v. Massachusetts*, which has since served as the foundation for public health laws, the U.S. Supreme Court endorsed the rights of states to pass and enforce compulsory vaccination laws.[17] In 1922, deciding a case filed by a girl excluded from a public school (and later a private school) in San Antonio, Texas, the U.S. Supreme Court found school immunization requirements to be constitutional.[18] Since then, courts have been generally supportive of the states' power to enact and implement immunization requirements.

Difficulties with efforts to control measles in the 1960s and 1970s ushered in the modern era of immunization laws in the United States.[12] In 1969, seventeen states had laws that required children to be vaccinated against measles before entering school, and twelve states had legally mandated requirements for vaccination against all six diseases for which routine immunization was carried out at the time.[13] During the 1970s, efforts were made to strengthen and strictly enforce immunization laws.[12,13] During measles outbreaks, some state and local health officials excluded from school those students who did not comply with immunization requirements, resulting in minimal backlash, quick improvement in local coverage, and control of outbreaks.[19–22] Efforts by the public health community and other immunization advocates to increase measles vaccine coverage among school-age children resulted in enforcement of immunization requirements for all vaccines and the introduction of such requirements in states that did not already have them. By the beginning of the 1980s, all fifty states had school immunization requirements.

Recent School Immunization Requirements

Because laws concerning immunization are state-based, there are substantial differences in requirements across the country. The requirements from state to state differ in terms of the school grades covered, the vaccines included, the processes and authority used to introduce new vaccines, reasons for exemptions (medical reasons, religious reasons, philosophical or personal beliefs), and the procedures for granting exemptions.[23]

State immunization laws contain provisions for certain exemptions. As of March 2008, all states permitted medical exemptions from school immunization requirements, 48 states allowed religious exemptions, and 21 states allowed exemptions based on philosophical or personal beliefs.[23] Several states (New York, Arkansas, and Texas) have recently expanded eligibility for exemptions.

Secular and Geographic Trends in Immunization Refusal

Between 1991 and 2004, the mean state-level rate of nonmedical exemptions increased from 0.98% to 1.48%. The increase in exemption rates was not uniform.[11] Exemption rates for states that allowed only religious exemptions remained at approximately 1% between 1991 and 2004; however, in states that allowed exemptions for philosophical or personal beliefs, the mean exemption rate increased from 0.99% to 2.54%.[11]

Like any average, the mean exemption rate presents only part of the picture because geographic clustering of nonmedical exemptions can result in local accumulation of a critical mass of susceptible children that increases the risk of outbreaks. There is evidence of substantial geographic heterogeneity in nonmedical-exemption rates between and within states.[24] For example, in the period from 2006 through 2007, the state-level nonmedical-exemption rate in Washington was 6%; however, the county-level rate ranged from 1.2% to 26.9%.[25] In a spatial analysis of Michigan's exemption data according to census tracts, twenty-three statistically significant clusters of increased exemptions were identified.[26] Similar heterogeneity in exemption rates has been identified in Oregon[27] and California (unpublished data).

The reasons for the geographic clustering of exemptions from school vaccination requirements are not fully understood, but they may include characteristics of the local population (e.g., cultural issues, socioeconomic status, or educational level), the beliefs of local healthcare providers and opinion leaders (e.g., clergy and politicians), and local media coverage. The factors known to be associated with exemption rates are heterogeneity in school policies[28] and the beliefs of school personnel who are responsible for compliance with the immunization requirements.[29]

Instead of refusing vaccines, some parents delay vaccination of their children.[30–32] Many parents follow novel vaccine schedules proposed by individual physicians (rather than those developed by expert committees with members representing multiple disciplines).[32,33] Most novel schedules involve administering vaccines over a longer period than that recommended by the Advisory Committee on Immunization Practices and the American Academy of Pediatrics or skipping the administration of some vaccines.

Individual Risk and Vaccine Refusal

Children with nonmedical exemptions are at increased risk for acquiring and transmitting vaccine-preventable diseases.[34,35] In a retrospective cohort study based on nationwide surveillance data from 1985 through 1992, children with exemptions were thirty-five times as likely to contract measles as nonexempt children (relative risk, 35; 95% confidence interval [CI], 34 to 37).[34] In a retrospective cohort study in Colorado based on data for the years 1987 through 1998, children with exemptions, as compared with unvaccinated children, were twenty-two times as likely to have had measles (relative risk, 22.2; 95% CI, 15.9 to 31.1) and almost six times as likely to have had pertussis (relative risk, 5.9; 95% CI, 4.2 to 8.2).35 Earlier data showed that lower incidences of measles and mumps were associated with the existence and enforcement of immunization requirements for school entry.[12,36–38]

The consequences of delayed vaccination, as compared with vaccine refusal, have not been studied in detail. However, it is known that the risk of vaccine-preventable diseases and the risk of sequelae from vaccine-preventable diseases are not constant throughout childhood. Young children are often at increased risk for illness and death related to infectious diseases, and vaccine delays may leave them vulnerable at ages with a high risk of contracting several vaccine-preventable diseases. Moreover, novel vaccine schedules that recommend administering vaccines over a longer period may exacerbate health inequities because parents with high socioeconomic status are more likely to make the extra visits required under the alternative schedules than parents with low socioeconomic status.[39]

Clustering of Vaccine Refusals and Community Risk

Multiple studies have shown an increase in the local risk of vaccine-preventable diseases when there is geographic aggregation of persons refusing vaccination. In Michigan, significant overlap between geographic clusters of nonmedical exemptions and pertussis clusters was documented.[26] The odds ratio for the likelihood that a census tract included in a pertussis cluster would also be included in an exemptions cluster was 2.7 (95% CI, 2.5 to 3.6) after adjustment for demographic factors.

In Colorado, the county-level incidence of measles and pertussis in vaccinated children from 1987 through 1998 was associated with the frequency of exemptions in that county.[35] At least 11% of the nonexempt children who acquired measles were infected through contact with an exempt child.[35] Moreover, school-based outbreaks in Colorado have been associated with increased exemption rates; the mean exemption rate among schools with outbreaks was 4.3%, as compared with 1.5% for the schools that did not have an outbreak ($P = 0.001$).[35]

High vaccine coverage, particularly at the community level, is extremely important for children who cannot be vaccinated, including children who have medical contraindications to vaccination and those who are too young to be vaccinated. These groups are often more susceptible to the complications of infectious diseases than the general population of children and depend on the protection provided by the vaccination of children in their environs.[40-42]

Vaccine Refusal and the Recent Increase in Measles Cases

Measles vaccination has been extremely successful in controlling a disease that previously contributed to considerable morbidity and mortality. In the United States, the reported number of cases dropped from an average of 500,000 annually in the era before vaccination (with reported cases considered to be a fraction of the estimated total, which was more than 2 million) to a mean of sixty-two cases per year from 2000 through 2007.[43-45] Between January 1, 2008, and April 25, 2008, there were five measles outbreaks and a total of sixty-four cases reported.[45] All but one of the persons with measles were either unvaccinated or did not have evidence of immunization. Of the twenty-one cases among children and adolescents in the vaccine-eligible age group (16 months to 19 years) with a known reason for nonvaccination, fourteen, or 67%, had obtained a nonmedical exemption, and all of the ten school-age children had obtained a nonmedical exemption.[45] Thirteen cases occurred in children too young to be vaccinated, and in more than one-third of the cases (eighteen of forty-four) occurring in a known transmission setting the disease was acquired in a healthcare facility.[45]

Outbreaks of vaccine-preventable disease often start among persons who refused vaccination, spread rapidly within unvaccinated populations, and also spread to other subpopulations. For example, of the four outbreaks with discrete index cases (one outbreak occurred by means of multiple importations) reported January through April 2008, three out of four index cases occurred in people who had refused vaccination due to personal beliefs; vaccination status could not be verified for the remaining cases.[45,46] In Washington State, a recent outbreak of measles occurred between April 12, 2008, and May 30, 2008, involving nineteen cases. All of the persons with measles were unimmunized with the exception of the last case, a person who had been vaccinated. Of the other eighteen cases, one was an infant who was too young to be vaccinated, two were younger than 4 years of age, and the remaining fifteen were of school age (unpublished data).

Who Refuses Vaccines and Why

Using data from the National Immunization Survey for the period from 1995 through 2001, Smith et al. compared the characteristics of children between the ages of 19 and 35 months who did not receive any vaccine (unvaccinated) with the characteristics of those who were partially vaccinated (undervaccinated).[47] As compared with the undervaccinated children, the unvaccinated children were more likely to be male, to be white, to belong to households with higher income, to have a married mother with a college education, and to live with four or more children.[47] Other studies have shown that children who are unvaccinated are likely to belong to families that intentionally refuse vaccines, whereas children who are undervaccinated are likely to have missed some vaccinations because of factors related to the healthcare system or sociodemographic characteristics.[48-51]

In a case-control study of the knowledge, attitudes, and beliefs of parents of exempt children as compared with parents of vaccinated children, respondents rated their views of their children's vulnerability to specific diseases, the severity of these diseases, and the efficacy and safety of the specific vaccines available for them. Composite scores were created on the basis of these vaccine-specific responses. As compared with parents of vaccinated children, significantly more parents of exempt children thought their children had a low susceptibility to the diseases (58% vs. 15%; $P < 0.05$), that the severity of the diseases was low (51% vs. 18%; $P < 0.05$), and that the efficacy and safety of the vaccines was low (54% vs. 17% for efficacy and 60% vs. 15% for safety; $P < 0.05$

for both comparisons).[52] Moreover, parents of exempt children were more likely than parents of vaccinated children both to have providers who offered complementary or alternative health care and to obtain information from the Internet and groups opposed to aspects of immunization.[52] The most frequent reason for nonvaccination, stated by 69% of the parents, was concern that the vaccine might cause harm.[52]

Other studies have also reported the importance of parents' concerns about vaccine safety when they decide against vaccination.[53–56] A national survey of parents from 2001 through 2002 showed that although only 1% of respondents thought vaccines were unsafe, the children of these parents were almost three times as likely to not be up to date on recommended vaccinations as the children of parents who thought that vaccines were safe.[54] In a separate case-control study with a national sample, under-immunization was associated with negative perceptions of vaccine safety (odds ratio, 2.0; 95% CI, 1.2 to 3.4).[55] In another case-control study, Bardenheier et al. found that although concerns regarding general vaccine safety did not differ between the parents of vaccinated children and the parents of undervaccinated or unvaccinated children, more than half of the case and control parents did express concerns about vaccine safety to their child's healthcare provider.[57] Moreover, parents of undervaccinated or unvaccinated children were more likely to believe that children receive too many vaccines.[57]

The Role of Healthcare Providers

Clinicians and other healthcare providers play a crucial role in parental decision making with regard to immunization. Health care providers are cited by parents, including parents of unvaccinated children, as the most frequent source of information about vaccination.[52]

In a study of the knowledge, attitudes, and practices of primary care providers, a high proportion of those providing care for children whose parents have refused vaccination and those providing care for appropriately vaccinated children were both found to have favorable opinions of vaccines.[58] However, those providing care for unvaccinated children were less likely to have confidence in vaccine safety (odds ratio, 0.37; 95% CI, 0.19 to 0.72) and less likely to perceive vaccines as benefitting individuals and communities.[58] Moreover, there was overlap between clinicians' unfavorable opinions of vaccines and the likelihood that they had unvaccinated children in their practice.[58]

There is evidence that healthcare providers have a positive overall effect on parents' decision making with regard to vaccination of their children. In a study by Smith et al., parents who reported that their immunization decisions were influenced by their child's healthcare provider were almost twice as likely to consider vaccines safe as parents who said their decisions were not influenced by the provider.[59]

In focus-group discussions, several parents who were not certain about vaccinating their child were willing to discuss their immunization concerns with a healthcare provider and wanted the provider to offer information relevant to their specific concerns.[56] These findings highlight the critical role that clinicians can play in explaining the benefits of immunization and addressing parental concerns about its risks.

Clinicians' Response to Vaccine Refusal

Some clinicians have discontinued or have considered discontinuing their provider relationship with families that refuse vaccines.[60,61] In a national survey of members of the American Academy of Pediatrics, almost 40% of respondents said they would not provide care to a family that refused all vaccines, and 28% said they would not provide care to a family that refused some vaccines.[61]

The academy's Committee on Bioethics advises against discontinuing care for families that decline vaccines and has recommended that pediatricians "share honestly what is and is not known about the risks and benefits of the vaccine in question."[62] The committee also recommends that clinicians address vaccine refusal by respectfully listening to parental concerns, explaining the risk of nonimmunization, and discussing the specific vaccines that are of most concern to parents.[62] The committee advises against more serious action in a majority of cases: "Continued refusal after adequate discussion should be respected unless the child is put at significant risk of serious harm (e.g., as might be the case during an epidemic). Only then should state agencies be involved to override parental discretion on the basis of medical neglect."[62]

Policy-Level Determinants of Vaccine Refusal

Immunization requirements and the policies that ensure compliance with the requirements vary considerably among the states; these variations have been associated with state-level exemption rates.[11,63] For example, the complexity of procedures for obtaining exemption has been shown to be inversely associated with rates of exemption.[63] Moreover, between 1991 and 2004, the mean annual incidence of pertussis was almost twice as high in states with administrative procedures that made it easy to obtain exemptions as in states that made it difficult.[11]

One possible way to balance individual rights and the greater public good with respect to vaccination would be to institute and broaden administrative controls. For example, a model law proposed for Arkansas suggested that parents seeking nonmedical exemptions be provided with counseling on the hazards of refusing vaccination.[64]

States also differ in terms of meeting the recommendations for age-appropriate coverage for children younger than 2 years of age.[65] School immunization requirements ensure completion by the time of school entry, but they do not directly influence the timeliness of vaccination among preschoolers. However, there is some evidence that school immunization laws have an indirect effect on preschool vaccine coverage. For example, varicella vaccine was introduced in the United States in 1995 and has played an important role in reducing the incidence of chickenpox.[66] In 2000, states that had implemented mandatory immunization for varicella by the time of school entry had coverage among children 19 to 35 months old that was higher than the average for all states. Having an immunization requirement could be an indicator of the effectiveness of a state's immunization program, but the effect of school-based requirements on coverage among preschoolers cannot be completely discounted.

Conclusions

Vaccine refusal not only increases the individual risk of disease but also increases the risk for the whole community. As a result of substantial gains in reducing vaccine-preventable diseases, the memory of several infectious diseases has faded from the public consciousness, and the risk–benefit calculus seems to have shifted in favor of the perceived risks of vaccination in some parents' minds. Major reasons for vaccine refusal in the United States are parental perceptions and concerns about vaccine safety and a low level of concern about the risk of many vaccine-preventable diseases. If the enormous benefits to society from vaccination are to be maintained, increased efforts will be needed to educate the public about those benefits and to increase public confidence in the systems we use to monitor and ensure vaccine safety. Because clinicians have an influence on parental decision making, it is important that they understand the benefits and risks of vaccines and anticipate questions that parents may have about safety. There are a number of sources of information on vaccines that should be useful to both clinicians and parents (e.g., Appendix 1 in the fifth edition of Vaccines, edited by Plotkin et al.; the list of Web sites on vaccine safety posted on the World Health Organization's Web site; and the Web site of the National Center for Immunization and Respiratory Diseases).[67–69]

References

1. Chen, R. T., and B. Hibbs. 1998. Vaccine safety: Current and future challenges. *Pediatr Ann* 27:445–455.

2. Chen, R. T., and F. DeStefano. 1998. Vaccine adverse events: Causal or coincidental? *Lancet* 351:611–612.

3. DeStefano, F. 2007. Vaccines and autism: Evidence does not support a causal association. *Clin Pharmacol Ther* 82:756–759.

4. Doja, A., and W. Roberts. 2006. Immunizations and autism: A review of the literature. *Can J Neurol Sci* 33:341–346.

5. Fombonne, E., and E. H. Cook. 2003. MMR and autistic enterocolitis: Consistent epidemiological failure to find an association. *Mol Psychiatry* 8:133–134.

6. Fombonne, E. 2008. Thimerosal disappears but autism remains. *Arch Gen Psychiatry* 65:15–16.

7. Schechter, R, and J. K. Grether. 2008. Continuing increases in autism reported to California's developmental services system: Mercury in retrograde. *Arch Gen Psychiatry* 65:19–24.

8. Thompson, W. W., C. Price, B. Goodson, D. K. Shay, P. Benson, V. L. Hinrichsen, et al. 2007. Early thimerosal exposure and neuropsychological outcomes at 7 to 10 years. *N Engl J Med* 357: 1281–1292.

9. Offit, P. A. 2008. Vaccines and autism revisited—the Hannah Poling case. *N Engl J Med* 358:2089–2091.

10. Smith, M. J., S. S. Ellenberg, L. M. Bell, and D. M. Rubin. 2008. Media coverage of the measles-mumps-rubella vaccine and autism controversy and its relationship to MMR immunization rates in the United States. *Pediatrics* 121:e836–e843.

11. Omer, S. B., W. K. Pan, N. A. Halsey, S. Stokley, L. H. Moulton, A. M. Navar, et al. 2006. Nonmedical exemptions to school immunization requirements: Secular trends and association of state policies with pertussis incidence. *JAMA* 296:1757–1763.

12. Orenstein, W. A., and A. R. Hinman. 1999. The immunization system in the United States—the role of school immunization laws. *Vaccine* 17(Suppl 3):S19–S24.

13. Jackson, C. L. 1969. State laws on compulsory immunization in the United States. *Public Health Rep* 84:787–795.

14. Colgrove, J., and R. Bayer. 2005. Could it happen here? Vaccine risk controversies and the specter of derailment. *Health Aff (Millwood)* 24:729–739.

15. Kaufman, M. 1967. The American anti-vaccinationists and their arguments. *Bull Hist Med* 41:463–478.

16. Stern, B. J. 1927. *Should We Be Vaccinated? A Survey of the Controversy in Its Historical and Scientific Aspects.* New York: Harper & Brothers.

17. Jacobson v. Massachusetts, 197 U.S. 11 (1905).

18. Zucht v. King, 260 U.S. 174 (Nov. 13, 1922).

19. Middaugh, J. P., and L. D. Zyla. 1978. Enforcement of school immunization law in Alaska. *JAMA* 239:2128–2130.

20. Lovejoy, G. S., J. W. Giandelia, and M. Hicks. 1974. Successful enforcement of an immunization law. *Public Health Rep* 89:456–458.

21. Fowinkle, E. W., S. Barid, and C. M. Bass. 1981. A compulsory school immunization program in Tennessee. *Public Health Rep* 96:61–66.

22. Centers for Disease Control and Prevention. 1981. Measles—Florida. *MMWR Morb Mortal Wkly Rep* 30:593–596.

23. Vaccine Exemptions. 2008. Johns Hopkins Bloomberg School of Public Health—Institute for Vaccine Safety. Available at: http://www.vaccinesafety.edu/ccexem.htm. Accessed April 16, 2009.

24. National Center for Immunization and Respiratory Diseases. 2007, May. School and childcare vaccination surveys. Available at: http://www.cdc.gov/vaccines/stats-surv/schoolsurv/default.htm. Accessed April 13, 2009.

25. School Status Data Reports. 2009. Washington State Department of Health. Available at: http://www.doh.wa.gov/DataandStatisticalReports/HealthBehaviors/Immunization/SchoolReports/. Accessed April 16, 2009.

26. Omer, S. B., K. S. Enger, L. H. Moulton, N. A. Halsey, S. Stokley, and D. A. Salmon. 2008. Geographic clustering of nonmedical exemptions to school immunization requirements and associations with geographic clustering of pertussis. *Am J Epidemiol* 168:1389–1396.

27. Attitudes, networking and immunizations in a community with a high rate of religious exemptions. Presented at the 37th National Immunization Conference, Chicago, March 17–20, 2003.

28. Salmon, D. A., S. B. Omer, L. H. Moulton, S. Stokley, M. P. Dehart, S. Lett, et al. 2005. Exemptions to school immunization requirements: The role of school-level requirements, policies, and procedures. [Erratum, *Am J Public Health* 2005;95:551.] *Am J Public Health* 95:436–440.

29. Salmon, D. A., L. H. Moulton, S. B. Omer, L. M. Chace, A. Klassen, P. Talebian, and N. A. Halsey. 2004. Knowledge, attitudes, and beliefs of school nurses and personnel and associations with nonmedical immunization exemptions. *Pediatrics* 113:e552–e559.

30. Luman, E. T., L. E. Barker, K. M. Shaw, M. M. McCauley, J. W. Buehler, and L. K. Pickering. 2005. Timeliness of childhood vaccinations in the United States: Days undervaccinated and number of vaccines delayed. *JAMA* 293:1204–1211.

31. Luman, E. T., K. M. Shaw, and S. K. Stokley. 2008. Compliance with vaccination recommendations for U.S. children. [Erratum, *Am J Prev Med* 2008:35:319.] *Am J Prev Med* 34:463–470.

32. Cohen, E. 2008. Should I vaccinate my baby? Cable News Network. Available at: http://www .cnn.com/2008/HEALTH/family/06/19/ep.vaccines/index.html. Accessed April 13, 2009.

33. Sears, R. Dr. Bob's blog categories: alternative vaccine schedule. Available at: http:// askdrsears.com/thevaccinebook/labels/Alternative%20Vaccine%20Schedule.asp. Accessed April 13, 2009.

34. Salmon, D. A., M. Haber, E. J. Gangarosa, L. Phillips, N. J. Smith, and R. T. Chen. 1999. Health consequences of religious and philosophical exemptions from immunization laws: Individual and societal risk of measles. [Erratum, *JAMA* 2000;283:2241.] *JAMA* 282:47–53.

35. Feikin, D. R., D. C. Lezotte, R. F. Hamman, D. A. Salmon, R. T Chen, and R. E. Hoffman. 2000. Individual and community risks of measles and pertussis associated with personal exemptions to immunization. *JAMA* 284:3145–3150.

36. Centers for Disease Control and Prevention. 1977. Measles—Unites States. *MMWR Morb Mortal Wkly Rep* 26:109–111.

37. Robbins, K. B., D. Brandling-Bennett, and A. R. Hinman. 1981. Low measles incidence: Association with enforcement of school immunization laws. *Am J Public Health* 71:270–274.

38. van Loon, F. P., S. J. Holmes, B. I. Sirotkin, W. W. Williams, S. L. Cochi, S. C. Hadler, and M. L. Lindegren. 1995. Mumps surveillance—United States, 1988–1993. *Mor Mortal Wkly Rep CDC Surveill Summ* 44:1–14.

39. Williams, I. T., J. D. Milton, J. B. Farrell, and N. M. Graham. 1995. Interaction of socioeconomic status and provider practices as predictors of immunization coverage in Virginia children. *Pediatrics* 96:439–446.

40. Bisgard, K. M., F. B. Pascual, K. R. Ehresmann, C. A. Miller, C. Cianfrini, C. E. Jennings, et al. 2004. Infant pertussis: Who was the source? *Pediatr Infect Dis J* 23:985–989.

41. Deen, J. L., C. A. Mink, J. D. Cherry, P. D. Christenson, E. F. Pineda, K. Lewis, et al. 1995. Household contact study of Bordetella pertussis infections. *Clin Infect Dis* 21:1211–1219.

42. Poehling, K. A., T. R. Talbot, M. R. Griffin, A. S. Craig, C. G. Whitney, E. Zell, et al. 2006. Invasive pneumococcal disease among infants before and after introduction of pneumococcal conjugate vaccine. *JAMA* 295:1668–1674.

43. Bloch, A. B., W. A. Orenstein, H. C. Stetler, S. G. Wassilak, R. W. Amler, K. J. Bart, et al. 1985. Health impact of measles vaccination in the United States. *Pediatrics* 76:524–532.

44. Orenstein, W. A., M. J. Papania, and M. E. Wharton. 2004. Measles elimination in the United States. *J Infect Dis* 189(Suppl 1):S1–S3.

45. Measles—United States. 2008. January 1–April 25, 2008. *MMWR Morb Mortal Wkly Rep* 57:494–498.

46. Centers for Disease Control and Prevention. 2008. Update: Measles—United States, January-July 2008. *MMWR Morb Mortal Wkly Rep* 57:893–896.

47. Smith, P. J., S. Y, Chu, and L. E. Barker. 2004. Children who have received no vaccines: Who are they and where do they live? *Pediatrics* 114:187–195.

48. Allred, N. J., K. G. Wooten, and Y. Kong. 2007. The association of health insurance and continuous primary care in the medical home on vaccination coverage for 19- to 35-month-old children. *Pediatrics* 119(Suppl 1):S4–S11.

49. Daniels, D., R. B. Jiles, R. M. Klevens, and G. A. Herrera. 2001. Undervaccinated African-American preschoolers: A case of missed opportunities. *Am J Prev Med* 20(Suppl):61–68.

50. Luman, E. T., McCauley, M. M., A. Shefer, and S. Y. Chu. 2003. Maternal characteristics associated with vaccination of young children. *Pediatrics* 111:1215–1218.

51. Smith, P. J., J. M. Santoli, S. Y. Chu, D. Q. Ochoa, and L. E. Rodewald. 2005. The association between having a medical home and vaccination coverage among children eligible for the Vaccines for Children program. *Pediatrics* 116: 130–139.

52. Salmon, D. A., L. H. Moulton, S. B. Omer, M. P. Dehart, S. Stokley, and N. A. Halsey. 2005. Factors associated with refusal of childhood vaccines among parents of school-aged children: A case-control study. *Arch Pediatr Adolesc Med* 159:470–476.

53. Humiston, S. G., E. B. Lerner, E. Hepworth, T. Blythe, and J. G. Goepp. 2005. Parent opinions about universal influenza vaccination for infants and toddlers. *Arch Pediatr Adolesc Med* 159:108–112.

54. Allred, N. J., K. M. Shaw, T. A Santibanez, D. L. Rickert, and J. M. Santoli. 2005. Parental vaccine safety concerns: Results from the National Immunization Survey, 2001–2002. *Am J Prev Med* 28:221–224.

55. Gust, D. A., T. W. Strine, E. Maurice, P. Smith, H. Yusuf, M. Wilkinson, et al. 2004. Under-immunization among children: Effects of vaccine safety concerns on immunization status. *Pediatrics* 114:e16–e22.

56. Fredrickson, D. D., T. C. Davis, C. L. Arnould, E. M. Kennen, S. G. Hurniston, J. T. Cross, and J. A. Bocchini, Jr. 2004. Childhood immunization refusal: Provider and parent perceptions. *Fam Med* 36:431–439.

57. Bardenheier, B., H. Yusuf, B. Schwartz, D. Gust, L. Barker, and L. Rodewald. 2004. Are parental vaccine safety concerns associated with receipt of measles-mumps-rubella, diphtheria and tetanus toxoids with acellular pertussis, or hepatitis B vaccines by children? *Arch Pediatr Adolesc Med* 158:569–575.

58. Salmon, D. A., W. K. Pan, S. B. Omer, A. M. Navar, W. Orenstein, E. K. Marcuse, et al. 2008. Vaccine knowledge and practices of primary care providers of exempt vs. vaccinated children. *Hum Vaccin* 4:286–291.

59. Smith, P. J., A. M. Kennedy, K. Wooten, D. A. Gust, and L. K. Pickering. 2006. Association between health care providers' influence on parents who have concerns about vaccine safety and vaccination coverage. *Pediatrics* 118:e1287–e1292.

60. Freed, G. L., S. J. Clark, B. F. Hibbs, and J. M. Santoli. 2004. Parental vaccine safety concerns: The experiences of pediatricians and family physicians. *Am J Prev Med* 26:11–14.

61. Flanagan-Klygis, E. A., L. Sharp, and J. E. Frader. 2005. Dismissing the family who refuses vaccines: A study of pediatrician attitudes. *Arch Pediatr Adolesc Med* 159:929–934.

62. Diekema, D. S. 2005. Responding to parental refusals of immunization of children. *Pediatrics* 115:1428–1431.

63. Rota, J. S., D. A. Salmon, L. E. Rodewald, R. T. Chen, B. F. Hibbs, and E. J. Gangarosa. 2001. Processes for obtaining nonmedical exemptions to state immunization laws. *Am J Public Health* 91:645–648.

64. Salmon, D. A., and A. W. Siegel. 2001. Religious and philosophical exemptions from vaccination requirements and lessons learned from conscientious objectors from conscription. *Public Health Rep* 116:289–295.

65. Luman, E. T., L. E. Barker, M. M. McCauley, and C. Drews-Botsch. 2005. Timeliness of childhood immunizations: A state-specific analysis. *Am J Public Health* 95:1367–1374.

66. Seward, J. F., B. M. Watson, C. L. Peterson, L. Mascola, J. W. Pelosi, J. X. Zhang, et al. 2002. Varicella disease after introduction of varicella vaccine in the United States, 1995–2000. *JAMA* 287:606–611.

67. Wexler, D. L., and T. A. Anderson. 2008. Web Sites That Contain Information About Immunization. In: *Vaccines*, 5th ed., eds. S. Plotkin, W. A. Orenstein, and P. A. Offit, 1685–1690. Philadelphia: Saunders.

68. World Health Organization. 2008, September. *Vaccine Safety Web Sites Meeting Credibility and Content Good Information Practices Criteria*. Geneva: World Health Organization.

69. National Center for Immunization and Respiratory Diseases. 2009. Centers for Disease Control and Prevention. Available at: http://www.cdc.gov/ncird/. Accessed April 16, 2009.

22 Fatal Exemption

Paul A. Offit*

The *Journal of the American Medical Association* (*JAMA*) recently published a study that received little attention from the press and, as a consequence, from the public. The study examined the incidence of whooping cough (pertussis) in children whose parents had chosen not to vaccinate them. The results were concerning.

Vaccines are recommended by the Centers for Disease Control and Prevention (CDC) and professional societies, such as the American Academy of Pediatrics. But these organizations cannot enforce their recommendations. Only states can do that—usually when children enter day-care centers and elementary schools—in the form of mandates. State vaccine mandates have been on the books since the early 1900s, but they weren't aggressively enforced until much later, as a consequence of tragedy.

In 1963, the first measles vaccine was introduced in the United States. Measles is a highly contagious disease that can infect the lungs, causing fatal pneumonia, or the brain, causing encephalitis. Before the vaccine, measles caused 100,000 American children to be hospitalized and 3,000 to die every year. In the early 1970s, public health officials found that states with vaccine mandates had rates of measles that were 50% lower than states without mandates. As a consequence, all states worked toward requiring children to get vaccines. Now every state has some form of vaccine mandates.

But not all children are subject to these mandates. All fifty states have medical exemptions to vaccines, such as a serious allergy to a vaccine component. Some forty-eight states also have religious exemptions. Amish groups, for example, traditionally reject vaccines, believing that clean living and a healthy diet are all that are needed to avoid vaccine-preventable diseases. Twenty states have philosophical exemptions. In some states, these exemptions are easy to obtain by simply signing your name to a form; in others, they are much harder, requiring notarization, annual renewal, a signature from a local health official, or a personally written letter from a parent.

* Originally published in *The Wall Street Journal,* January 20, 2007. Reprinted with permission.

The *JAMA* study examined the relationship between vaccine exemptions and rates of disease. The authors found that between 1991 and 2004, the percentage of children whose parents had chosen to exempt them from vaccines increased by 6% per year, resulting in a 2.5-fold increase. This increase occurred almost solely in states where philosophical exemptions were easy to obtain. Worse, states with easy-to-obtain philosophical exemptions had twice as many children suffering from pertussis—a disease that causes inflammation of the windpipe and breathing tubes, pneumonia, and, in about twenty infants every year, death—than states with hard-to-obtain philosophical exemptions.

The finding that lower immunization rates caused higher rates of disease should not be surprising. In 1991, a massive epidemic of measles in Philadelphia centered on a group that chose not to immunize its children; as a consequence, nine children died from measles. In the late 1990s, severe outbreaks of pertussis occurred in Colorado and Washington among children whose parents feared pertussis vaccine. In 2005, a 17-year-old unvaccinated girl, unknowingly having brought measles with her from Romania, attended a church gathering of 500 people in Indiana and caused the largest outbreak of measles in the United States in 10 years—an outbreak limited to children whose parents had chosen not to vaccinate them. These events showed that, for contagious diseases such as measles and pertussis, it is hard for unvaccinated children to successfully hide among herds of vaccinated children.

Some would argue that philosophical exemptions are a necessary pop-off valve for a society that requires children to be injected with biological agents for the common good. But as anti-vaccine activists continue to push more states to allow for easy philosophical exemptions, more and more children will suffer and occasionally die from vaccine-preventable diseases.

When it comes to issues of public health and safety, we invariably have laws. Many of these laws are strictly enforced and immutable. We don't allow philosophical exemptions to restraining young children in car seats, to smoking in restaurants, or to stopping at stop signs. The notion of requiring vaccines for school entry, although it seems to tear at the very heart of a country founded on the basis of individual rights and freedoms, saves lives. Given the increasing number of states allowing philosophical exemptions to vaccines, at some point we will to be forced to decide whether it is our inalienable right to catch and transmit potentially fatal infections.

23 Politics, Parents, and Prophylaxis—Mandating HPV Vaccination in the United States

R. Alta Charo[*]

Cancer prevention has fallen victim to the culture wars. Throughout the United States, state legislatures are scrambling to respond to the availability of Merck's human papillomavirus (HPV) vaccine, Gardasil, and to the likely introduction of GlaxoSmithKline's not-yet-approved HPV vaccine, Cervarix, which have been shown to be effective in preventing infection with HPV strains that cause about 70% of cases of cervical cancer. At the Centers for Disease Control and Prevention (CDC), the Advisory Committee on Immunization Practices (ACIP) has voted unanimously to recommend that girls 11 and 12 years of age receive the vaccine, and the CDC has added Gardasil to its Vaccines for Children Program, which provides free immunizations to impoverished or underserved children.

Yet despite this federal imprimatur, access to these vaccines has already become more a political than a public health question. Although the more important focus might be on the high cost of the vaccines—a cost that poses a genuine obstacle to patients, physicians, and insurers—concern has focused instead on a purported interference in family life and sexual mores. This concern has resulted in a variety of political efforts to forestall the creation of a mandated vaccination program. In Florida and Georgia, for example, efforts to increase adoption of the vaccine have been stalled by legislative maneuvering. The Democratic governor of New Mexico has announced that he will veto a bill that mandates vaccinations. The Republican governor of Texas came under fire (and under legal attack from his own attorney general) when he issued an executive order to the same effect, mandating that all girls entering the sixth grade receive the vaccine; the policy was attacked as an intrusion on parental discretion and an invitation to teenage promiscuity. But all these measures included a parental right

* From *New England Journal of Medicine*, Charo, R. A., Politics, parents, and prophylaxis—Mandating HPV vaccination in the United States, 356:1905–1908. Copyright © 2007 Massachusetts Medical Society. Reprinted with permission from Massachusetts Medical Society.

to opt out, whether on religious or secular grounds. The opposition seemed more about acknowledging the realities of teenage sexuality than about the privacy and autonomy of the nuclear family.

For more than a century, it has been settled law that states may require people to be vaccinated, and both federal and state court decisions have consistently upheld vaccination mandates for children, even to the extent of denying unvaccinated children access to the public schools. State requirements vary as to the range of communicable diseases but are often based on ACIP recommendations. School-based immunization requirements represent a key impetus for widespread vaccination of children and adolescents[1] and are enforceable even when they allegedly conflict with personal or religious beliefs.[2] In practice, however, these requirements usually feature exceptions that include individual medical, religious, and philosophical objections.

HPV-vaccination mandates, which are aimed more at protecting the vaccinee than at achieving herd immunity, have been attacked as an unwarranted intrusion on individual and parental rights. The constitutionality of vaccination mandates is premised on the reasonableness of the risk–benefit balance, the degree of intrusion on personal autonomy, and, most crucial, the presence of a public health necessity. On the one hand, to the extent that required HPV vaccination is an example of state paternalism rather than community protection, mandatory programs lose some of their justification. On the other hand, the parental option to refuse vaccination without interfering in the child's right to attend school alters this balance. Here the mandates act less as state imperatives and more as subtle tools to encourage vaccination. Whereas an opt-in program requires an affirmative effort by a parent, and thus misses many children whose parents forget to opt in, an opt-out approach increases vaccination rates among children whose parents have no real objection to the program while perfectly preserving parental autonomy.

Opposition to HPV vaccination represents another chapter in the history of resistance to vaccination and, on some levels, reflects a growing trend toward parental refusal of a variety of vaccines based on the (erroneous) perception that many vaccines are more risky than the diseases they prevent. In most cases, pediatricians have largely restricted themselves to educating and counseling objecting families because it is rare that the risks posed by going unvaccinated are so substantial that refusal is tantamount to medical neglect. In the case of HPV vaccine, parents' beliefs that their children will remain abstinent (and therefore uninfected) until marriage render it even more difficult to make the case for mandating a medical form of prevention. Even with an opt-out program, critics may argue that the availability of a simple and safe alternative—that is, abstinence—undermines the argument for a state initiative that encourages vaccination through mandates coupled with an option for parental refusal.

But experience shows that abstinence-only approaches to sex education do not delay the age of sexual initiation, nor do they decrease the number of sexual encounters.[3] According to the CDC, although only 13% of American girls are sexually experienced by 15 years of age, by age 17, the proportion grows to 43%, and by age 19, to 70%.[4] School-based programs are crucial for reaching those at highest risk of contracting sexually transmitted diseases, and despite the relatively low rate of sexual activity before age 15, the programs need to begin with children as young as 12 years: the rates at which adolescents drop out of school begin to increase at 13 years of age,[1] and younger dropouts have been shown to be especially likely to engage in earlier or riskier sexual activity.

Another fear among those who oppose mandatory HPV vaccination is that it will have a disinhibiting effect and thus encourage sexual activity among teens who might otherwise have remained abstinent. This outcome, however, seems quite unlikely. The threat of pregnancy or even AIDS is far more immediate than the threat of cancer, but sex education and distribution of condoms have not been shown to increase sexual activity. Indeed, according to a study conducted by researchers at the University of Pennsylvania, it is the comprehensive sex-education approaches that include contraceptive training that "delay initiation of sexual intercourse, reduce frequency of sex, reduce frequency of unprotected sex, and reduce the number of sexual partners."[5] Opposition to the HPV-vaccination mandates, then, would seem to be based more on an inchoate concern: that to recognize the reality of teenage sexual activity is implicitly to endorse it.

Public health officials may have legitimate questions about the merits of HPV vaccine mandates, in light of the financial and logistic burdens these may impose on families and schools, and also may be uncertain about adverse-event rates in mass-scale programs. But given that the moral objections to requiring HPV vaccination are largely emotional, this source of resistance to mandates is difficult to justify. Because, without exception, the proposed laws permit parents to refuse to have their daughters vaccinated, the only valid objection is that parents must actively manifest such refusal. Such a slight burden on parents can hardly justify backing away from the most effective means of protecting a generation of women, and in particular, poor and disadvantaged women, from the scourge of cervical cancer. To lighten that burden even further, the Virginia governor has proposed that refusals need not even be put in writing. Perhaps it is time for parents who object to HPV vaccinations to take a lesson from their children and heed the words of Nancy Reagan: Just say no.

References

1. National Foundation for Infectious Diseases. 2005. *Adolescent Vaccination: Bridging From a Strong Childhood Foundation to a Healthy Adulthood.* Bethesda, MD: National Foundation for Infectious Diseases. Available at: http://www.nfid.org/pdf/publications/adolescentvacc.pdf. Accessed April 19, 2007.

2. Hodges, J., and L. Gostin. 2001. School vaccination requirements: Historical, social, and legal perspectives. *KY Law J* 90: 831–890.

3. Trenholm, C., B. Devaney, K. Fortson, L. Quay, J. Wheeler, and M. Clark. 2007, April. *Impacts of Four Title V, Section 510 Abstinence Education Programs: Final Report.* Princeton, NJ: Mathematica Policy Research Available at: http://www.mathematica-mpr.com/publications/PDFs/impactabstinence.pdf. Accessed April 19, 2007.

4. Dailard, C. 2006. Legislating against arousal: The growing divide between federal policy and teenage sexual behavior. *Guttmacher Policy Rev* 9:12–16.

5. Bleakley, A., M. Hennessy, and M. Fishbein. 2006. Public opinion on sex education in US schools. *Arch Pediatr Adolesc Med* 160:1151–1156.

24 Lessons from the Failure of Human Papillomavirus Vaccine State Requirements

Jason L. Schwartz, Arthur L. Caplan, Ruth R. Faden, and Jeremy Sugarman[*]

The licensure in 2006 of a vaccine against the subtypes of human papillomavirus (HPV) responsible for the majority of cervical cancers and genital warts was heralded as a watershed moment for vaccination, cancer prevention, and global health.[1] A safe and effective vaccine against HPV has long been viewed as an enormous asset to cervical cancer prevention efforts worldwide. This is particularly true for places lacking robust Pap screening programs where cervical cancer has the greatest prevalence and mortality.[2] Well before its licensure, however, some observers noted significant obstacles that would need to be addressed for an HPV vaccination program to succeed. These included the vaccine's relatively high cost, availability, and opposition from socially conservative groups.[3] Such concerns associated with the implementation of HPV vaccination were soon overwhelmed by the furor that followed the unexpectedly early efforts by the U.S. state governments to require the vaccine as a condition of attendance in public schools, proposals imprecisely referred to as "mandates."[4] In this chapter, we review the controversy surrounding this debate and its effects on important ethical and public health issues that still need to be addressed.

Gardasil, the trade name of the HPV vaccine developed by Merck, was licensed by the U.S. Food and Drug Administration (FDA) on June 8, 2006. Using virus-like particle technology, the vaccine protects against HPV subtypes 16 and 18, which are responsible for approximately 70% of cervical cancer cases in the United States and Europe and 60% in the rest of the world.[5] The quadrivalent vaccine also includes protection against subtypes 6 and 11, the overwhelming causes of genital warts in both sexes. Internationally, Gardasil is licensed in seventy countries as of May 2007, with additional applications pending.[6] A second vaccine developed by GlaxoSmithKline under the trade name Cervarix was submitted to the FDA for licensure on March 29, 2007,

* Originally published in *Clinical Pharmacology & Therapeutics*, 2007, 82 (6):760–763. Reprinted with permission of John Wiley and Sons.

with approval expected in early 2008. This bivalent vaccine provides protection against HPV subtypes 16 and 18 only.

In clinical testing, Gardasil had impressive safety and efficacy profiles. In more than 20,000 research subjects, it was shown to be 100% effective in preventing the precursor lesions caused by HPV subtypes 16 and 18, with a highly favorable adverse event profile.[7] Within a month of its licensure, the Advisory Committee on Immunization Practices (ACIP) of the U.S. Centers for Disease Control and Prevention (CDC) recommended that all girls receive a three-dose series of Gardasil at ages 11–12 years or as early as 9 years of age based on a physician's judgment.[8] The ACIP also recommended that girls and women ages 13–26 years receive the vaccine. Priced at $120 per dose, Gardasil became the most expensive vaccine ever marketed.

Experts in vaccine policy generally agree regarding the activities crucial to the safe and appropriate introduction of a new vaccine.[9,10] For instance, it is critical that long-term monitoring of safety and effectiveness of a new vaccine begin as soon as it is introduced. This is necessary because far more people will now receive the vaccine than did so during clinical testing, and they will do so in relatively uncontrolled settings. Financing issues are also addressed during this period. For childhood vaccines in the United States, this includes the establishment of government-supported programs providing low-cost or free vaccines to uninsured and underinsured children. Additionally, private payers add the vaccine to their coverage portfolio and set reimbursement rates for providers. Perhaps most important, the initial months following the licensure of a new vaccine signal the beginning of comprehensive educational efforts, informing healthcare providers and parents about the new vaccine, the disease it protects against, and the vaccine's safety, risks, and benefits.[11]

For most vaccines, each of the activities described above gradually increases in size and scope. Well before the licensure of Gardasil, it became clear that its timetable would likely be dramatically accelerated. By fall 2005, major publications were previewing the licensure of the first "cancer vaccine" and the public debate likely to occur surrounding the administration of a vaccine against a sexually transmitted infection to teenage and pre-teenage girls.[12,13] Gardasil's licensure and the ACIP recommendation in June 2006 similarly appear to have received unprecedented media coverage compared to analogous moments for other new vaccines.

Throughout the summer, editorials and op-eds regarding the vaccine were overwhelmingly positive. They cited the vaccine's life-saving potential and encouraged swift efforts at increasing the vaccine's availability and addressing the limitations on access created as a result of its cost.[14,15] Even the socially conservative groups viewed as likely opponents of the vaccine against a sexually transmitted infection were supportive.[16] In general, these groups believed that the vaccine was a valuable tool against cervical cancer that should be widely available, but that decisions regarding who receives it should be left to parents alone.

This momentum and goodwill for the vaccine began to stall in September 2006 following the introduction of a bill in the Michigan state legislature that would require the vaccination of girls attending public schools. Such requirements are the mainstay of state childhood vaccination efforts, and proponents of vaccines point to them as the only proven way to ensure high rates of vaccination in the United States.[17] The proposed Michigan legislation and that of the many states that took similar steps in the ensuing months were remarkable for the speed with which they arrived. (A list of state action on HPV vaccination can be found at http://www.ncsl.org/research/health/ hpv-vaccine-state-legislation-and-statutes.aspx.) With less than a year having passed since the vaccine's licensure, the activities associated with the rollout of new vaccines had scarcely begun, much less matured to the point at which discussions of state requirements are typically initiated.

The possibility of state HPV vaccination requirements led to an unlikely alliance of civil libertarians and social conservatives, whose opposition to government interference with parental decision making trumped their general support for the vaccine, and self-described "vaccine safety" groups that are vocal critics of most U.S. vaccine policies. Joining them were prominent voices from the infectious disease, vaccine policy, and public health communities who were responding to perceived hastiness in the unprecedented pace from licensure to school requirements.[4] Together, individuals from these varied groups argued that it was either too soon to consider an HPV vaccine requirement, as there had not been adequate opportunities for public education or consensus building, or the sexual transmission of the virus did not warrant the kind of school mandate generally, although not exclusively, reserved for diseases easily transmitted in a school setting. (Hepatitis B and tetanus vaccines are notable exceptions. All fifty U.S. states and the District of Columbia require tetanus vaccination as a condition of school or day-care attendance, as do forty-seven states plus the District of Columbia for hepatitis B vaccine.)[18]

An ill-fated February 2007 executive order from Texas governor Rick Perry requiring HPV vaccination for all girls entering sixth grade dramatically increased the level of criticism toward state requirements and the processes by which they came about.[19] Lost in the coverage of possible political favors, conflicts of interest, and the power of corporate lobbying in Texas by Merck were any substantive arguments in favor of the executive order (since overturned by the Texas legislature) and the remarkable good that could be achieved by the vaccine independent of any state actions to promote its use.

Some critics of state HPV requirements emphasized how such policies violated obligations to respect parental autonomy. Imprecisely referring to state proposals as "mandates," these critics overlooked the opt-out provisions included by legislators that would have allowed a parent to obtain an exemption, even without a medical, philosophical, or religious justification. Instead, they critiqued the ethics of state HPV requirement proposals as though the broad opt-out provisions included in the proposed policies were nonexistent or unimportant.[4,20,21] In fact, although there have been calls to limit or even eliminate exemptions from state vaccination requirements because of links found between exemptions and additional mortality and morbidity from other vaccine-preventable diseases, there has not been a mandate—an absolute requirement to be vaccinated without exception—for any vaccine in the United States since World War I.[22,23]

Quite apart from whether it was prudent public health policy to implement state requirements for HPV vaccination so soon after the vaccine's licensure, these attacks on the state initiatives may have exacted a real ethical price in terms of the public's understanding of the justifications for state vaccination requirements generally, as well as the public's understanding of the merits of the HPV vaccine itself.

State vaccination requirements can provide the necessary stimulus to ensure that a vaccine reaches the populations who would benefit most from it, particularly those with limited access to health care. In the case of HPV, ensuring widespread availability of the vaccine is critical, as, for example, cervical cancer incidence and mortality are disproportionately greater in African Americans, a group with reduced Pap screening rates compared to the national average.[24] Although by no means a comprehensive solution to systemic disparities in the U.S. healthcare system, a state requirement incorporating opt-out provisions could be a useful approach to addressing disparities in cervical cancer incidence and mortality without infringing on the rights and prerogatives of others. The controversy created by state action in Texas and elsewhere may make it more difficult for states to reintroduce HPV vaccination requirements in the future, should a consensus emerge that such a policy makes good public health sense and is needed to ensure that the girls most in need of the vaccine receive it.

Part of the "staying power" of this controversy is that it is not only about "mandates" but also includes allegations about price gouging, corporate profits, and political motives behind the vaccine policy. Consider, for example, the role of Merck in advance of and since Gardasil's licensure. Even before the vaccine was licensed, the company was remarkably active in promoting awareness of HPV and its link to cervical cancer.[25] These public activities were later revealed to coexist with far less publicized lobbying of state legislatures and governors in support of school-entry requirements.[26] With Merck less than 3 years removed from the withdrawal of Vioxx and its accompanying financial and public relations damage, it is not surprising that many responded negatively to what appeared to be a company overly interested in influencing the opinions of policymakers, physicians, and the public regarding its new vaccine.

As some of the public health experts who opposed state requirements observed, there is value in the gradual development of vaccination programs over several years despite the understandable desire to maximize the vaccine's potential benefits as quickly as possible. Rare vaccine-related conditions can never be ruled out based on clinical trial data alone. The rapid distribution of any new product to millions of patients, particularly children, before the accumulation of some large-scale safety data could be devastating in the event, however unlikely, that a safety-related concern emerges in a vaccine's first few years. For this reason, prudence suggests the temporary postponement of implementing state requirements, given the surge in vaccine administration that would quickly follow.

In the specific case of HPV vaccine, it is also crucial for policymakers to evaluate the still emerging data on its short- and long-term efficacy. In a healthcare environment that limits spending on prevention, a vaccine series totaling more than $300 is a significant burden on public funds that subsidize vaccine costs for uninsured or underinsured children. It is still unknown whether booster vaccinations will be required and, if so, how often. Currently, long-term follow-up from Merck's clinical trials has shown 5 years of protection from the initial vaccine series.[27] The extent of longer term protection is uncertain, as is the vaccine's level of cross-protection, the additional benefit provided against HPV subtypes not included in the vaccine.[28] Although these data continue to emerge, legislators and other policymakers would be wise to resist making definitive assessments of the priority assigned to HPV vaccination efforts relative to other public health and healthcare programs.

As these data are compiled, efforts should be refocused on building public understanding and support for the value of HPV vaccination. Despite the frequent discussion of mandates and school-entry requirements, the success of U.S. vaccination efforts—for Gardasil or any vaccine—depends on maintaining public confidence in the fundamental value of vaccination and trust in the individuals responsible for the design and implementation of vaccination programs. Without widespread support, it is unrealistic to think that any system of state requirements could be enforced by an already overburdened and understaffed public health system.

It remains to be seen how much confusion and public distrust has been created by seemingly well-intended but premature efforts in the United States to impose state requirements for vaccination of girls against HPV. Although the majority of respondents in one recent study opposed HPV vaccine requirements, the more important question, still unanswered, is what level of enthusiasm still exists for the vaccine itself.[29]

At the same time, the outcry surrounding the proposed state vaccination requirements in the United States is of little relevance to the rest of the world, particularly those countries where cervical cancer is a far greater cause of suffering and death. With an HPV vaccine badly needed in parts of Africa, Asia, and South America, time and energy would be better spent designing and implementing programs aimed at the affordable and effective vaccination of developing world populations. Given the potentially enormous worldwide benefit of a safe and effective HPV vaccine, every critique, however articulate, of the U.S. state requirement debate should be viewed as another missed opportunity to call attention to the far more pressing need for the vaccine internationally. Annually, 493,000 new cases of cervical cancer are diagnosed and 274,000 deaths are caused by the disease, most of which occur in the developing world.[2]

Even if ways are found to make HPV vaccine available to girls and women in the developing world, hesitancy about vaccine requirements in the United States may well be seized on by vaccine critics in poor nations as a reason for not utilizing the vaccine to prevent these deaths. HPV vaccination efforts in the developing world should grow incrementally in a manner similar to the gradual introduction of a vaccine in the United States. The gradual implementation of vaccine programs permits close monitoring of potential adverse events as well as an opportunity to identify ways to improve even successful programs over time.

This process must also recognize the additional challenges unique to vaccinating populations in the developing world. Although efforts to introduce HPV vaccine to the developing world have begun, the pace of activity around this and earlier vaccines suggests that a hasty, large-scale rollout of the vaccine in those nations is extremely unlikely to occur. However, the reverse scenario—years of delays as pricing, delivery, and administrative issues are resolved—remains a significant and inexcusable possibility.

Provided that the events of the past year have not done irreparable damage to cervical cancer prevention efforts overall, attention should be directed toward the careful assessment of long-term vaccine safety and effectiveness as increasing numbers of girls and women are vaccinated. At the same time, sound programs remain crucial to educate providers and parents about the scope and severity of the HPV-related diseases and the risks and benefits of the vaccine. Such a model would follow the long successful pattern for the steady growth of a new vaccination program. Finally, policymakers must not lose sight of the unique challenges and remarkable value that HPV vaccines are highly likely to have outside the United States. This would justify additional efforts being directed toward studying and fulfilling this potential.

References

1. U.S. Food and Drug Administration. 2006. FDA licenses new vaccine for prevention of cervical cancer and other diseases in females caused by human papillomavirus. FDA press release. Available at: http://www.fda.gov/NewsEvents/Newsroom/PressAnnouncements/2006/ucm108666 .htm. Accessed August 20, 2007.

2. Parkin, D. M., and F. Bray. 2006. Chapter 2: The burden of HPV-related cancers. *Vaccine* 24 (suppl 3):S11–S25.

3. McNeil, C. 2006. Coming soon: Cervical cancer vaccines, and an array of public health issues. *J Natl Cancer Inst* 98:432–434.

4. Gostin, L. O., and C. D. DeAngelis. 2007. Mandatory HPV vaccination: Public health vs private wealth. *JAMA* 297:1921–1923.

5. Clifford, G. M., J. S. Smith, M. Plummer, N. Munoz, and S. Franceschi. 2003. Human papillomavirus types in invasive cervical cancer worldwide: A meta-analysis. *Br J Cancer* 88:63–73.

6. Merck. 2007. Data published in *The Lancet* show Gardasil was 100 percent effective in preventing high-grade vulvar and vaginal lesions caused by HPV types 16 and 18. Merck press release. Available at: http://www.businesswire.com/news/home/20070517006085/en/Data-Published -Lancet-Show-GARDASIL-100-Percent/. Accessed June 5, 2007.

7. Gardasil [Quadrivalent Human Papillomavirus (Types 6, 11, 16, 18) Recombinant Vaccine]. Package insert. Available at: http://www.merck.com/product/usa/pi_circulars/g/gardasil/gardasil _pi.pdf. Accessed August 20, 2007.

8. U.S. Centers for Disease Control and Prevention. 2007. Quadrivalent human papillomavirus vaccine: Recommendations of the Advisory Committee on Immunization Practices (ACIP). *MMWR Morb Mortal Wkly Rep* 56 (RR-2):1–24.

9. Institute of Medicine. 2000. *Calling the Shots: Immunization Finance Policies and Practices*. Washington, DC : National Academies Press.

10. Orenstein, W. A., L. E. Rodewald, and A. R. Hinman. Immunization in the United States. In: *Vaccines*, 4th ed., eds. S. A. Plotkin and W. A. Orenstein, 1357–1386. Philadelphia: Saunders.

11. Sherris, J., A. Friedman, S. Wittet, P. Davies, M. Steben, and M. Sariya. 2006. Chapter 25: Education, training, and communication for HPV vaccines. *Vaccine* 24 (suppl 3):S210–S218.

12. Rubin, R. 2005, October 19. Injected into a controversy. *USA Today*.

13. Guyon, J. 2005, October 31. The coming storm over a cancer vaccine. *Fortune*.

14. Preventing a cancer. Editorial. 2006, June 18. *Boston Globe*.

15. A major advance in women's health. Editorial. 2006, June 19. *Philadelphia Inquirer* .

16. Sprigg, P. 2006, July 15. Pro-family, pro-vaccine—but keep it voluntary. *Washington Post*.

17. Hinman, A. R., W. A. Orenstein, D. E. Williamson, and D. Darrington. 2002. Childhood immunization: Laws that work. *J Law Med Ethics* 30 (suppl):122–127.

18. Immunization Action Coalition. 2007. State mandates on immunization and vaccine-preventable diseases. Immunization Action Coalition. Available at: http://www.immunize.org/laws. Accessed June 11, 2007.

19. Saul, S., and A. Pollack. 2007, February 17. Furor on rush to require cervical cancer vaccine. *New York Times.*

20. Zimmerman, R. K. 2006. Ethical analysis of HPV vaccine policy options. *Vaccine* 24:4812–4820.

21. Colgrove, J. 2006. The ethics and politics of compulsory HPV vaccination. *N Engl J Med* 355:2389–2391.

22. Omer, S. B., W. K. Pan, N. A. Halsey, S. Stokley, L. H. Moulton, A. M. Navar, et al. 2006. Nonmedical exemptions to school immunization requirements: Secular trends and association of state policies with pertussis incidence. *JAMA* 296:1757–1763.

23. Offit, P. A. 2007, January 20. Fatal exemption. *Wall Street Journal.*

24. Bonney, L. E., M. Lally, D. R. Williams, M. Stein, and T. Flanigan. 2006. Where to begin human papillomavirus vaccination? *Lancet Infect Dis* 6:389.

25. Zimm, A., and J. Blum. 2006. Merck promotes cervical cancer shot by publicizing viral cause. *Bloomberg News.* Available at: http://www.bloomberg.com/apps/news?pid=10000103&sid=amVj.y3Eynz8&refer=us. Accessed June 26, 2007.

26. Pollack, A., and S. Saul. 2007, February 21. Merck to halt lobbying for vaccine for girls. *New York Times.*

27. Villa, L. L., R. L. Costa, C. A. Petta, R. P. Andrade, J. Paavonen, O. E. Iversen, et al. 2006. High sustained efficacy of a prophylactic quadrivalent human papillomavirus types 6/11/16/18 L1 virus-like particle vaccine through 5 years of follow-up. *Br J Cancer* 95:1459–1466.

28. Koutsky, L. A., and Harper, D. M. 2006. Chapter 13: Current findings from prophylactic HPV vaccine trials. *Vaccine* 24 (suppl 3):S114–S121.

29. CS Mott Children's Hospital. 2007. Majority of US parents not in favor of state HPV vaccine mandates. CHEAR—National Poll on Children's Health (2007). Available at: http://www.med.umich.edu/opm/newspage/2007/poll3.htm. Accessed June 5, 2007.

25 Responding to Parental Refusals of Immunization of Children

Douglas S. Diekema and the American Academy of Pediatrics Committee on Bioethics[*]

The immunization of children against a multitude of infectious agents has been hailed as one of the most important health interventions of the twentieth century.[1-3] Immunizations have eliminated smallpox infection worldwide, driven polio from North America, and made formerly common infections such as diphtheria, tetanus, measles, and invasive *Hemophilus influenzae* infections rare occurrences. By one account, pediatric immunizations are responsible for preventing 3 million deaths in children each year worldwide.[3] Despite this success, some parents continue to refuse immunizations for their children. The number of pertussis cases has increased steadily in the United States over the past 20 years, and Web sites critical of immunization are prominent on the Internet, a source that many parents rely on for health information.[4] It is ironic that the remarkable success of vaccine programs has resulted in a situation in which most parents have no memory of the devastating effects of illnesses such as poliomyelitis, measles, and other vaccine-preventable diseases, making it more difficult for them to appreciate the benefits of immunization.

According to a periodic survey of fellows of the American Academy of Pediatrics (AAP) on immunization-administration practices, seven out of ten pediatricians reported that they had had a parent refuse an immunization on behalf of a child in the 12 months preceding the survey.[5] The measles-mumps-rubella (MMR) vaccine was refused most frequently, followed by varicella vaccine, pneumococcal conjugate vaccine, hepatitis B vaccine, and diphtheria and tetanus toxoids and pertussis vaccines. Further, 4% of pediatricians had refused permission for an immunization for their own children younger than 11 years. When faced with parents who refuse immunization, almost all pediatricians reported that they attempt to educate parents regarding the importance of immunization and document the refusal in the patient's medical record.

A small number of pediatricians reported that they always (4.8%) or sometimes (18.1%) tell parents that they will no longer serve as the child's physician if, after educational efforts, the parents continue to refuse permission for an immunization.[5]

The AAP strongly endorses universal immunization. However, for universal childhood immunization programs to be successful, parents must comply with immunization recommendations. The problem of parental refusal of immunization for children is an important one for pediatricians. Parents may have many reasons for refusing immunization. Some parents may object to immunization on religious or philosophical grounds, some may object to what seems to be a painful assault on their child, and others may believe that the benefits of immunization do not justify the risks to their child. Many commonly held beliefs about the risks of immunization are not supported by available data, and they frequently originate from the unsupported claims of organizations that are critical of immunization. These antivaccine information sources not only propagate unproven claims regarding vaccines but also may undermine the physician–family relationship by challenging the parents' trust of the medical profession.

What should the pediatrician do when faced with a parent who refuses to consent to immunizations for a child? The goal of this clinical report is to provide guidance to the pediatrician faced with this difficult situation. The physician faced with a parent who refuses to immunize a child faces three important and distinct issues that will be addressed in this chapter. First, are there situations in which parents who withhold immunizations from their children risk harming them sufficiently that their decision constitutes actionable medical neglect and should be reported to state child protective services agencies? Second, are there situations in which a parental decision to withhold immunization from a child puts other individuals at risk of harm sufficient to justify public health intervention? Finally, how should the pediatrician respond to a parent who refuses immunizations for his or her child?

Parental Refusals and the Best Interests of Children

Healthcare professionals and parents are bound by the duty to seek medical benefit for and minimize harm to children in their care. When faced with the decision to immunize a child, the welfare of the child should be the primary focus. However, parents and physicians may not always agree on what constitutes the best interest of an individual child. In those situations, physicians may need to tolerate decisions they disagree with if those decisions are not likely to be harmful to the child.[6] Although decision making involving the health care of children should be shared between physicians and parents, parental permission must be sought before children receive medical interventions, including immunizations.[7] Parents are free to make choices regarding medical care unless those choices place their child at substantial risk of serious harm.

Whether parents place their children at substantial risk of serious harm by refusing immunization will depend on several factors, including the probability of contracting the disease if unimmunized and the morbidity and mortality associated with infection. The results of such an analysis will also vary depending on the prevalence of disease in the community in which the child resides or the areas in which the child is likely to travel. The balance between the risks and benefits to a given individual favors immunization most strongly when rates of immunization in the community are low and disease prevalence is high. In most cases, however, as immunization rates increase and disease prevalence decreases, the balance may tip the other way.[8,9] Although the benefits of a measles vaccine program, for example, clearly outweigh the risks at a population level,[10] an unimmunized child living in a well-immunized community derives significant indirect protection from herd immunity.[11] Even in a community with high immunization rates, the risk assumed by an unimmunized child is likely to be greater than the risks associated with immunization. However, the risk remains low, and in most cases, the parent who refuses immunizations on behalf of his or her child living in a well-immunized community does not place the child at substantial risk of serious harm.

The role of the physician in these situations is to provide parents with the risk and benefit information necessary to make an informed decision and attempt to correct any misinformation or misperceptions that may exist. For example, in a national survey of parents, 25% believed falsely that their child's immune system could become weakened as a result of too many immunizations.[12] Exploring and addressing parental concerns may be an effective strategy with reluctant parents. Only in rare cases in which the decision of a parent places a child at substantial risk of serious harm may the healthcare professional be obligated to involve state agencies in seeking to provide the necessary immunization over the parents' objections. For example, for the situation in which a child has sustained a deep and contaminated puncture wound, it might be justifiable to challenge the decision of a child's parents to refuse treatment with tetanus vaccine. In these situations, the healthcare professional would involve the appropriate state child protective services agency because of the concern about medical neglect. It would be up to the state agency to decide whether immunization would be required. Although this state role has been recognized as constitutionally valid in the United States, courts have closely examined such actions, showing reluctance to require medical treatment over the objection of parents "except where immediate action is necessary or where the potential for harm is rather serious."[13]

Community Interests and Public Health

The benefits provided by most vaccines extend beyond benefit to the individual who is immunized. There is also a significant public health benefit. Parents who choose not to immunize their own children increase the potential for harm to other persons in four important ways.[14] First, should an unimmunized child contract a disease, that child poses a potential threat to other unimmunized children. Second, even in a fully immunized population, a small percentage of immunized individuals will either remain or become susceptible to disease. These individuals have done everything they can to protect themselves through immunization, yet they remain at risk. Third, some children cannot be immunized because of underlying medical conditions. These individuals derive important benefit from herd immunity and may be harmed by contracting disease from those who remain unimmunized. Finally, immunized individuals are harmed by the cost of medical care for those who choose not to immunize their children and whose children then contract vaccine-preventable disease.

A parent's refusal to immunize his or her child also raises an important question of justice that has been described as the problem of "free riders."[14–16] Parents who refuse immunization on behalf of their children are, in a sense, free riders who take advantage of the benefit created by the participation and assumption of immunization risk or burden by others while refusing to participate in the program themselves. The decision to refuse to immunize a child is made less risky because others have created an environment in which herd immunity will likely keep the unimmunized child safe. These individuals place family interest ahead of civic responsibility. Although such parents do reject what many would consider to be a moral duty, coercive measures to require immunization of a child over parental objections are justified only in cases in which others are placed at substantial risk of serious harm by the parental decision.

Compulsory immunization laws in the United States have been upheld repeatedly as a reasonable exercise of the state's police power in the absence of an epidemic or even a single case.[17,18] They also have been found to be constitutional even for cases in which the laws conflict with the religious beliefs of individuals.[19]

When others are placed at substantial risk of serious harm, the range of choices of the individual may be restricted. With regard to immunization, the key question becomes whether the harms associated with unimmunized individuals are great enough to make restrictions permissible. In times of epidemic disease, when an effective vaccine can end the epidemic and protect those individuals who have not yet contracted the disease, the answer clearly is yes.

In a highly immunized population in which disease prevalence is low, the risk of disease from the small number of children who remain unimmunized does not usually pose a significant enough health risk to others to justify state action.[20] Diseases with high morbidity and mortality (such as smallpox), however, might create a situation in which even a single case of infection would justify mandatory immunization of the population. For most routine vaccines, less forcible alternatives can be used justifiably to encourage parents to immunize children because of the public health benefit. In the case of vaccines routinely recommended for children, the AAP supports the use of appropriate public health measures, education, and incentives for immunization.[7] Because unimmunized children do pose a risk to other children who lack immunity to vaccine-preventable infections, the AAP also supports immunization requirements for school entry.

Responding to Parents Who Refuse Immunization for Their Children

What is the pediatrician to do when faced with a parent who refuses immunization for his or her child? First and most important, the pediatrician should listen carefully and respectfully to the parents' concerns, recognizing that some parents may not use the same decision criteria as the physician and may weigh evidence differently than the physician does.[21] Vaccines are very safe, but they are not risk free, nor are they 100% effective.[22] This fact poses a dilemma for many parents and should not be minimized. The pediatrician should share honestly what is and is not known about the risks and benefits of the vaccine in question, attempt to understand the parents' concerns about immunization, and attempt to correct any misperceptions and misinformation.[23–25] Pediatricians should also assist parents in understanding that the risks of any vaccine should not be considered in isolation but in comparison to the risks of remaining unimmunized. For example, although the risk of encephalopathy related to the measles vaccine is 1 in 1 million, the risk of encephalopathy from measles illness is 1,000 times greater.[22] Parents can also be referred to one of several reputable and data-based Web sites for additional information on specific immunizations and the diseases they prevent (see pages 52 and 53 of the Red Book[25] for a list of Internet resources related to immunization).

Many parents have concerns related to one or two specific vaccines. A useful strategy in working with families that refuse immunization is to discuss each vaccine separately. The benefits and risks of vaccines differ, and parents who are reluctant to accept the administration of one vaccine may be willing to allow others.

Parents also may have concerns about administering multiple vaccines to a child in a single visit. In some cases, taking steps to reduce the pain of injection, such as those suggested in the Red Book,[26] may be sufficient. In other cases, parents may be willing to permit a schedule of immunization that does not require multiple injections at a single visit.

Physicians should also explore the possibility that cost is a reason for refusing immunization. For parents whose child does not have adequate preventive care insurance coverage, even the administrative costs and copayments associated with immunization can pose substantial barriers. In such cases, the physician should work with the family to help them obtain appropriate immunizations for the child.

For all cases in which parents refuse vaccine administration, pediatricians should take advantage of their ongoing relationship with the family and revisit the immunization discussion on each subsequent visit. As respect, communication, and information build over time in a professional relationship, parents may be willing to reconsider previous vaccine refusals.

Continued refusal after adequate discussion should be respected unless the child is put at significant risk of serious harm (e.g., during an epidemic). Only then should state agencies be involved to override parental discretion on the basis of medical neglect. Physician concerns about liability should be addressed by good documentation of the discussion of the benefits of immunization and the risks associated with remaining unimmunized. Physicians also may wish to consider having the parents sign a refusal waiver (a sample refusal-to-immunize waiver can be found at https://www.aap.org/en-us/Documents/immunization_refusaltovaccinate.pdf). In general, pediatricians should endeavor not to discharge patients from their practices solely because a parent refuses to immunize a child. However, when a substantial level of distrust develops, significant differences in the philosophy of care emerge, or poor quality of communication persists, the pediatrician may encourage the family to find another physician or practice. Although pediatricians have the option of terminating the physician–patient relationship, they cannot do so without giving sufficient advance notice to the patient or custodial parent or legal guardian to permit another health care professional to be secured.[27] Such decisions should be unusual and generally made only after attempts have been made to work with the family. Families with doubts about immunization should still have access to good medical care, and maintaining the relationship in the face of disagreement conveys respect and at the same time allows the child access to medical care. Furthermore, a continuing relationship allows additional opportunity to discuss the issue of immunization over time.

References

1. Centers for Disease Control and Prevention. 1999. Impact of vaccines universally recommended for children—United States, 1990–1998. *MMWR Morb Mortal Wkly Rep* 48:243–248.

2. Centers for Disease Control and Prevention. 1999. Ten great public health achievements—United States, 1990–1999. *MMWR Morb Mortal Wkly Rep* 48:241–243.

3. Bonanni, P. 1999. Demographic impact of vaccination: A review. *Vaccine* 17 (suppl 3): S120–S125.

4. Davies, P., S. Chapman, and J. Leask. 2002. Antivaccination activists on the World Wide Web. *Arch Dis Child* 87:22–25.

5. American Academy of Pediatrics, Division of Health Policy Research. 2001. *Periodic Survey of Fellows No. 48: Immunization Administration Practices*. Elk Grove Village, IL: American Academy of Pediatrics.

6. Buchanan, A. E., and D. W. Brock. 1990. *Deciding for Others: The Ethics of Surrogate Decision Making*. New York, NY: Cambridge University Press.

7. American Academy of Pediatrics, Committee on Bioethics. 1995. Informed consent, parental permission, and assent in pediatric practice. *Pediatrics* 95:314–317.

8. 1981. Pertussis vaccine. *Br Med J (Clin Res Ed)* 282:1563–1564.

9. 1981. Vaccination against whooping cough. *Lancet* 1 (8230):1138–1139.

10. Hinman, A. R., and J. P. Koplan. 1984. Pertussis and pertussis vaccine: Reanalysis of benefits, risks, and costs. *JAMA* 251:3109–3113.

11. Fox, J. P., L. Elveback, W. Scott, L. Gatewood, and E. Ackerman. 1971. Herd immunity: Basic concept and relevance to public health immunization practices. *Am J Epidemiol* 94:179–189.

12. Gellin, B. G., E. W. Maibach, and E. K. Marcuse. 2000. Do parents understand immunizations? A national telephone survey. *Pediatrics* 106:1097–1102.

13. Wing, K. R. 1990. *The Law and the Public's Health*. 3rd ed. Ann Arbor, MI: Health Administration Press.

14. Veatch, R. M. 1987. The ethics of promoting herd immunity. *Fam Community Health* 10:44–53.

15. Menzel, P. T. 1995. The pros and cons of immunisation—paper four: Non-compliance: Fair or free-riding. *Health Care Anal* 3:113–115.

16. Ball, L. K., G. Evans, and A. Bostrom. 1998. Risky business: Challenges in vaccine risk communication. *Pediatrics* 101:453–458.

17. McMenamin, J. P., and W. B. Tiller. 1991. Children as patients. In: *Legal Medicine: Legal Dynamics of Medical Encounters*. 2nd ed., *American College of Legal Medicine*. 282–317. St Louis, MO: Mosby Year Book.

18. Dover, T. E. 1979. An evaluation of immunization regulations in light of religious objections and the developing right of privacy. *Univ Dayton Law Rev* 4:401–424.

19. Jacobson v. Massachusetts, 197 US 11 (1905).

20. Ross, L. F., and T. J. Aspinwall. 1997. Religious exemptions to the immunization statutes: balancing public health and religious freedom. *J Law Med Ethics* 25:202–209, 283.

21. Meszaros, J. R., D. A. Asch, J. Baron, J. C. Hershey, H. Kunreuther, and J. Schwartz-Buzaglo. 1996. Cognitive processes and the decisions of some parents to forego pertussis vaccination for their children. *J Clin Epidemiol* 49:697–703.

22. Maldonado, Y. A. 2002. Current controversies in vaccination: Vaccine safety. *JAMA* 288:3155–3158.

23. Wilson, C. B., and E. K. Marcuse. 2001. Vaccine safety–vaccine benefits: Science and the public's perception. *Nat Rev Immunol* 1:160–165.

24. Pattison, S. 2001. Ethical debate: Vaccination against mumps, measles, and rubella: Is there a case for deepening the debate? Dealing with uncertainty. *BMJ* 323:840.

25. American Academy of Pediatrics. 2003. Parental misconceptions about immunization. In: *Red Book: 2003 Report of the Committee on Infectious Diseases,* 26th ed., eds. L. K. Pickering, 50–53. Elk Grove Village, IL: American Academy of Pediatrics.

26. American Academy of Pediatrics. 2003. Managing injection pain. In: *Red Book: 2003 Report of the Committee on Infectious Diseases,* 26th ed., eds. L. K. Pickering, 20–21. Elk Grove Village, IL: American Academy of Pediatrics.

27. American Medical Association, Council on Ethical and Judicial Affairs. 2002. Termination of the physician-patient relationship. In: *Code of Medical Ethics: Current Opinions, 2002–* 2003 ed., 110. Chicago, IL: American Medical Association.

26 Influenza Vaccination of Healthcare Personnel: Revised Society for Healthcare Epidemiology of America (SHEA) Position Paper (*Excerpt*)

Thomas R. Talbot, Hilary Babcock, Arthur L. Caplan, Deborah Cotton, Lisa L. Maragakis, Gregory A. Poland, Edward J. Septimus, Michael L. Tapper, and David J. Weber[*]

Vaccination of healthcare personnel (HCP) serves several purposes: (1) prevent transmission to patients, including those with a lower likelihood of vaccination response themselves; (2) reduce the risk that the HCP will become infected with influenza; (3) create "herd immunity" that protects both HCP and patients who are unable to receive vaccine or unlikely to respond with a sufficient antibody response; (4) maintain a critical societal workforce during disease outbreaks; and (5) set an example concerning the importance of vaccination for every person.

Unfortunately, despite tremendous efforts to promote HCP influenza vaccination by government agencies, regulatory groups, professional societies, and visible vaccination champions, influenza vaccination rates among HCP remain unacceptably low. In a 2009 report by the Research and Development (RAND) Corporation, only 53% of surveyed HCP reported receipt of influenza vaccination during the 2008–2009 influenza season.[1] In addition, in 2009, 39% of HCP stated they had no intention of getting vaccinated even with the heightened concern surrounding influenza with the novel H1N1 influenza A pandemic.[2] These data mirror findings from the National Health Interview Survey, in which HCP influenza vaccination rates did not change significantly from the 2003–2004 influenza season (44.8%) through the 2007–2008 season (49.0%).[3]

Much discussion has occurred surrounding the ethics and legality of mandatory influenza vaccination programs for HCP.[4–10] Those against mandatory programs argue that the data supporting the impact of HCP influenza vaccination on patients are inconclusive, voluntary programs have not been given enough time to have an impact or have not addressed attitudinal barriers to vaccination effectively, and such policies may place patient protection above HCP autonomy and do not respect HCP autonomy. These practical and moral arguments are not persuasive.

* Originally published in *Infection Control and Hospital Epidemiology*, 2010, 31 (10):987–995. Republished with permission.

Voluntary vaccination programs have been in place for decades, with little evidence for an overall increase in HCP vaccination rates. Furthermore, multifaceted mandatory vaccination programs have been tried and tested and have been found to be the single most effective strategy to increase HCP vaccination rates, with multiple facilities and systems achieving vaccination coverage of more than 95%.[11]

Those in support of mandatory programs argue that influenza vaccination is an ethical responsibility of HCP because HCP have a duty to act in the best interests of their patients (beneficence), to not place their patients at undue risk of harm (nonmaleficence), and to protect the vulnerable and those at high risk of infection. The duty to put patient interests first is outlined in nearly every professional code of ethics in medicine, nursing, and other healthcare fields. Because the likelihood of a serious adverse reaction to influenza vaccine is extremely low, the duty to protect vulnerable patients and to put their interest above the personal interest of the healthcare worker does not demand undue sacrifice. Finally, the use of mandatory vaccination programs for the public health and protection of the greater population has clear legal precedents.[12]

Revised SHEA Position on Influenza Vaccination of HCP

SHEA views influenza vaccination of HCP as a *core patient and HCP safety practice* with which noncompliance should not be tolerated. We believe it is the professional and ethical responsibility of HCP and the institutions within which they work to prevent the spread of infectious pathogens to their patients by following evidence-based infection prevention practices. Just as HCP would not be allowed to participate in a surgical procedure without first performing an appropriate surgical hand scrub or wearing appropriate sterile attire, failure to perform a basic patient safety intervention, such as influenza vaccination, is unacceptable. Therefore, for the safety of patients and HCP, SHEA endorses a policy in which influenza vaccination is an ongoing condition of HCP employment, unpaid service, or receipt of professional privileges.

Because the types of HCP included in vaccination programs may vary, with contract staff, private physicians, students, and volunteers often excluded, this recommendation applies to all HCP practicing in all healthcare settings (including contract workers, independent practitioners, volunteers, students, and product vendors), regardless of whether the HCP have direct patient contact or the HCP are directly employed by the facility.[13,14]

Exemptions to influenza vaccination mandates should be allowed only for medical contraindications to vaccination, specifically allergy to eggs and prior allergic or severe adverse reactions to influenza vaccine. Such exemptions should be adequately documented and reviewed before allowing exemption from this requirement. Some facilities have allowed religious exemptions as part of HCP vaccination programs requiring that those requesting a religious exemption demonstrate a deeply held conviction, as determined by review by an institutional panel. However, most religions do not prohibit vaccination. Legal pressures to avoid discrimination implied by allowing religious exemptions for only one religion or requiring an individual to belong to an organized religion to get a religious exemption have broadened the use of religious exemptions to others. Because vaccination of HCP is a patient safety and public health intervention, SHEA does not endorse the use of religious exemptions to influenza vaccination because failure to be vaccinated results in an unacceptable risk to patients and other HCP. Legal support for such policies has been noted with school-entry vaccination requirements, in which the absence of religious exemptions has been legally upheld against objections that such policies infringed on individuals' religious principles.[8]

Personal belief or philosophical exemptions (e.g., for those who do not believe in the need for influenza vaccination or for those who are opposed to the concept of *mandatory* vaccination) should not be allowed. The allowance of personal belief exemptions for school-entry vaccination requirements has been associated with an increased risk of the acquisition and transmission of vaccine-preventable diseases.[13] Although a few facilities and systems have been successful in achieving high vaccination rates in the setting of personal belief exemptions,[14,15] allowance of personal belief exemptions runs counter to the concept that HCP influenza vaccination is a core patient safety intervention from which the HCP cannot merely opt out, particularly given the known safety and efficacy of influenza vaccination.

Influenza vaccination of HCP is an important and key component of infection prevention programs designed to reduce healthcare-associated influenza. As with any core patient safety practice, low rates of compliance that place patients and HCP at risk are unacceptable. Because HCP influenza vaccination rates in the setting of voluntary programs have remained low over the nearly three decades that HCP influenza vaccination has been recommended, SHEA endorses policies that require influenza vaccination as a condition of employment as part of a comprehensive influenza infection control program.

References

1. Harris, K. M., J. Maurer, and N. Lurie. 2009. Influenza vaccine use by adults in the USA: Snapshot from the end of the 2008–2009 vaccination season. Rand Health. Available at: http://www.rand.org/pubs/occasional_papers/2009/RAND_OP270.pdf. Accessed February 19, 2010.

2. Ibid.

3. Caban-Martinez, A. J., D. J. Lee, E. P. Davila, W. G. LeBlanc, K. L. Arheart, K. E. McCollister, et al. 2010. Sustained low influenza vaccination rates in US healthcare workers. *Prev Med* 50 (4):210–212.

4. Anikeeva, O., A. Braunack-Mayer, and W. Rogers. 2009. Requiring influenza vaccination for healthcare workers. *Am J Public Health* 99 (1):24–29.

5. Helms, C. M., and P. M. Polgreen. 2008. Should influenza immunisation be mandatory for healthcare workers? Yes. *BMJ* 337:a2142.

6. Isaacs, D., and J. Leask. 2008. Should influenza immunisation be mandatory for healthcare workers? No. *BMJ* 337:a2140.

7. Steckel, C. M. 2007. Mandatory influenza immunization for healthcare workers: An ethical discussion. *AAOHN J* 55 (1):34–39.

8. Stewart, A. M. 2009. Mandatory vaccination of healthcare workers. *N Engl J Med* 361 (21):2015–2017.

9. Tilburt, J. C., P. S. Mueller, A. L. Ottenberg, G. A. Poland, and B. A. Koenig. 2008. Facing the challenges of influenza in healthcare settings: The ethical rationale for mandatory seasonal influenza vaccination and its implications for future pandemics. *Vaccine* 26 (suppl 4):D27–D30.

10. van Delden, J. J., R. Ashcroft, A. Dawson, G. Marckmann, R. Upshur, and M. F. Verweij. 2008. The ethics of mandatory vaccination against influenza for healthcare workers. *Vaccine* 26 (44):5562–5566.

11. Lindley, M. C., J. Yonek, F. Ahmed, J. F. Perz, and G. Williams Torres. 2009. Measurement of influenza vaccination coverage among healthcare personnel in US hospitals. *Infect Control Hosp Epidemiol* 30 (12):1150–1157.

12. Talbot, T. R., T. H. Dellit, J. Hebden, D. Sama, and J. Cuny. 2010. Factors associated with increased healthcare worker influenza vaccination rates: Results of a national survey of university hospitals and medical centers. *Infect Control Hosp Epidemiol* 31 (5):456–462.

13. Omer, S. B., D. A. Salmon, W. A. Orenstein, M. P. deHart, and N. Halsey. 2009. Vaccine refusal, mandatory immunization, and the risks of vaccine-preventable diseases. *N Engl J Med* 360 (19):1981–1988.

14. Cormier, S. B., E. Septimus, J. A. Moody, J. D. Hickok, and J. B. Perlin. 2010, March 20. Implementation of a successful seasonal influenza vaccine strategy in a large healthcare system. In: Program and abstracts of Fifth Decennial International Conference on Healthcare-Associated Infections, Atlanta, GA. Abstract 385.

15. Palmore, T. N., J. P. Vandersluis, J. Morris, A. Michelin, L. M. Ruprecht, J. M. Schmitt, and D. K. Henderson. 2009. A successful mandatory influenza vaccination campaign using an innovative electronic tracking system. *Infect Control Hosp Epidemiol* 30 (12):1137–1142.

V Pandemics and Bioterrorism: The Role of Vaccines in Preparedness and Response

In addition to their ongoing role in day-to-day disease prevention efforts in the United States and worldwide, vaccines figure prominently in efforts to prepare for and respond to public health emergencies such as naturally occurring pandemics and manmade acts of bioterrorism. Pandemic influenza of avian origin, "bird flu," was a primary concern of governments in the initial years of the twenty-first century. Those planning efforts were adapted when a novel H1N1 influenza pandemic emerged in 2009–2010. A vaccination program was quickly launched as part of the global response, but the pandemic had already begun to wane by the time large-scale vaccination was ready to commence.

During this same period, bioterrorism—particularly using smallpox or anthrax—was a focus of substantial planning, research, and investment. Attention to the threat of bioterrorism followed the terrorist events of September 11, 2001, and the anthrax attacks by mail later that fall. Although vaccines had long existed against both primary potential agents of bioterrorism, hundreds of millions of dollars were spent refining and stockpiling existing vaccines and seeking to develop new, improved vaccines to strengthen preparedness for a potential bioterror attack.

More recently, the value of vaccines has been a central component of discussions regarding newly emerging infectious threats to public health, as occurred during the global Ebola outbreak centered in West Africa that began in 2013 (discussed in Part VII). The Zika outbreak starting in South and Central America prompted similar attention to what role a vaccine could play in long-term response plans as well as scrutiny of how long it takes for such a vaccine to become available.

The specifics of any potential new outbreak and the particular pathogen involved would bring unique circumstances and demand new attention as more is learned about them. But efforts to study, develop, and eventually distribute vaccines in response to public health emergencies such as pandemics and bioterrorism raise many common issues of policy and ethics, as chapters in this section illustrate. We begin with several chapters on an issue that would affect the public quite directly—the distribution of vaccine doses and the prioritization of various groups in these health emergencies when vaccine supplies are inadequate to meet demand. Ezekiel Emanuel and Alan Wertheimer propose an approach that assigns value to individuals moving through the various stages of life and having made investments in their futures, a view that places the very young and very old behind those in the middle years of life in receiving scarce vaccine doses. Kristy Buccieri and Stephen Gaetz review many proposals about allocation before suggesting an alternative of their own, the prioritization of groups such as the homeless, which are already underserved by the healthcare system and thereby more likely to be susceptible to health threats and their effects.

Turning to issues of vaccine distribution across the international community, Tadataka Yamada examines the responsibilities of rich countries and multinational vaccine manufacturers to work to ensure that vaccines for global health emergencies are available to all populations that could benefit from them, not simply allocated based on countries' wealth, the locations of vaccine manufacturing facilities, or similar factors. David Fidler continues on these questions of equity in global vaccine access, noting the important role and limitations of international law in shaping agreements to share viral specimens and resources such as vaccine supplies.

These questions of the best distribution of scarce vaccines are only possible following successful research and development programs. Given the risks associated with the pathogens involved in this work, research in these areas, whether in the laboratory or in human subjects, raises ethical and policy issues of its own, as the final pair of chapters in this section illustrate. The Presidential Commission for the Study of Bioethical Issues was asked to evaluate potential clinical trials of anthrax vaccines in healthy children, an effort to provide valuable information to guide the potential use of this vaccine in younger individuals in the event of an attack. The Commission expressed considerable concerns about the risks that these pediatric research subjects would be exposed to and recommended that research could only proceed in a limited, incremental fashion. Tia Powell offers a competing perspective, arguing that well-controlled pediatric research of anthrax vaccines prior to a potential attack is essential, so as to avoid conducting what would in essence be a large, uncontrolled experiment of an untested product in children if an actual attack were to happen.

Further Reading

Kendall Hoyt. 2012. Long Shot: Vaccines for National Defense. Cambridge, MA: Harvard University Press.

Richard E. Neustadt and Harvey V. Fineberg. 1978. The Swine-Flu Affair: Decision-Making on a Slippery Disease. Washington, DC: National Academies Press.

U.S. Department of Health and Human Services. 2005. HHS Pandemic Influenza Plan. Available at: http://www.flu.gov/planning-preparedness/federal/hhspandemicinfluenzaplan.pdf.

World Health Organization. 2007. Ethical Considerations in Developing a Public Health Response to Pandemic Influenza. Available at: http://www.who.int/entity/ethics/publications/who-cds -epr-gip-2007-2/en/index.html.

27 Who Should Get Influenza Vaccine When Not All Can?

Ezekiel J. Emanuel and Alan Wertheimer[*]

The potential threat of pandemic influenza is staggering: 1.9 million deaths, 90 million people sick, and nearly 10 million people hospitalized, with almost 1.5 million requiring intensive-care units (ICUs) in the United States.[1] The National Vaccine Advisory Committee (NVAC) and the Advisory Committee on Immunization Practices (ACIP) have jointly recommended a prioritization scheme that places vaccine workers, health-care providers, and the ill elderly at the top and healthy people ages 2 to 64 at the very bottom, even under embalmers (see table 27.1).[1] The primary goal informing the recommendation was to "decrease health impacts including severe morbidity and death"; a secondary goal was to minimize societal and economic impacts.[1] As the NVAC and ACIP acknowledge, such important policy decisions require broad national discussion. In this spirit, we believe an alternative ethical framework should be considered.

The Inescapability of Rationing

Because of current uncertainty of its value, only "a limited amount of avian influenza A (H5N1) vaccine is being stockpiled."[1] Furthermore, it will take at least 4 months from identification of a candidate vaccine strain to production of the first vaccine.[1] At present, few production facilities worldwide make influenza vaccine, and only one does so completely in the United States. Global capacity for influenza vaccine production is just 425 million doses per annum, if all available factories would run at full capacity after a vaccine was developed. Under currently existing capabilities for manufacturing vaccine, it is likely that more than 90% of the U.S. population will not be vaccinated in the first year.[1] Distributing the limited supply will require determining priority groups.

* From *Science*, Emanuel, E. J., and A. Wertheimer, 312 (5775):854–855, 2006. Reprinted with permission from AAAS.

Table 27.1

Priorities for Distribution of Influenza Vaccine

Tier[a]	NVAC and ACIP Recommendations (subtier)[b]	Life-Cycle Principle (LCP)	Investment Refinement of LCP Including Public Order
1	Vaccine production and distribution workers	Vaccine production and distribution workers	Vaccine production and distribution workers
	Frontline healthcare workers	Frontline healthcare workers	Frontline healthcare workers
	People 6 months to 64 years old with ≥2 high-risk conditions or history of hospitalization for pneumonia or influenza		
	Pregnant women		
	Household contacts of severely immunocompromised people		
	Household contacts of children ≤6 months of age		
	Public health and emergency response workers		
	Key government leaders		
2	Healthy people ≥65 years old	Healthy 6-month-olds	People 13 to 40 years old with <2 high-risk conditions, with priority to key government leaders; public health, military, police, and fire workers; utility and transportation workers; telecommunications and IT workers; funeral directors
	People 6 months to 64 years old with 1 or more high-risk conditions	*Healthy 1-year-olds*	
	Healthy children 6 months to 23 months old	Healthy 2-year-olds	

Table 27.1 (Continued)

Tier[a]	NVAC and ACIP Recommendations (subtier)[b]	Life-Cycle Principle (LCP)	Investment Refinement of LCP Including Public Order
	Other public health workers, emergency responders, public safety workers (police and fire), utility workers, transportation workers, telecommunications and IT workers	*Healthy 3-year-olds, etc.*	*People 7 to 12 years old and 41 to 50 years old with <2 high-risk conditions with priority as above*
			People 6 months to 6 years old and 51 to 64 years old with <2 high-risk conditions, with priority at above[c]
			People ≥65 years old with <2 high-risk conditions
3	Other health decision makers in government	People with life-limiting morbidities or disabilities, prioritized according to expected life years	People 6 months to 64 years old with ≥2 high-risk conditions
	Funeral directors		
4	Healthy people 2 to 64 years old		People ≥65 years old with ≥2 high-risk conditions

[a]Tiers determine priority ranking for the distribution of vaccine if limited in supply. [b]Subtiers in italicized text establish who gets priority within the tier (starting from the top of the tier) if limited vaccine cannot cover everyone in the tier; prioritization may occur within subtiers as well. [c]Children 6 months to <13 years would not receive vaccine if they can be effectively confined to home or otherwise isolated.

Who will be at highest risk? Our experience with three influenza pandemics presents a complex picture. The mortality profile of a future pandemic could be U-shaped, as it was in the mild-to-moderate pandemics of 1957 and 1968 and interpandemic influenza seasons, in which the very young and the old are at highest risk. The mortality profile could be an attenuated W shape, as it was during the devastating 1918 pandemic, in which the highest risk occurred among people between 20 and 40 years of age, whereas the elderly were not at high excess risk.[2,3] Even during pandemics, the elderly appear to be at no higher risk than during interpandemic influenza seasons.[4]

Clear ethical justification for vaccine priorities is essential to the acceptability of the priority ranking and any modifications during the pandemic. With limited vaccine supply, uncertainty over who will be at highest risk of infection and complications, and questions about which historic pandemic experience is most applicable, society faces a fundamental ethical dilemma: Who should get the vaccine first?

The NVAC and ACIP Priority Rankings

Many potential ethical principles for rationing health care have been proposed. "Save the most lives" is commonly used in emergencies, such as burning buildings, although "women and children first" played a role on the Titanic. "First come, first served" operates in other emergencies and in ICUs when admitted patients retain beds despite the presentation of another patient who is equally or even more sick. "Save the most quality life years" is central to cost-effectiveness rationing. "Save the worst-off" plays a role in allocating organs for transplantation. "Reciprocity"—giving priority to people willing to donate their own organs—has been proposed. "Save those most likely to fully recover" guided priorities for giving penicillin to soldiers with syphilis in World War II. Save those "instrumental in making society flourish" through economic productivity or by "contributing to the well-being of others" has been proposed by Murray and others.[5,6]

The save-the-most-lives principle was invoked by NVAC and ACIP. It justifies giving top priority to workers engaged in vaccine production and distribution and health-care workers. They get higher priority not because they are intrinsically more valuable people or of greater "social worth," but because giving them first priority ensures that maximal life-saving vaccine is produced and health care is provided to the sick.[7] Consequently, it values all human life equally, giving every person equal consideration in who gets priority regardless of age, disability, social class, or employment.[7] After these groups, the save-the-most-lives principle justifies priority for those predicted to be at highest risk of hospitalization and dying. We disagree with this prioritization.

Life-Cycle Principle

The save-the-most-lives principle may be justified in some emergencies when decision urgency makes it infeasible to deliberate about priority rankings and impractical to categorize individuals into priority groups. We believe that a life-cycle allocation principle (see table 27.1) based on the idea that each person should have an opportunity to live through all the stages of life is more appropriate for a pandemic.[8,9] There is great value in being able to pass through each life stage—to be a child, a young adult, and to then develop a career and family, and to grow old—and to enjoy a wide range of the opportunities during each stage.

Multiple considerations and intuitions support this ethical principle. Most people endorse this principle for themselves.[8,9] We would prioritize our own resources to ensure that we could live past the illnesses of childhood and young adulthood and would allocate fewer resources to living ever longer once we reached old age.[9] People strongly prefer maximizing the chance of living until a ripe old age, rather than being struck down as a young person.[10,11]

Death seems more tragic when a child or young adult dies than an elderly person—not because the lives of older people are less valuable but because the younger person has not had the opportunity to live and develop through all stages of life. Although the life-cycle principle favors some ages, it is also intrinsically egalitarian.[7] Unlike being productive or contributing to others' well-being, every person will live to be older unless their life is cut short.

The Investment Refinement

A pure version of the life-cycle principle would grant priority to 6-month-olds over 1-year-olds who have priority over 2-year-olds, and on. An alternative, the investment refinement, emphasizes gradations within a life span. It gives priority to people between early adolescence and middle age on the basis of the amount the person invested in his or her life balanced by the amount left to live.[12] Within this framework, 20-year-olds are valued more than 1-year-olds because the older individuals have more developed interests, hopes, and plans but have not had an opportunity to realize them.[11,12] Although these groupings could be modified, they indicate ethically defensible distinctions among groups that can inform rationing priorities.

One other ethical principle relevant for priority ranking of influenza vaccine during a pandemic is public order. It focuses on the value of ensuring safety and the provision of necessities, such as food and fuel. We believe the investment refinement combined with the public-order principle (IRPOP) should be the ultimate objective of all pandemic response measures, including priority ranking for vaccines and interventions to limit the course of the pandemic, such as closing schools and confining people to their homes. These two principles should inform decisions at the start of an epidemic, when the shape of the risk curves for morbidity and mortality are largely uncertain.

Like the NVAC and ACIP ranking, the IRPOP ranking would give high priority to vaccine production and distribution workers, as well as healthcare and public health workers with direct patient contact. However, contrary to the NVAC and ACIP prioritization for the sick elderly and infants, IRPOP emphasize people between 13 and 40 years of age. The NVAC and ACIP priority ranking comports well with those groups at risk during the mild-to-moderate 1957 and 1968 pandemics. IRPOP prioritizes those age cohorts at highest risk during the devastating 1918 pandemic. Depending on patterns of flu spread, some mathematical models suggest that following IRPOP priority ranking could save the most lives overall.[13]

Conclusions

The life-cycle ranking is meant to apply to the situation in the United States. During a global pandemic, there will be fundamental questions about sharing vaccines and other interventions with other countries. This raises fundamental issues of global rationing that are too complex to address here.

Fortunately, although we are worried about an influenza pandemic, it is not upon us. Indeed, the current H5N1 avian flu may never develop into a human pandemic. This gives us time to both build vaccine production capacity to minimize the need for rationing and rationally assess policy and ethical issues about the distribution of vaccines.

References

1. U.S. Department of Health and Human Services. 2005. HHS Pandemic Influenza Plan. Washington, DC: U.S. Department of Health and Human Services. Available at: www.flu.gov/planning -preparedness/federal/hhspandemicinfluenzaplan.pdf. Accessed March 29, 2006.

2. Collin, S. D. Influenza and pneumonia excess mortality at specific ages in the epidemic of 1943–44, with comparative data for preceding epidemics. *Public Health Reports* 60 (1945):853.

3. Olson, D. R., L. Simonsen, P. J. Edelson, and S. S. Morse. Epidemiological evidence of an early wave of the 1918 influenza pandemic in New York City. *Proceedings of the National Academy of Sciences of the United States of America* 102 (2005):11059.

4. Simonsen, L., D. R. Olson, C. Viboud, E. Heiman, R. J. Taylor, M. A. Miller, et al. 2004. Pandemic influenza and mortality: Past evidence and projections for the future. In: *The Threat of Pandemic Influenza: Are We Ready?* ed. S. L. Knobler, et al. Washington, DC: National Academies Press.

5. Murray, C. J. L., and A. D. Lopez, eds. 1996. *The Global Burden of Disease*. Geneva: World Health Organization.

6. Murray, C. J. L., and A. K. Acharya. Understanding DALYs (disability-adjusted life years). *Journal of Health Economics* 16 (1997):710.

7. Dworkin, R. 1978. *Taking Rights Seriously*. Cambridge, MA: Harvard University Press.

8. Williams, A. Intergenerational equity: an exploration of the "fair innings" argument. *Health Economics* 6 (1997):117.

9. Daniels, N. 1988. *Am I My Parents' Keeper?* New York: Oxford University Press.

10. Cropper, M. L., S. K. Aydede, and P. R. Portney. Public preferences for life saving: Discounting for time and age. *Journal of Risk and Uncertainty* 8 (1994):243.

11. Johannesson, M., and P. O. Johansson. Is the valuation of a QALY gained independent of age? Some empirical evidence. *Journal of Health Economics* 16 (1997):589.

12. Dworkin, R. 1993. *Life's Dominion*. New York: Knopf.

13. Halloran, M. E., and I. M. Longini, Jr. Public health: Community studies for vaccinating schoolchildren against influenza *Science* 311 (2006):615.

28 Ethical Vaccine Distribution Planning for Pandemic Influenza: Prioritizing Homeless and Hard-to-Reach Populations (*Excerpt*)

Kristy Buccieri and Stephen Gaetz[*]

Pandemic planning contains a moral dimension, such that certain values, principles, norms, and interests take priority over others (Kotalik, 2005). In the event of a public health crisis, such as the recent H1N1 pandemic, ethical dilemmas arise over the allocation of limited resources when the needs of a society overwhelm the supply of human and material resources that are immediately available. In such instances, public health officials are tasked with making swift decisions about how, where, and to whom these limited resources are to be distributed (Thompson et al., 2006). These decisions are among the most difficult of the ethical dilemmas faced by the government officials, policymakers, and healthcare providers in such situations (McGorty et al., 2007). The allocation of resources during a pandemic can become a highly contentious issue, especially if evidence-based decision making does not coincide with the popular public opinion. Disagreements may arise, with some of the most heatedly debated pertaining to the allocation of a scarce vaccine supply.

In this chapter, we discuss ethical pandemic planning practices in relation to the need for an equitable vaccination distribution strategy. Specifically, we argue that following the immunization of healthcare and emergency workers, priority should be given to high-risk and hard-to-reach populations, such as people who are homeless, based on the ethical principles of equity and utility (WHO, 2007). It has been noted by Kaposy and Bandrauk (2012) that vaccine strategies which give priority to vulnerable, yet stigmatized groups may be met with resistance. Alongside these researchers, we argue that there is a need for strategic immunization responses that prioritize the medically and socially vulnerable in times of pandemic outbreak. This kind of strategy not only benefits these individuals but also serves the collective good of society as a whole.

* Reprinted from Buccieri, K., and S. Gaetz. 2013. Ethical vaccine distribution planning for pandemic influenza: Prioritizing homeless and hard-to-reach populations. *Public Health Ethics* 6 (2):185–196, by permission of Oxford University Press.

We begin this chapter by reviewing the ongoing debates around vaccine distribution and the principles of equity and utility that inform these decisions. We then discuss the need for a focus on homeless and hard-to-reach populations as medically, socially, and structurally at-risk persons during a pandemic influenza outbreak. This is not to suggest that homeless individuals should be the first persons to be vaccinated; rather we argue that they should receive priority status, alongside other vulnerable groups such as children and those with chronic health conditions, following the immunization of healthcare and essential service workers, such as emergency responders. The homeless are a subset of vulnerable populations, and we argue that the order in which they are immunized (in relation to others) be considered based on the epidemiology of individual pandemic strains. We conclude by calling on pandemic planners to not only prioritize homeless individuals after healthcare and essential workers but also invest in connecting homeless individuals to stable health care as a preventive measure.

Prioritizing Vaccine Distribution: Ethical Principles

According to the World Health Organization (2009a, 2009b), pandemic planning must always be founded on ethical principles that assist policymakers in balancing a range of interests while protecting and respecting the rights of all citizens. However, experience has shown that decision makers often disagree on what principles should be followed in making fair priority setting decisions (Upshur et al., 2005). Unfortunately, the inability to predict which influenza virus will result in a pandemic, combined with limited national and global capacity to mass produce vaccines in a relatively short time essentially guarantees that an effective vaccine will not be available to most or all persons during the early stages of any pandemic influenza outbreak (Blumenshine et al., 2008). Difficult decisions need to be made quickly with regard to which citizens will be eligible to receive this limited supply.

There should be no surprise that any rationing strategy will experience opposition from many people (Emanuel and Wertheimer, 2006a). The questions of how to obtain the greatest benefit and how to do so fairly with limited vaccination supplies have been of considerable debate among policymakers and researchers. Most pandemic plans give priority for the use of antivirals and vaccines to healthcare workers and people employed in emergency services (Upshur et al., 2005). This is called the utility principle because it suggests that resources should be used to provide the maximum possible health benefit by saving the most lives (WHO, 2007).

Under the utility principle, preference is given to certain persons based on clinical factors, the epidemiology of the spread of the disease, and ensuring the functioning of society (McGorty et al., 2007). This usually means that essential healthcare workers, especially those who work with the elderly and other medically high-risk populations, are given priority in an effort to prevent the spread of the virus to the patients they are in contact with (May, 2005). In addition, the utility principle also encourages preferential vaccination for individuals who provide other critical services necessary for society to function, for instance, utilities, police, transportation, and food supply (WHO, 2007).

Kass et al. (2008) argue that alongside healthcare workers, a cross-section of the population should be immunized (such as truck drivers, water maintenance support people, and police officers, among others) to maintain the functioning of society. Under this proposed strategy, these individuals would have first access to immunization for themselves and possibly their families in exchange for agreeing to work during the pandemic and maintaining the operation of essential services for other citizens.

Emanuel and Wertheimer (2006b) also propose an adapted version of the utility principle, which they identify as the life-cycle principle. They suggest that vaccinations should be distributed favoring younger over older persons with an investment refinement that emphasizes gradations within a life span. This principle would give priority to those who are between early adolescence and middle age, based on the amount of time invested in life balanced by the amount of time left to live.

When considering allocation decisions, prioritizing homeless and hard-to-reach individuals may be met with resistance based on common misconceptions and biases toward homeless individuals. Our concern with models such as this one is that the public-order principle (Emanuel and Wertheimer, 2006b) could be used to argue that homeless individuals neither substantially contribute to maintaining public order nor are they necessarily in a strong position to realize their life investments. Here, the issue of fairness becomes central. Public health officials must consider a range of factors, such as a person's risk of becoming infected, severity of the illness, and/or complications that could arise.

However, they must also consider the ability of individuals to distance themselves from others who are or could become infected. Housed citizens have the option of finding seclusion in their homes (for at least part of the day), whereas homeless individuals are constantly in contact with others through social service agencies. Those who choose to seclude themselves and not access service agencies do so at the cost of not having food, safety and shelter. Thus, given the vulnerable nature of this population, a decision not to allocate part of the vaccine supply could only be based on sociopolitical factors, such as public disapproval of factors such as poverty and joblessness.

The utility principle is insufficient to address the pressing needs of vulnerable individuals in times of pandemic influenza. As such, the principle of equity states that the distribution of benefits and burdens must be fair and that when conflict arises, the appropriate response should be determined in an open and transparent process that takes into account local circumstances and cultural values (WHO, 2007). This may at times cause conflict. For instance, Kaposy and Bandrauk (2012) argue that vaccine strategies that prioritize vulnerable yet stigmatized groups may face resistance. In situations such as these, policymakers need to weigh the benefits of immunizing vulnerable populations against the potential for public disapproval. They are tasked with making decisions that may be unpopular but are in the best interest of public health. Granting priority vaccination to homeless populations is an equitable strategy.

Equity can be generally understood as a rejection of various forms of discrimination, attempts at minimizing unfairness, the granting of priority status to those who have a relatively strong claim to life-saving treatments based on young age, being at high risk of severe disease or death, and possibly those who are primary pandemic responders, such as healthcare workers (Verweij, 2009). Vaccinating the homeless early in a pandemic outbreak fulfils the principle of equity for three key reasons. First, as individuals, they are medically at risk due to chronic health conditions that could cause complications. Second, as a population, they are socially at risk, living in poverty with few resources to aid in prevention and/or rehabilitation. Third, they are dependent on social service agencies, forcing them into contact with others and only providing isolation to those who are willing to forfeit access to food, shelter, and security. In addition to being an anti-discriminatory measure, priority vaccination is fair because it would decrease the medical risks, connect this population with supports, and lower the risk of transmission within congregate settings.

The equity principle suggests that in a pandemic influenza outbreak, those who are more vulnerable due to medical and/or social risks may be considered a priority for vaccination. However, as previously stated, most pandemic influenza plans instead employ the principle of utility by assigning vaccination priority to healthcare workers and those employed in emergency services (Upshur et al., 2005). Yet as Lee et al. (2008) have argued, if decision makers are aware that those who are less well-off will likely be burdened more during a pandemic, then this may create a moral imperative for pandemic influenza plans to ensure that these individuals do not suffer in unfair and unjust ways.

Verweij (2009) has argued that allocating scarce resources to those who are economically disadvantaged must not be predicated solely on this factor alone. In the following section, we argue that prioritizing vaccination for those who are medically, socially, and structurally at high risk—and in particular those who are homeless or under-housed—is an ethical and a strategic response that incorporates both the utility and equity principles. High-risk populations, such as the homeless, often suffer from a myriad of health conditions that make them susceptible to infections and negative adverse effects. Immunizing them early is an important way to reduce the chances that they will become infected and infect others, including persons in the general population.

Homeless individuals often spend considerable amounts of time in congregate settings, such as shelters and drop-in centers, with other high-risk individuals. Without access to stable housing and private spaces, many homeless individuals are highly mobile throughout the day, potentially exposing everyone they come into contact with to the influenza virus and creating vectors of disease throughout a given city. Immunizing high-risk populations, such as the homeless, is not only an equitable strategy for ensuring their well-being but also draws on the utility principle to save most of the lives through limiting public exposure.

We are not arguing that homeless persons must be the first persons to be immunized in a pandemic outbreak, but they should be given special consideration and priority status as a public health measure. Our model coincides with proposals made by researchers such as Kass et al. (2008), who argue that healthcare workers and a cross-section of essential workers should be immunized first. However, we contend that following the immunization of these key personnel, homeless, and hard-to-reach populations should be considered for priority over other healthy, low-risk populations. When establishing a priority sequence, planners should consider their generally poor health and mental health status, their close proximity with others who may be ill, and their constant public mobility as reasons for granting them priority status based on the principles of utility and equity. Additionally, those who work with the homeless should be given priority vaccination as well in order to maintain the functioning of critical infrastructure, such as shelters and drop-in centers.

Vaccine Distribution: Prioritizing Homeless and Underhoused Individuals

Despite the recognition of substantial health inequities and increased calls to reduce health disparities (Beiser and Stewart, 2005; Appleyard, 2009), some populations continue to be particularly vulnerable to illness and injury and at the same time experience considerable discrimination within the healthcare system. It is argued that the vulnerability of homeless individuals to disease, their socially marginal status, and, significantly, weaknesses in many current national responses to homelessness present key challenges to effective pandemic preparedness.

Although the health of homeless persons is undoubtedly compromised by situational factors (e.g., poor nutrition) and preexisting health conditions (e.g., comprised immunity), one must also take into account how the infrastructural response to homelessness contributes to their vulnerability. The Canadian response to homelessness, for instance, continues to emphasize the provision of community-based emergency services, including shelters, drop-ins, and soup kitchens (Gaetz, 2009; Hurtubise et al., 2009). In Toronto, there are more than sixty emergency shelters and sixty drop-ins, the latter of which serve not only homeless populations but also underhoused and otherwise marginalized individuals. Such emergency services may unintentionally promote disease transmission as a result of limited space and the subsequent close proximity of clients as they sleep, eat, and engage in other activities (Daiski, 2005). The highly mobile nature of many homeless persons means that as they move through the city, they produce networks of contamination. As largely unvaccinated persons (Bucher et al., 2006), the homeless may act as undetected reservoirs of infection and an important bridge population (Coady et al., 2008).

Compromised health and well-being are thus consequences of overcrowded living conditions, lack of access to safe and private spaces, reliance on shelters and drop-ins to meet daily needs, and barriers to accessing services. Complicating matters is the fact that people who are homeless often experience considerable barriers in accessing health care (Hwang et al., 2001; O'Connell, 2004; Frankish et al., 2009).

As a result of being largely disconnected from the healthcare system, hard-to-reach populations, such as the homeless, may be less likely than the general public to receive immunizations (Vlahov et al., 2007). In one study, researchers analyzed 4,319 medical charts of persons from three different homeless shelters in New York during influenza seasons from 1997 to 2004 (Bucher et al., 2006). They found that less than one-fourth of all persons examined and one-third of those over 65 years of age had evidence of influenza vaccination noted in their charts. Likewise, researchers found that within eight Bronx and Harlem neighborhoods, there is an unmet need for influenza vaccine among those who have experienced homelessness (Bryant et al., 2006). These findings are troubling, given that hard-to-reach populations are particularly vulnerable when immunization rates are low (Weatherill et al., 2004). Decreased vaccination rates, poor health, and barriers to accessing health care all increase the risk for acquiring influenza and for attendant morbidity (Coady et al., 2008).

All of this research supports our assertion that people who are homeless may be particularly vulnerable to infection in the event of an influenza pandemic, highlighting the necessity of implementing effective strategies to ensure that homeless populations have access to vaccination during a pandemic. Research from Tijuana, Mexico, has shown that the isolation of hard-to-reach populations can be protective (Rodwell et al., 2010). However, vaccination is important for those who are homeless, not only because many are at increased risk for complications due to poor health, but it is also a critical way to prevent influenza transmission through the general population. Dushoff et al. (2007) note that it is imperative to distinguish between the direct effect of vaccination—protecting the vaccinated individual from contracting the disease—and indirect vaccination—protecting unvaccinated people by reducing the level of infectiousness in the population. Vaccinating for influenza within shelters and drop-in centers arguably may reduce the general population infection rates in similar ways as has been noted with targeted tuberculosis initiatives (Bucher et al., 2006).

The H1N1 pandemics of 2009 and 2010 allowed Toronto Public Health (TPH) the chance to hold pH1N1 vaccination clinics in homeless shelters and drop-in centers with the objective of vaccinating as many homeless and underhoused persons as possible. Given the low vaccination rates among homeless populations during regular influenza seasons (Bucher et al., 2006), TPH aimed to facilitate access to immunization by offering clinics in agencies frequented by homeless individuals. The increased vaccination rates benefit not only homeless individuals but also the general public, suggesting that prioritizing community vaccination programs for homeless individuals is a beneficial approach that brings together the principles of equity by protecting homeless individuals and utility by preventing the spread of the virus.

Conclusions

In a pandemic situation, decision makers have to make difficult choices, often with limited time, resources, and information at their disposal. How and to whom vaccinations are to be allocated are among the most challenging of these decisions, as the financial and social costs can be high. A number of principles have been suggested for guiding this decision-making process. Although the utility principle of administering vaccine to those who come into contact with people who are ill, such as healthcare workers, has generally been favored in national plans, others argue that the equity principle is more ethical. The equity principle states that the most vulnerable individuals and/or those who would suffer the greatest effects of illness should get priority for vaccination.

In this chapter, we have argued that homeless individuals are among the most medically and socially high-risk persons. Their generally poor physical and mental health and high mobility rates make them specifically susceptible to infection, suffering ill effects, and transmitting the virus to others in the homeless and general populations. However, it is not just the personal characteristics of individuals that need to be taken account of. We must also consider how we institutionally organize our response to homelessness as contributing to the problem. Although there is a great deal of variation in how shelters, day programs, and soup kitchens are configured and operated, it is safe to say that most services regularly place homeless people in congregate settings, often in very close quarters, for eating, sleeping, and resting. Not all services have adequate ventilation or care facilities. If individuals become ill, quarantine and respite care become a challenge and can pose a risk to other homeless individuals. In other words, our institutional response to homelessness in fact produces an increased risk of the spread of infectious disease, and organizational practice of moving homeless persons out of such settings during much of the day means greater contact with the general public. Finally, one has to question what might follow in the case of state-mandated mandatory quarantine—what would be the ethical considerations and impact of forcing homeless people into staying in these same congregate settings during a pandemic?

Because our structural response to homelessness in fact produces vulnerability, a consideration of equity not only demands nondiscrimination against this population, but also the vulnerability of this population requires prioritization. Focusing efforts on immunizing homeless individuals is a sound public health strategy that relies on both the utility and equity principles of vaccine distribution. We agree with Kass et al. (2008) that immediate priority should be given to healthcare and essential workers, but we add that homeless and other high-risk, hard-to-reach individuals should be vaccinated before other populations in accordance with the principles of utility and equity. Implementing a strategy of this nature is possible and encouraged, although we emphasize that it must be approached with discretion and care. Homelessness is often a source of stigmatization, and public health officials must be cautious to not perpetuate this. Educating the public about why homeless and other hard-to-reach populations would be prioritized must not be done in such a way as to send the message that they are diseased and/or that they spread disease. Communicating to the public that priority vaccination is a fair response to address medical, social, and structural factors that place the homeless at risk could help to improve the public's support for the initiative. To this end, ensuring a transparent and informed public communication strategy that locates the cause within a broader sociopolitical context—rather than an individual one—could aid in creating public support without creating further stigmatization.

Homeless and hard-to-reach populations are at high risk for adverse medical and social effects during emergency situations, such as a pandemic. However, our discussion throughout this chapter is also meant to highlight the daily vulnerability these individuals experience. A thorough discussion of how this vulnerability could be prevented or addressed prior to an emergency (e.g., through shelter design) is beyond the scope of this chapter. Limiting ourselves to the present topic of vaccination, we return to our findings and re-state that connecting homeless individuals with stable healthcare provision, whether through general practitioners, nurse outreach workers, or community health centers, is a primary means of prevention. Ensuring that these individuals are connected with healthcare workers may serve to improve their general physical and mental health, reducing their risk of vulnerability in times of emergencies, and it may also encourage seasonal vaccination.

We have also argued that community outreach initiatives are an effective way to access homeless and hard-to-reach individuals, who have historically low influenza vaccination rates. Our research shows that TPH's community-based strategy was effective not only at raising the immunization rate of homeless and underhoused individuals but also at increasing the rate to match the provincial and national levels as a whole. The strength of this program was its ability to bring accessible immunization clinics to homeless persons in Toronto, resulting in stronger relationships between TPH and the clients and staff within the homelessness sector.

Given the success of this program during the H1N1 pandemic, future efforts should be made to provide community-based vaccine clinics of this scale during seasonal influenza periods as well. As Baylis et al. (2008) write, "Social justice directs us to explore the context in which certain political and social structures are created and maintained, and in which certain policy decisions are made and implemented. It asks us to look beyond effects on individuals and to see how members of different social groups may be collectively affected by private and public practices that create inequalities in access and opportunity" (203).

The decision to give priority vaccination to homeless individuals is an ethically sound social justice strategy. It incorporates the principle of equity by immunizing highly vulnerable individuals and the principle of utility by preventing widespread disease transmission. Reaching out through community-based vaccine initiatives is an effective way to connect homeless individuals with much needed health care, develop trust within the community, promote vaccination, and protect society in a public health emergency.

References

Appleyard, T. 2009. *Bridging the Preparedness Divide: A Framework for Health Equity in Ontario's Emergency Management Programs.* Toronto: Wellesley Institute.

Baylis, F., N. P. Kenny, and S. Sherwin. 2008. A relational account of public health ethics. *Public Health Ethics* 1:196–209.

Beiser, M., and M. Stewart. 2005. Reducing health disparities: A priority for Canada. *Can J Public Health* 96:S4–S7.

Blumenshine, P., A. Reingold, S. Egerter, R. Mockenhaupt, P. Braveman, and J. Marks. 2008. Pandemic influenza planning in the United States from a health disparities perspective. *Emerg Infect Dis* 14:709–715.

Bryant, W. K., D. C. Ompad, S. Sisco, S. Blaney, K. Glidden, E. Phillips, D. Vlahov, S. Galea, and the Project VIVA Intervention Working Group. 2006. Determinants of influenza vaccination in hard-to-reach urban populations. *Prev Med* 43:60–70.

Bucher, S. J., P. W. Brickner, and R. L. Vincent. 2006. Influenzalike illness among homeless persons. *Emerg Infect Dis* 12:1162–1163.

Coady, M. H., S. Galea, S. Blaney, D. C. Ompad, S. Sisco, D. Vlahov and the Project VIVA Intervention Working Group. 2008. Project VIVA: A multilevel community-based intervention to increase influenza vaccination rates among hard-to-reach populations in New York City. *Am J Public Health* 98:1314–1321.

Daiski, I. 2005. The health bus: Healthcare for marginalized populations. *Policy Polit Nurs Pract* 6:30–38.

Dushoff, J., J. B. Plotkin, C. Viboud, L. Simonsen, M. Miller, M. Loeb, and D. J. D. Earn. 2007. Vaccinating to protect a vulnerable subpopulation. *PLoS Med* 4:921–927.

Emanuel, E. J., and A. Wertheimer. 2006a. Response. *Science* 314:1539–1540.

Emanuel, E. J., and A. Wertheimer. 2006b. Who should get influenza vaccine when not all can? *Science* 312:854–855.

Frankish, J., S. Hwang, D. Quantz. 2009. The relationship between homelessness and health: An overview of research in Canada. In: *Finding Home: Policy Options for Addressing Homelessness in Canada,* rev. ed., eds. J. D Hulchanski, P. Campsie, S. Chau, S. Hwang, and E. Paradis, 1–21. Toronto: Cities Centre, University of Toronto.

Gaetz, S. 2009. The struggle to end homelessness in Canada: How we created the crisis, and how we can end it. *Open Health Serv Policy J* 2:94–99.

Hurtubise, R., P. O. Babin, and C. Grimard. 2009. Shelters for the homeless: Learning from research. In: *Finding Home: Policy Options for Addressing Homelessness in Canada,* rev. ed., eds. J. D. Hulchanski, P. Campsie, S. Chau Hwang, and E. Paradis, 1–24. Toronto: Cities Centre, University of Toronto.

Hwang, S. W., J. J. O'Connell, J. M. Lebow, M. F. Bierer, E. J. Orav, and T. A. Brennan. 2001. Health care utilization among homeless adults prior to death. *J Health Care Poor Underserved* 12:50–58.

Kaposy, C., and N. Bandrauk. 2012. Prioritizing vaccine access for vulnerable but stigmatized groups. *Public Health Ethics* 5:283–295.

Kass, N. E., J. Otto, D. O'Brien, and M. Minson. 2008. Ethics and severe pandemic influenza: Maintaining essential functions through a fair and considered sesponse. *Biosecur Bioterror* 6:227–236.

Kotalik, J. 2005. Preparing for an influenza pandemic: Ethical issues. *Bioethics* 19:422–431.

Lee, C., W. A. Rogers, and A. Braunack-Mayer. 2008. Social justice and pandemic influenza planning: The role of communication strategies. *Public Health Ethics* 1:223–234.

McGorty, E. K., L. Devlin, R. Tong, N. Harrison, M. Holmes, and P. Silberman. 2007. Ethical guidelines for an influenza pandemic. *N C Med J* 68:38–42.

O'Connell, J. 2004. Dying in the shadows: The challenge of providing health vare for homeless people. *CMAJ* 170:1251–1252.

Rodwell, T. C., A. M. Robertson N. Aguirre, A. Vera, C. M. Anderson, R. Lozada, L. Chait, R. T. Schooley, Z. Q. Zhang, and S. A. Strathdee. 2010. Pandemic (H1N1) 2009 surveillance in marginalized populations, Tijuana, Mexico. *Emerg Infect Dis* 16:1292–1295.

Thompson, A. K., K. Faith, J. L. Gibson, and R. E. G. Upshur. 2006. Pandemic influenza preparedness: An ethical framework to guide decision-making. *BMC Med Ethics* 7:E12.

Upshur, R. E. G., K. Faith, J. L. Gibson, A. K. Thompson, C. S. Tracy, K. Wilson, and P. A. Singer. 2005. *Stand on Guard for Thee: Ethical Considerations in Preparedness for Pandemic Influenza: A Report of the University of Toronto Centre for Bioethics Pandemic Influenza Working Group.* Toronto: University of Toronto Joint Centre for Bioethics.

Verweij, M. 2009. Moral principles for allocating scarce medical resources in an influenza pandemic. *J Bioeth Inq* 6:159–169.

Vlahov, D., M. H. Coady, D. C. Ompad, and S. Galea. 2007. Strategies for improving influenza immunization rates among hard-to-reach populations. *J Urban Health* 84:615–631.

Weatherill, S. A., J. A. Buxton, and P. C. Daly. 2004. Immunization programs in non-traditional dettings. *Can J Public Health* 95:133–137.

World Health Organization. 2007. *Ethical Considerations in Developing a Public Health Response to Pandemic Influenza.* Geneva: World Health Organization.

World Health Organization. 2009a. *Pandemic Influenza Preparedness and Response: A WHO Guidance Document.* Geneva: World Health Organization.

World Health Organization. 2009b. *Whole-of-Society Pandemic Readiness: WHO Guidelines for Pandemic Preparedness and Response in the Non-Health Sectors.* Geneva: World Health Organization.

29 Poverty, Wealth, and Access to Pandemic Influenza Vaccines

Tadataka Yamada[*]

On June 11, 2009, Margaret Chan, director general of the World Health Organization (WHO), declared that the status of the influenza A (H1N1) pandemic had reached phase 6—active transmission on a global scale. Until now, the case fatality rate of this influenza has been quite low, but history teaches us that the situation could take a turn for the worse during the next wave of the pandemic. If a 1918-like pandemic were to occur today, tens of millions of people could die, the vast majority of them in the world's poorest countries.

Fortunately, the prospects for developing an effective vaccine to prevent infection with the current H1N1 virus are excellent, and the world's pharmaceutical companies are working diligently at this task. In contemplating equal access to such a vaccine, it is important to consider three key issues: manufacturing capacity, cost, and delivery.

Only a few countries in the world have plants for manufacturing influenza vaccine, and three companies—GlaxoSmithKline, Sanofi-Aventis, and Novartis—account for most of the world's manufacturing capacity. The number of doses of vaccine against H1N1 influenza that could be produced with the existing capacity is large, but the sobering truth is that even if production were switched over completely from seasonal influenza vaccine to pandemic influenza vaccine, there would not be nearly enough for everyone in the world. The size of the gap in potential supply depends greatly on the dose that is required, and it may be possible to reduce the necessary dose by as much as 75% with the use of an adjuvant. The challenging problem is that much, if not most, of the manufacturing capacity is already spoken for through purchasing contracts held by many of the world's wealthy countries.

The second issue is cost. Despite the enormous technological investment required to create a vaccine, the traditional cost of seasonal influenza vaccines even in wealthy countries is quite low. For the pandemic H1N1 influenza vaccine, the major manufacturers have indicated a willingness to offer tiered pricing, with affordable prices for poor countries. Going even further, Sanofi-Aventis has committed to donating 100 million doses of its vaccine to a stockpile for poor countries, and GlaxoSmithKline has committed to donating 50 million doses. Nevertheless, financial commitments from wealthy countries will be needed to help poorer countries purchase vaccines—cost should not be a barrier to access.

Finally, the scope of access to vaccines will in part be determined by the infrastructure required to deliver them to all citizens in mass campaigns. Ironically, poor countries may have an advantage on this front because many have recent experience with mass campaigns involving vaccines against polio, measles, and hepatitis B; delivery may therefore be less of a challenge for them, provided that the vaccines reach them in a timely fashion. By contrast, in many wealthier countries, such campaigns have not been undertaken for some time. Getting the vaccine to large numbers of young adults, in particular, may be a formidable task for which preparations must surely be made as soon as possible.

Our limited capacity for producing potentially lifesaving vaccines presents a pressing moral challenge. I believe wholeheartedly that all lives have equal value (this is the basic principle motivating the Bill and Melinda Gates Foundation, where I work), and I believe that every stakeholder has a responsibility to ensure that the pandemic does not take a 1918-like toll on the world. We have therefore worked with partner stakeholders to develop a proposed set of principles to guide the global allocation of pandemic vaccine (see Principles to Guide Global Allocation of Pandemic Vaccine).

Rich countries have a responsibility to stand in line and receive their vaccine allotments alongside poor countries, even if they have paid for their vaccine before others could do so. It would be inexcusable to force poor countries to wait until the rich have been served under their existing contracts with vaccine manufacturers. Moreover, rich countries must also consider how they can provide contributions to offset the cost of vaccines for countries that cannot afford to pay for them. Countries that are home to influenza-vaccine manufacturing plants have a special responsibility to avoid nationalizing those facilities in an effort to reserve their output for their own citizens before others. All countries must prepare now for the rapid delivery of the vaccines as soon as they become available.

Manufacturers have a responsibility to apply their full capabilities to creating the greatest possible quantity of vaccine doses. Despite contractual obligations to supply many wealthy countries with their vaccines, manufacturers must resist the temptation to commit all their capacity to those who can pay the most. This is not a time to adhere to the "first come, first served" model of business because we may be facing a health crisis of global proportions in which all people and countries are equally at risk. To ensure fairness, full adherence to a tiered pricing scheme in which the cost to the purchaser is proportionate to its ability to pay is essential. The generous donations made by Sanofi-Aventis and GlaxoSmithKline set an example that all manufacturers should emulate. In return for their responsible actions, it would be reasonable for manufacturers to be indemnified against liability from potential adverse reactions to their vaccines.

Regulatory agencies have an important responsibility in this impending crisis because they stand between the manufacturers of pandemic influenza vaccines and the people who will benefit from them. It is critically important that regulators apply their usual rigorous standards in approving the new vaccines—but also that they do so in a timely fashion. A special task facing them is the rapid review and consideration of the safety and efficacy of adjuvants, whose use could greatly reduce the required dose of vaccine and thereby expand the number of doses that could be manufactured.

The WHO has provided strong leadership as the world has contemplated the prospect of an influenza pandemic. We are counting on the organization to guide us, wisely and fairly, through the complex challenges that lie ahead.

The prospect of a worsening global influenza pandemic is real and will not go away anytime soon. I cannot imagine standing by and watching if, at the time of crisis, the rich live and the poor die. It will take collective commitment and action by all of us to prevent this from happening.

Principles to Guide Global Allocation of Pandemic Vaccine

1. The global community should take steps to protect all populations, including those without resources to protect themselves.
2. Vaccination should be considered in the context of comprehensive pandemic preparedness and response efforts in all nations.
3. Developed countries and vaccine manufacturers should urgently agree on a mechanism to ensure access to vaccine by developing countries.
4. Influenza vaccine manufacturers should identify strategies such as tiered pricing and donations to make pandemic vaccine more accessible to developing nations.
5. Pandemic vaccines allocated to developing nations should become available in the same time frame as vaccines for developed nations.

6. The global community should obtain data to help establish a consensus on the safety and efficacy of adjuvants, and efforts should be made to ensure the fullest use of this and other dose-sparing strategies.

7. All countries obtaining pandemic vaccine should ensure that mechanisms are in place to provide the vaccine to their populations, to ensure that this scarce resource is not wasted, and donors should be prepared to provide resources and technical assistance to help countries bolster these mechanisms.

8. The WHO is uniquely positioned to lead the global response to a pandemic virus and should support governments and industry in their efforts to implement these principles.

From the Pneumonia and Flu Web site of the Bill and Melinda Gates Foundation (www.gatesfoundation.org/topics/Pages/pneumonia-flu.aspx).

30 Negotiating Equitable Access to Influenza Vaccines: Global Health Diplomacy and the Controversies Surrounding Avian Influenza H5N1 and Pandemic Influenza H1N1

David P. Fidler[*]

One of the most controversial areas of global health diplomacy over the past 5 years has involved negotiations to increase equitable access to vaccines for highly pathogenic avian influenza A (H5N1) (HPAI-H5N1) and pandemic 2009 influenza A (H1N1) (2009-H1N1). The limited results produced by these negotiations have stimulated calls for a new global framework to improve equitable access to influenza vaccines. The prospects for such a framework are not, however, promising because the national interests of most developed states vis-à-vis dangerous influenza strains favor retaining the existing imbalanced, reactive, and ad hoc approach to vaccine access. This chapter examines why negotiating equitable access to influenza vaccines in the context of HPAI-H5N1 and 2009-H1N1 has been, and promises to continue to be, a difficult diplomatic endeavor.

Influenza Vaccine Access Controversies: HPAI-H5N1 and 2009-H1N1

The re-emergence of HPAI-H5N1 in 2004 and its spread triggered fears that the world was on the brink of a potentially devastating influenza pandemic.[1] Preparations for pandemic influenza frantically began and included plans to develop a vaccine for a pandemic H5N1 strain. These plans ran headlong into developing-country concerns that their populations would not have access to H5N1 vaccines. These concerns, and the lack of any mechanism to ensure equitable access to vaccines and other benefits from research on influenza viruses, prompted Indonesia, in 2007, to refuse to share H5N1 virus samples with the World Health Organization (WHO) that would be used for surveillance.[2,3] Supported by many developing countries, Indonesia's action questioned the legitimacy of WHO's Global Influenza Surveillance Network and forced

* Originally published in *PLoS Medicine*, 2010; 7 (5):e1000247. Reprinted under the terms of a Creative Commons Attribution License.

WHO and its member states to begin negotiations to create a new system of influenza virus and benefits sharing.[4] Although WHO member states agreed to establish a stockpile of H5N1 vaccine,[5] the negotiations have, to date, failed to reach agreement.[6]

Concerns about equitable access flared again in 2009 when a novel strain of influenza A (H1N1) emerged and spread around the world. The speed and ease with which the 2009-H1N1 strain moved meant that a vaccine was the only practical means of preventing infection, and efforts to produce a vaccine began in the late spring and early summer.[7] Developed countries placed large advance orders for 2009-H1N1 vaccine and bought virtually all the vaccine that companies could manufacture.[8,9] Developing countries and WHO identified the lack of equity in how developed countries were securing access to the vaccine.[10] WHO entered talks with manufacturers and developed-country governments to secure some vaccine for developing countries,[11] and WHO and the United Nations (UN) appealed for monetary donations to purchase vaccines and other supplies to help developing countries address the 2009-H1N1 virus.[12] These efforts yielded donation pledges from manufacturers[13] and developed countries,[14] but the donations still left the developing world with limited supplies[15] compared to developed countries, which would retain, even after donations, sufficient vaccine to cover their populations.

Feared and actual problems with 2009-H1N1 vaccine production, however, affected the amount and timing of vaccine available for developing countries. As of this writing, Canada had not joined other developed countries in pledging to donate vaccines because of shortages within Canada,[16] and Canada awarded its vaccine contract to a Canadian company because it feared that foreign governments might restrict exports to Canada because of vaccine shortages within their territories.[17] The Australian government made it clear to the Australian manufacturer CSL that it must fulfill the government's domestic needs before exporting vaccine to the United States.[18] On September 17, 2009, the United States pledged to donate 10% of its vaccine purchases to WHO, but on October 28, U.S. Secretary of Health and Human Services Kathleen Sebelius stated that the United States would not donate H1N1 vaccine as promised until all at-risk Americans had access because production problems had created shortages in the United States.[19] These fears and actions reinforced the sense that the status quo concerning equitable access to influenza vaccines for developing countries was flawed.

Moving Beyond Strain-Specific Responses: The Call for a Global Access Framework

The unsatisfactory nature of vaccine access concerning HPAI-H5N1 and 2009-H1N1 has created interest in the creation of a global framework for equitable access that would become operational before the next influenza crisis. In a presentation to the Forum of Microbial Threats of the Institute of Medicine in September 2009, WHO's lead influenza specialist, Keiji Fukuda, described the problems experienced with the negotiations on HPAI-H5N1 virus and benefits sharing and on obtaining donations from manufacturers and developed countries for 2009-H1N1 vaccine.[20] Fukuda emphasized that the process and outcomes of the negotiations were suboptimal in terms of both public health and global equity and justice. Other experts have made similar claims concerning the moral and social justice issues at stake in equitable access to 2009-H1N1 vaccines.[21,22] In the interests of global health and global solidarity, Fukuda argued that a framework was needed to support global responses to influenza threats and ensure equitable access to vaccines for developing countries.[16] He asserted that improving access is the central global governance issue of our times, which gives the need for a global access framework importance beyond the world of public health.

Getting to Access: Negotiating Equitable Access to Influenza Vaccines

Negotiations to increase access to vaccines for HPAI-H5N1 and 2009-H1N1 have not proved successful for many reasons. In the Intergovernmental Meeting (IGM) on Pandemic Influenza Preparedness Framework for the Sharing of Influenza Viruses and Access to Vaccines and Other Benefits, WHO member states failed to reach agreement because they could not agree on benefit sharing.[23] Developing countries want obligatory benefit sharing in return for virus sharing, with binding terms spelled out in a Standard Material Transfer Agreement (SMTA). In contrast, developed countries want to avoid binding obligations to provide benefits (e.g., vaccines, antivirals) in exchange for access to virus samples provided by developing countries. At least one news report indicated that developed countries wanted to avoid losing their ability to place advance orders for influenza vaccine because of a binding SMTA.[19]

Interestingly, the 2009-H1N1 outbreak was underway when the IGM negotiations concluded unsuccessfully, meaning that this latest influenza threat was not a "game changer" for the positions staked out by WHO member states. In fact, the manner in which the outbreak and vaccine development and use proceeded favored developed countries for two reasons. First, countries with cases of 2009-H1N1 shared virus samples with WHO for surveillance and vaccine development without a quid pro quo for benefit sharing. To date, Indonesia remains the only country that has refused to share virus samples; other developing countries, even those that have supported Indonesia, share their samples without requiring benefits in return. Second, developed countries were able, through advance purchase contracts, to access almost all the vaccine that existing manufacturing facilities can produce[8,9] to ensure they would have 2009-H1N1 vaccine for their populations—precisely the option developed countries do not want the proposed SMTA to affect.

In terms of vaccine for 2009-H1N1, donations from manufacturers and developed countries were not the product of real negotiations, given that WHO and developing countries had little leverage to influence developed countries other than rhetoric about equity, justice, and solidarity. As experts noted, the donations from manufacturers were initially made without a fixed delivery date, meaning that the donated vaccines might arrive too late to be of much benefit in developing countries.[24] Developed countries only agreed to make donations after (1) they learned, unexpectedly, that a one-dose regimen would immunize adults, which doubled the amount of vaccine available[25]; and (2) data from the Northern and Southern hemispheres revealed that the 2009-H1N1 virus was behaving as a mild virus and not as a killer strain,[15] which reduced the threat the virus posed. In addition, developed countries pledging donations made sure that they had enough vaccine to cover their populations or, as happened with the United States, postponed donations to address national needs. In essence, manufacturers and developed countries incurred minimal financial, national public health, or political costs in pledging and, if necessary, delaying vaccine donations.

Vaccine and Resource Access in International Law

What has transpired in the contexts of HPAI-H5N1 and 2009-H1N1 reflects patterns seen in other efforts to create equitable access for vaccines and drugs. Existing international legal regimes that support global health, such as the WHO Constitution, the "right to health" in human rights treaties, and the International Health Regulations 2005, do not contain specific, binding provisions on equitable access to vaccines and drugs for developing countries. WHO's interest in creating a new global framework rather than relying on existing legal agreements reinforces the lack of any specific equitable access regime. Efforts to generate equitable access are not operated through purpose-built international legal instruments, and these efforts include WHO's adoption of a nonbinding global strategy on public health, innovation, and intellectual property[26]; provision of vaccines and drugs by intergovernmental organizations (e.g., WHO, UNICEF); bilateral donation schemes (e.g., the President's Emergency Plan for AIDS Relief); and public–private and nongovernmental mechanisms that make vaccines and drugs more available to developing countries (e.g., the Global Fund to Fight AIDS, Tuberculosis, and Malaria; the GAVI Alliance; Clinton Global Initiative; Médecins Sans Frontières' Campaign for Access to Essential Medicines; the International

Finance Facility for Immunization; UNITAID; and Advance Market Commitments for Vaccines).

This reality provides insight into why negotiations on virus and benefit sharing in connection with HPAI-H5N1 have, to date, failed, and why negotiations on a global access framework in the wake of the problems surrounding 2009-H1N1 would face obstacles. In short, states have not agreed to binding arrangements on more equitable access but, rather, attempt to increase such access through ad hoc, reactive, and non-binding activities that preserve national freedom of action while demonstrating some humanitarian concern.

Moreover, the situation concerning access to vaccines and drugs reflects how states generally allocate control of and access to resources. The central principles for allocating resources in international law are (1) sovereignty for resources found within a state's territory,[27] and (2) exclusive jurisdiction or control for resources found seawards from coastal states (e.g., the Exclusive Economic Zone in the law of the sea).[28] International relations provide few, if any, examples of states establishing a global framework to allocate resources, or the benefits derived from their exploitation, equitably. The most famous effort occurred in the negotiation of the UN Convention on the Law of the Sea (UNCLOS) in the 1970s and early 1980s, and it involved designating mineral resources found beyond 200 nautical miles from coastal states as the "common heritage of mankind," which would be exploited under jurisdiction of an International Seabed Authority, with benefits accruing to developing countries.[29] However, the United States and other developed countries opposed this aspect of UNCLOS, which, because of this opposition, has been revised to reflect what these developed countries prefer concerning exploitation of these mineral resources.[30]

The problems of equitable access to vaccines and drugs reflect these larger patterns in international law and international relations. As Indonesia's assertion of "viral sovereignty" demonstrates, states have sovereignty over biological samples isolated within their territories. Negotiations within the WHO[5] and the IGM[19] have re-emphasized that states have sovereignty over biological resources found within their jurisdictions. Similarly, states in which vaccines and drugs are manufactured have sovereignty over the manufacturing process and the products themselves until they are exported. States that import vaccines and drugs then have sovereignty over such resources and, absent a binding obligation, may allocate them however they wish. Negotiations to create a global access framework that more equitably distributes influenza vaccines would need to navigate through triple claims of sovereignty—a very tall order, without even factoring in the divergence of national interests seen in the IGM negotiations on virus and benefit sharing and the access problems associated with vaccine for 2009-H1N1.

Conclusion

Increasing equitable access to vaccines for dangerous influenza strains represents a difficult challenge for global health diplomacy, a challenge this chapter has addressed in only a preliminary manner. Efforts to recalibrate virus and benefit sharing in connection with HPAI-H5N1 through intergovernmental negotiations so far have not been successful. The manner in which access to vaccine for 2009-H1N1 played out highlights why the interests of developed and developing countries diverge in this context, and the reasons behind this divergence deserve deeper study. Existing international legal regimes on global health provide no templates for negotiating the new global access framework that WHO and others perceive is necessary. Similarly, negotiations for equitable access to resources, or the benefits of their exploitation, have generally failed in other areas of international relations, dimming prospects that precedents for a global access framework for pandemic influenza vaccines can be found outside the global health context. The default rules for allocating resources in international law rely on the principle of sovereignty, and these rules hold in the context of virus samples and vaccine supplies, as demonstrated with HPAI-H5N1 and 2009-H1N1.

Even the emergence of the first pandemic strain of influenza in 40 years in 2009 did not break the pattern of state behavior with respect to equitable access to a valuable but scarce resource. The appearance of a more severe influenza strain will reinforce rather than overcome this pattern because developed countries will prize their power and flexibility of action more in a severe pandemic than in a mild one, thus making hope for a crisis-sparked breakthrough misguided. The negotiating path that could lead to a new global access framework for influenza vaccines is not apparent, especially in a context in which aggregate global production capacity is woefully inadequate, the geographic location of production facilities is concentrated in developed countries, timelines for developing new vaccines create problems for rapid prevention strategies, and existing manufacturing technologies and distribution systems require improvements.

The need to increase global production capacity, diversify locales for manufacturing facilities, decrease the time from "lab to jab," and reduce production and distribution uncertainties has been recognized for years without sufficient progress being made, as evidenced by the HPAI-H5N1 and 2009-H1N1 controversies. Further research is required on ways in which states and non-state actors can address these problems through negotiated collective action. The diplomatic environment may have been made more difficult by accusations made and hearings held by officials in the Council of Europe that WHO succumbed to pressure from the pharmaceutical industry to declare a "false pandemic" and support development and use of a vaccine.[31,32] In the environment that exists on these issues, diplomatic advances will not be made simply by repeated claims that an undefined "global framework" is required because more equitable access is the just and moral end all states should seek.

References

1. Garrett, L. 2005. The next pandemic? *Foreign Affairs* 84 (4):3–23.

2. Fidler, D. P. 2008. Influenza virus samples, international law, and global health diplomacy. *Emerging Infectious Diseases* 14 (1):88–94.

3. Garrett, L., and D. P. Fidler. 2007. Sharing H5N1 viruses to stop a global influenza pandemic. *PLoS Med* 4 (11):e330.

4. For documentation produced by the IGM, see Intergovernmental Meeting on Pandemic Influenza Preparedness: Sharing of Influenza Viruses and Access to Vaccines and Other Benefits, Documentation. Available at: http://apps.who.int/gb/pip/.

5. World Health Assembly. 2007, May 23. Pandemic influenza preparedness: Sharing of influenza viruses and access to vaccines and other benefits. *WHA* 60.28.

6. Third World Network. 2009. WHO: Negotiations to continue on influenza virus and benefit sharing. Available at: http://www.twnside.org.sg/title2/intellectual_property/info.service/2009/twn.ipr.info.090507.htm.

7. Collin, N., X. de Radigues, and WHO H1N1 Vaccine Task Force. 2009. Vaccine production capacity for seasonal and pandemic (H1N1) 2009 influenza. *Vaccine* 27:5184–5186.

8. Brown, D. 2009, May 7. Vaccine would be spoken for; rich nations have preexisting contracts. *Washington Post*.

9. Whalen, J. 2009, May 16. Rich nations lock in flu vaccine as poor ones fret. *Wall Street Journal*.

10. Chan, M. 2009, July 14. Director-General of the World Health Organization, Strengthening multilateral cooperation on intellectual property and public health. Address to the World Intellectual Property Organization Conference on Intellectual Property and Public Policy Issues, Geneva, Switzerland. Available at: http://www.who.int/dg/speeches/2009/intellectual_property_20090714/en/index.html.

11. Butler, D. 2009, May 13. Q&A with Marie-Paule Kieny, the vaccine research director of the World Health Organization, on swine flu. *Nature News*. Available at: http://www.nature.com/news/2009/090513/full/news.2009.478.html.

12. Evans, R. 2009, September 25. More H1N1 vaccines likely for poor countries. *U.N. Reuters*. Available at: http://www.reuters.com/article/healthNews/idUSTRE58O4LG20090925?feedType=RSS&feedName=healthNews&pageNumber=2&virtualBrandChannel=0&sp=true.

13. WHO. 2009, June 17. WHO welcomes Sanofi-Aventis' donation of vaccine. Available at: http://www.who.int/mediacentre/news/statements/2009/vaccine_donation_20090617/en/index .html.

14. White House. 2009, September 17. President announces plan to expand fight against global H1N1 pandemic. Available at: http://www.whitehouse.gov/the_press_office/President -Announces-Plan-to-Expand-Fight-Against-Global-H1N1-Pandemic/.

15. Poorer nations get swine flu jabs. 2009, October 12. *BBC News.* Available at: http://news.bbc .co.uk/2/hi/health/8302416.stm..

16. Branswell, H. 2009, November 27. With H1N1 vaccine shipments topping 20M, Canada mulls options for leftovers. *Canadian Press.*

17. Branswell, H. 2009, November 4. Fears that countries would hoard vaccine in pandemics behind single supplier. *Canadian Press.* Available at: http://ca.news.yahoo.com/s/capress/091104/ health/health_flu_vaccine_single_supplier.

18. McNeil, D. G., Jr. 2009, November 4. Nation is facing vaccine shortage for seasonal flu. *New York Times.*

19. Americans first before US gives H1N1 flu vaccine. 2009, October 29. *Agence France-Presse.*

20. Fukuda, K. 2009, September 15. 2009 influenza (H1N1) pandemic: Lessons for going forward. Presentation at the Forum of Microbial Threats Workshop on the Domestic and International Aspects of the 2009 Influenza A (H1N1) Pandemic: Global Challenges, Global Solutions. Available at: http://www.iom.edu/Object.File/Master/73/476/Fukuda%20revised%20for%20WEB.pdf.

21. Gostin, L. O. 2009, August 8. Global goal for swine flu vaccine quest. *The Australian.*

22. Yamada, T. 2009. Poverty, wealth, and access to pandemic influenza vaccines. *N Engl J Med* 361:1129–1131.

23. Third World Network. 2009, May 19. WHO: Key elements of virus and benefit-sharing frame-work still unresolved. Available at: http://www.twnside.org.sg/title2/intellectual_property/info .service/2009/twn.ipr.info.090506.htm

24. Garrett, L. 2009, October 7. Global health update.

25. Neuzil, K. M. 2009. Pandemic influenza vaccine policy: Considering the early evidence. *N Engl J Med* 361:e59.

26. World Health Assembly. 2008, May 24. Global strategy and plan of action on public health, innovation, and intellectual property. *WHA* 61.21.

27. Brownlie, I. 2008. *Principles of Public International Law*, 7th ed. Oxford: Oxford University Press.

28. Churchill, R. R., and A. V. Lowe. 1999. *The Law of the Sea*, 3rd ed. Manchester: Manchester University Press.

29. United Nations Convention on the Law of the Sea. 1982, December 10. Part XI. Available at: http://www.un.org/Depts/los/convention_agreements/texts/unclos/closindx.htm.

30. Agreement Relating to the Implementation of Part XI of the United Nations Convention on the Law of the Sea. 1994, July 28. Available at: http://www.un.org/Depts/los/convention _agreements/texts/unclos/closindxAgree.htm

31. Pollard, C. 2010, January 12. Swine flu "a false pandemic" to sell vaccines, expert says. *The Daily Telegraph.* Available at: http://www.dailytelegraph.com.au/news/world/swine-flu-a -false-pandemic-to-sell-vaccines-expert-says/story-e6frev00-1225818409903.

32. Fukuda, K. 2010, January 26. Statement by Dr. Keiji Fukuda on behalf of WHO at the Council of Europe on pandemic (H1N1) 2009. Available at: http://www.who.int/csr/disease/swineflu/ coe_hearing/en/index.html.

31 Safeguarding Children: Pediatric Medical Countermeasure Research (*Executive Summary*)

Presidential Commission for the Study of Bioethical Issues[*]

Safeguarding children is one of our nation's foremost obligations. We have both a fundamental duty to protect individual children from undue risk during research and an obligation to protect all children during an emergency—to the extent ethically and practically possible—by being prepared with both the fruits of scientifically and ethically sound research and a fulsome national readiness to respond.

In January 2012, the Secretary of Health and Human Services (HHS) asked the Presidential Commission for the Study of Bioethical Issues (the Bioethics Commission) to advise the U.S. government—in its mission to be fully prepared to mitigate the impact of bioterrorism attacks—on ethical considerations in evaluating and conducting pediatric medical countermeasure (MCM) research.[1] The Secretary also asked that the Bioethics Commission "include the ethical considerations in conducting a pre- and post-event study of [anthrax vaccine adsorbed (AVA) post-exposure prophylaxis] in children as part of its review."[2]

Pediatric MCM research involves testing interventions with children that will be used in response to an attack either before an attack occurs (i.e., pre-event research) or testing such interventions following an attack (i.e., post-event research). Pre- and post-event pediatric MCM research poses risks to the individual children enrolled in research who, in many cases, do not stand to benefit directly from the research.

Research with children differs from that with adults because children cannot consent in the relevant sense; they are substantially lacking in the developed capacities necessary for adequately informed and voluntary decision making, making them a vulnerable population. Although this incapacity is most often attributed to their level of cognitive development, the vulnerability of children can derive from multiple sources

* From the Presidential Commission for the Study of Bioethical Issues, *Safeguarding Children: Pediatric Medical Countermeasure Research*, 2013. Full report available at: http://bioethics.gov/node/833.

(such as expectations of deference to adult authority, lack of independent resources for autonomous decision making, and longstanding institutionalized relationships of adult authority and power). For this reason, extra protections are warranted to ensure that children are not placed at excessive risk for the benefit of others. These additional safeguards include: parental permission, meaningful child assent, and limits on the degree of permissible research-related risk.

The Bioethics Commission's ethical analysis lies at the intersection of the unique characteristics of MCM research and pediatric research. In its 1977 report, *Research Involving Children*, the National Commission for the Protection of Human Subjects of Biomedical and Behavioral Research (the National Commission) presciently described this type of challenge: "The ethical principles at stake are the moral obligation to protect the community ... and the moral prohibition against using unconsenting persons, at considerable risk to their well-being, for the promotion of the common good."[3]

The four ethical principles that guide the Bioethics Commission's discussion of pediatric research protections are respect for persons, beneficence, and justice—as outlined in the *Belmont Report*[4]—and democratic deliberation, which was implicit both in the way the National Commission carried out its work and also in its recommendations regarding the process of reviewing and approving pediatric research.

HHS (and later the U.S. Food and Drug Administration [FDA]) adopted the National Commission's recommendations almost verbatim, and the regulations subsequently promulgated concerning research with children remain largely the same today, comprising Subpart D of HHS regulations at 45 C.F.R. Part 46 and FDA regulations at 21 C.F.R. Part 50.[5]

The National Commission's most straightforward recommendations addressed research that poses only minimal risk or that offers the prospect of direct benefit to participants. These recommendations would subsequently be codified in sections 404 and 405 of the HHS regulations. More complicated but still ethically tractable was research posing greater than minimal risk but likely to yield generalizable knowledge about the participants' condition. Research that is greater than minimal risk with no prospect of direct benefit to subjects or benefit to others with their condition was considered decidedly more controversial and ethically problematic. In the regulations, this last type of research was reserved for evaluation and approval by a national panel of experts and the Secretary of HHS for HHS-supported research (section 407).[6]

Pre-event Research

Pediatric research that presents no prospect of direct benefit to participants or that is not likely to yield generalizable knowledge about the participants' condition generally can only be conducted if it presents no more than minimal risk, except in extraordinary circumstances. Thus, the Bioethics Commission concluded that pre-event pediatric MCM research—which presents no prospect of direct benefit because no children are affected by the condition being studied—generally cannot proceed unless it is minimal risk research. Pre-event research might in some cases be designed in a way that would permit it to be judged minimal risk through an age de-escalation process in which risks are assessed and evaluated at each step. Robust research with young adults might support the conclusion that research with the oldest children is minimal risk. Similarly, research with the oldest children that further characterizes research risk might support an inference that research with the next oldest group of children is minimal risk as well.

Recommendation 1: Pre-event Pediatric Medical Countermeasure Research Risk Limited to Minimal Except under Extraordinary Circumstances

Pre-event pediatric medical countermeasure testing should be conducted with a research design posing only a minimal level of research risk except under extraordinary circumstances. If pre-event pediatric medical countermeasure research cannot be conducted as a minimal risk study, research that exposes children to no more than a minor increase over minimal risk—a level that is still limited and poses no substantial risk to health or well-being—should proceed to a national-level review under HHS regulations at 45 C.F.R. § 46.407 and/or FDA regulations at 21 C.F.R. § 50.54.

Recommendation 2: Risk in Pre-event Pediatric Medical Countermeasure Research

Before beginning pre-event medical countermeasure studies with children, ethically sound modeling, testing with animals, and testing with the youngest adults must be completed to identify, understand, and characterize research risks. If pediatric research is determined to be minimal risk and is to be conducted, progressive age de-escalation should be employed whenever possible from the oldest age group of children to the youngest group necessary to provide additional protection to the youngest and most vulnerable children, and to ensure that data from an older age group can inform the research design and the estimate of risk level for the next younger age group.

There will be instances in which it will be impossible to design minimal risk pre-event MCM research. In such cases, national-level review under section 407 would be required, but review should proceed only if researchers can demonstrate that the research poses no more than a minor increase over minimal risk to participants.

Recommendation 3: Pre-conditions to National-Level Review of Pre-event Pediatric Medical Countermeasure Research

Pre-event pediatric medical countermeasure research may proceed to national-level review under HHS regulations at 45 C.F.R. § 46.407 and/or FDA regulations at 21 C.F.R. § 50.54 only when researchers have demonstrated and reviewers concur that a minimal risk study is impossible and the proposed study poses no more than a minor increase over minimal risk to research participants. In part because of the inherent uncertainty of a bioterrorism attack, pre-event pediatric medical countermeasure research posing greater than a minor increase over minimal risk should not be approved under 45 C.F.R. § 46.407 or 21 C.F.R. § 50.54.

The Bioethics Commission's recommended framework, structured around the three conditions for national-level review, clarifies the circumstances in which proposed research presents a "reasonable opportunity" to address a "serious problem," specifies a rigorous set of conditions necessary to determine whether the research would be conducted in accordance with "sound ethical principles," and reiterates the importance of informed parental permission and meaningful and developmentally appropriate child assent. Decision makers should assess proposed pre-event pediatric MCM research that poses more than minimal risk using this framework to ensure that all the necessary aspects of a study have been evaluated and found ethically permissible before moving forward.

Recommendation 4: Ethical Framework for National-Level Review of Pre-event Pediatric Medical Countermeasure Research

To ensure the thoroughness and ethical rigor of national-level review, reviewers should apply the Bioethics Commission's recommended ethical framework for reviewing pre-event pediatric medical countermeasure research that poses greater than minimal risk, but no more than a minor increase over minimal risk, under HHS regulations at 45 C.F.R. § 46.407 and/or FDA regulations at 21 C.F.R. § 50.54. A proposed protocol must meet the requirements of the framework outlined in this chapter to be approved.

The framework clarifies the circumstances in which proposed research presents a "reasonable opportunity" to address a "serious problem," in particular, that seriousness must be judged by the consequences of exposure, likelihood (or threat) of exposure, and the "vital importance" of the information to be gained. The framework also specifies a rigorous set of conditions necessary to determine whether the research would be conducted in accordance with the required "sound ethical principles" that fall into five general categories: (1) ethical threshold of acceptable risk and adequate protection from harm; (2) ethical research design, for example, scientific necessity, valid research plan using small trials and age de-escalation with appropriate monitoring, and planning for post-event research; (3) post-trial requirements to ensure ethical distribution of medical countermeasures in the event of an attack, as well as a plan for treatment or compensation for research-related injury; (4) community engagement; and (5) transparency and accountability. Finally, the framework reiterates the importance of informed parental permission and meaningful and developmentally appropriate child assent.

Application to Trials of AVA with Children: Pre-event Research

In confronting the ethical questions surrounding MCM testing in pediatric populations, the Bioethics Commission concluded that before ethical pre-event pediatric AVA trials can be considered, further steps must be taken, including additional minimal risk research with adult participants to determine whether the research risks to children—who do not stand to benefit directly from it—pose no substantial risk to their health or well-being.

Given the amount of safety, immunogenicity, and dosing information about AVA in young adults ages 18 to 25 years, and given the widespread distribution of AVA in this population, it is possible that with additional testing in adults ages 18 to 20 years—testing to determine adverse effects, alternative dosing methods, and immunogenicity—testing of AVA with the oldest children (e.g., adolescents who are 16 to 17 years of age) could be considered no more than minimal risk. Consequently, it would be reviewed under section 404.

Informed, careful age de-escalation might allow researchers to infer minimal risk studies down the age scale. However, if data suggest that the use of AVA is affected, for example, by a child's developmental stage (e.g., infancy or puberty), or if an inference of minimal risk from an older group of children to the next younger group is not possible, a study designed to pose a minor increase over minimal risk might be appropriate for national-level review.

Post-event Research

Public health officials must be prepared to conduct post-event research when a bioterrorism attack occurs regardless of whether pre-event pediatric MCM research trials were conducted. In contrast to pre-event testing, in which ethical deliberations focus on whether any research with children would be ethically permissible, in post-event circumstances, research is ethically required to safeguard the well-being of current and future children. If a pediatric MCM research trial were completed pre-event, data should be collected following the administration of the tested intervention to acquire necessary additional safety information. In the absence of a pre-event investigation, an emergency situation might warrant administering an untested MCM to children in an effort to save lives. When children receive an untested MCM, it is ethically imperative that health officials collect data to learn as much as possible about the use of the untested MCM from the event.

Recommendation 5: Post-event Pediatric Medical Countermeasure Research

Post-event research should be planned in advance and conducted when untested medical countermeasures are administered to children in an emergency or when limited pre-event medical countermeasure studies have already occurred. Institutional review boards must be cognizant of the exigencies imposed on research under emergency conditions, and when reviewing post-event medical countermeasure research proposals, ensure that adequate processes are in place for informed parental permission and meaningful child assent. Institutional review boards must also ensure that the research design is scientifically sound, children enrolled in research have access to the best available care, adequate plans are in place to treat or compensate children injured by research, and provisions are made to engage communities throughout the course of research.

In the event of a bioterrorism attack, the U.S. government has emergency preparedness plans to mobilize medical interventions, drugs, vaccines, and supplies from the Strategic National Stockpile for distribution to affected portions of the population. The federal government delivers supplies to the states, which have individualized distribution strategies based on localized need and infrastructure. In the event that the MCM needed is either still in clinical trials or has not yet been approved for the specified application, two mechanisms available—an emergency use authorization (EUA) and an investigational new drug application (IND)—allow the government to distribute an unapproved intervention to help people in an emergency. Underlying the motivation for these mechanisms are a host of ethical principles, including respect for persons, beneficence, and justice. Together, the EUA and IND provide mechanisms to supply necessary MCMs with varying levels of clinical and research protections to ensure adequate respect for persons, as appropriate.

Recommendation 6: Regulatory Mechanisms for Post-event Pediatric Medical Countermeasure Research and Distribution

When there are no data on the administration of a medical countermeasure to children and it will be provided to children in an emergency, the medical countermeasure should be provided under a treatment IND to ensure that rigorous pediatric research protections apply to safeguard those children who receive the medical countermeasure. When a medical countermeasure is distributed broadly to children using a treatment IND, it is essential that the U.S. government also conduct a concurrent small-scale study under an investigator IND to obtain data that can potentially be used to support an emergency use authorization for pediatric use of the medical countermeasure in a future event. To expedite post-event research and ensure the availability of appropriate medical countermeasures for children, a pre-IND consultation and approval should be put in place before an event.

Application to Trials of AVA with Children: Post-event Research

In an event involving the release of weaponized anthrax, or other large-scale release of spores, a plan exists to provide children, like adults, treatment with a 60-day course of antibiotics as well as AVA.[7] The FDA and the U.S. Centers for Disease Control and Prevention (CDC) have a treatment IND in place to allow for broad access to AVA for children in the event of an emergency. Work is ongoing to clarify the informed consent process. In addition, the FDA and CDC are collaborating to develop a nested proto-col that would involve research and surveillance to better understand immunogenic-ity and reactogenicity to the vaccine.[8] Both of these mechanisms require Institutional Review Board (IRB) approval.

Under the Bioethics Commission's ethical approach, even if a pre-event study of AVA with children is approved, post-event research would be necessary to gather additional safety and immunogenicity data beyond the limited amount a pre-event study could produce. If a pre-event study is not approved and AVA is nonetheless administered to children in the event of an attack, post-event research would be ethically required.

It is important that any post-event distribution of AVA to children, regardless of the specific mechanism, entail democratic deliberation in the form of extensive com-munity engagement. Community engagement should begin in pre-event research and continue through post-event activities. Moreover, it is critical that any post-event research protocol be scientifically sound, have adequate processes in place to ensure informed parental permission and meaningful child assent, provide for adequate treat-ment or compensation for research-related injuries, and ensure that enrolled children have access to the best available care.

•

Pediatric MCM research brings into sharp focus the fact that the health and security of children are paramount. It highlights the importance of both protecting children from unjustifiable research risks and ensuring their safety as far as possible in the event of an emergency. Grounding its work in the principles of respect for persons, beneficence, justice, and democratic deliberation, the Bioethics Commission reaffirmed the ethical foundations of pediatric research and applied them to the particularly complex and difficult case of pediatric MCM research. As exemplified by the Bioethics Commission's deliberations, such research warrants an ongoing national conversation to ensure the highest standards of protection for children that reflect an unwavering commitment to safeguard all children *from* unacceptable risks in research and *through* research that promotes their health and well-being.

Notes and References

1. For the purposes of this report, the Bioethics Commission defined medical countermeasures (MCMs) as U.S. Food and Drug Administration (FDA)-regulated products and interventions used to combat the effects of chemical, biological, radiological, or nuclear (CBRN) events. Given the Bioethics Commission's definition of MCM, it used the term *bioterrorism* to refer to chemical, biological, radiological, and nuclear attacks generally.

2. Letter from Secretary Kathleen Sebelius, Health and Human Services (HHS), to Amy Gutmann, Chair, Presidential Commission for the Study of Bioethical Issues (PCSBI). 2012, January 6. Available at: http://bioethics.gov/cms/sites/default/files/news/PediatricCountermeasures-LetterfromtheSecretary.pdf.

3. The National Commission for the Protection of Human Subjects of Biomedical and Behavioral Research. 1977. *Research Involving Children* (DHEW Publication OS 77–0004). Washington, DC: Department of Health, Education, and Welfare. Available at: http://bioethics.georgetown.edu/pcbe/reports/past_commissions/Research_involving_children.pdf.

4. The National Commission for the Protection of Human Subjects of Biomedical and Behavioral Research. 1978. *The Belmont Report: Ethical Principles and Guidelines for the Protection of Human Subjects of Research* (DHEW Publication OS 78–0012). Washington, DC: Department of Health, Education, and Welfare. Available at: http://www.hhs.gov/ohrp/humansubjects/guidance/belmont.html.

5. The language of the two sets of regulations is substantively identical. The Bioethics Commission refers only to HHS regulations in the text of this chapter, although the discussion encompasses the provisions of Subpart D as codified by both HHS and the FDA. See Additional Protections for Children Involved as Subjects in Research, 48 Fed. Reg. 9,814 (March 8, 1983) (codified at 45 C.F.R. §§ 46.401 et seq.) and Additional Safeguards for Children in Clinical Investigations of FDA-Regulated Products, 66 Fed. Reg. 20,589 (April 24, 2001) (codified at 21 C.F.R. §§ 50.50 et seq.).

6. In the case of FDA-regulated research, the Commissioner of Food and Drugs, in consultation with a national panel of experts, makes the final determination (21 C.F.R. § 50.54). When

research is governed by both FDA and HHS regulations, the Secretary of HHS makes the final determination. FDA. 2006, December. Guidance for Clinical Investigators, Institutional Review Boards, and Sponsors: Process for Handling Referrals to FDA Under 21 C.F.R. 50.54. Available at: http://www.fda.gov/downloads/RegulatoryInformation/Guidances/ucm127605.pdf.

7. U.S. Centers for Disease Control and Prevention. 2010. Use of anthrax vaccine in the United States: Recommendations of the Advisory Committee on Immunization Practices (ACIP), 2009. *Morbidity and Mortality Weekly Report: Recommendations and Reports* 59 (RR-06):21. Available at: http://www.cdc.gov/mmwr/preview/mmwrhtml/rr5906a1.htm; National Biodefense Science Board. 2011. *Challenges in the Use of Anthrax Vaccine Adsorbed (AVA) in the Pediatric Population as a Component of Post-Exposure Prophylaxis (PEP): A Report of the National Biodefense Science Board.* Available at: http://www.phe.gov/Preparedness/legal/boards/nbsb/recommendations/Documents/avwgrpt1103.pdf.

8. Maher, C. 2012, November 5. Regulatory landscape for providing MCMs to children in an emergency. Presentation to PCSBI. Available at: http://bioethics.gov/node/788.

32 Protecting Our Children from Bioterrorism Requires Testing of Anthrax Vaccine

Tia Powell*

Last month, the Presidential Commission for the Study of Bioethical Issues released a nuanced and thoughtful report recommending against studying the anthrax vaccine in children. I might have agreed—why put any child at unnecessary risk?—had I not spent a year co-chairing an Institute of Medicine report on protecting the public from a deadly anthrax attack.

Anthrax is considered the most likely threat for a bioterrorism attack because its hardy, microscopic spores are easily cultivated and make for a powerful weapon. Symptoms develop a few days after exposure, and once they do, the disease is usually fatal, and gruesomely so. (Death typically results from internal bleeding, pulmonary failure, and meningitis.) An exposed population also must be vaccinated to prevent the spores from reactivating and causing infection weeks after the original exposure.

Since the 2001 anthrax scare, when letters containing anthrax spores were mailed to media outlets and two U.S. senators, the government has gone to considerable lengths to improve our defenses, particularly in the event of a large-scale airborne attack. We have large stockpiles of drugs as well as a U.S. Federal Drug Administration (FDA)-approved vaccine ready for deployment. There have been numerous drills across the country to ensure we know how to respond—and quickly.

But here is the rub. Although the vaccine has long been approved and used in adults, it has never been studied in children. The President's Commission declined to permit anthrax vaccine research on children on the grounds that child participants have no prospect for direct benefit because they had not been exposed to anthrax. This distinction is crucial in research regulation because pediatric studies with "no direct benefit" face substantial barriers for approval. But this is a category error. Vaccines are preventive treatments, and vaccine research is preventive research. Such a study is not done on those who have been exposed to an agent but rather on those who are at risk

* Originally published in *The Huffington Post*, April 2013. Reprinted with permission.

of exposure. (The exception would be in case of exposure during a natural disaster.) If the population in the study is at risk, there is potential benefit to them from receiving the vaccine.

Bioterrorism experts are a gloomy lot. They're highly educated people, often with multiple advanced degrees, who spend their days pondering frightening worst-case scenarios. They take anthrax very seriously; many are already vaccinated. That's why a group of such experts, the National Biodefense Science Board, recommended studying the vaccine in children, pending ethics approval.

Here's how it could work: Query those who, based on their professional work, are highly informed about bioterrorism and who can meet a high standard for informed consent. Then within this group, identify those who are parents and live in high-risk cities (there is a list). Ask them whether they see a potential benefit for their children in vaccine trial participation. Based on an informal sample of my acquaintances from the world of bioterrorism preparedness, all would strongly consider enrolling their child in an anthrax vaccine trial—based on potential benefit. Even with requiring rigorous parental informed consent, child assent, limiting to children in high-risk cities and starting with the oldest, I am betting you would still have enough children to complete a solid study.

It is important to protect children from the risks of research. It is even more important to avoid exposing millions of children to untested vaccine in the ultimate clinical study—one that unfolds during a live public health disaster.

VI   Global Vaccination and Disease Eradication Programs

Vaccination programs in low- and middle-income countries typically differ enormously in design, scope, and character from those in the United States and other wealthy countries that were the principal focus of the chapters in parts III and IV of this volume. Particularly for developing countries, issues of access and affordability present profoundly difficult challenges to vaccination efforts. At the same time, vaccine delivery often must occur in settings where health infrastructures are lacking and the health needs of citizens and communities are many.

In the world's wealthiest nations, common goals may include sustaining vaccination rates of 90% or higher for existing vaccines and introducing newly approved vaccines as quickly as possible. But in many developing countries, vaccination coverage targets are often far more modest. Building vaccination programs against diseases for which vaccines have been available for years (or even decades, as in the cases of polio and measles vaccines) remains a foremost need and priority.

This section examines a few of the many critically important policy and ethical questions raised when considering vaccination activities in developing countries. The first two chapters underscore the challenges of ensuring global access to vaccines and consider potential solutions. Dave Chokshi and Aaron Kesselheim highlight some of the core obstacles with which global vaccination efforts must contend, including infrastructure, regulatory pathways, and funding. Seth Berkley extends this discussion of funding and financing in his examination of tiered pricing programs, through which countries pay different prices for the same vaccines based on their wealth.

Conducting vaccination programs in the context of humanitarian emergencies introduces additional complexity for health agencies and workers alike. Keymanthri Moodley, Kate Hardie, and colleagues discuss the ethical concerns raised by these activities, including when such programs are appropriate and how they should be designed and implemented.

The remainder of the section looks at various aspects of disease eradication efforts in the past, present, and future. The coordinated global campaign leading to the eradication of smallpox remains among the foremost triumphs in the history of public health. It is also a model for numerous ongoing and intended disease control efforts. D. A. Henderson, a leader of the smallpox eradication program, discusses that work and its lessons for the future in an interview with Petra Klepac.

Paul Greenough next presents accounts of deeply troubling actions that took place in the final stages of the eradication effort. These actions would appear to constitute clear violations of human rights on the part of healthcare workers participating in this work. Greenough acknowledges the difficulty of knowing how common the conduct he writes about was, a point echoed by William Foege, another leader of the smallpox eradication campaign. In his own account of the eradication effort, Foege (2011) writes:

Coercion was never program policy. A 1995 article by Paul Greenough gives the erroneous impression that coercion was required for containment to work in the final elimination of smallpox. He recount four instances in which two American epidemiologists used coercion plus a fifth instance in which an Indian government vaccinator used force to hold and vaccinate people. ... The cases cited are no doubt true, but they would have been aberrations, perhaps the result of the kind of frustration that anyone who has worked in the field can understand. Cultural sensitivity was emphasized in the training of smallpox workers in India and in the field was the norm rather than the exception. Certainly force was not needed for eradication. Greenough interpreted this aberration to be the norm. (p. 206)

Smallpox eradication has been both a model and an inspiration for the ongoing effort to eradicate polio, a program that has received extraordinary attention, investment, and energy from a broad partnership of public health advocates for more than two decades. Tremendous progress has been made in reducing the prevalence of the virus, but preventing the remaining few cases has been a costly, time-consuming, and as yet unsuccessful endeavor. The wisdom and ethics of continuing to pursue polio eradication, instead of prioritizing ongoing control of the virus while redirecting resources to other pressing global health needs, are debated in the next two chapters. Arthur Caplan offers a skeptical assessment of the ethics of disease eradication, while Claudia Emerson and Peter A. Singer provide a spirited ethical defense.

If polio eradication—or any vaccination program in developing countries—is to be successful, public trust in medical and public health personnel is essential, just as we have seen previously in the context of vaccination programs in wealthy countries. This trust was thought to have been jeopardized by a "sham" vaccination program organized by the U.S. Central Intelligence Agency to gain intelligence as part of its successful pursuit of Osama bin Laden. The deans of many leading U.S. schools of public health wrote to President Barack Obama to express their objection to these actions and their concerns for its consequences for future global health efforts. That letter and the response from a senior White House official providing assurance that such programs will not occur in the future conclude this section.

Further Reading

William Foege. 2011. *House on Fire: The Fight to Eradicate Smallpox.* Berkeley, CA: University of California Press.

Gavi: The Vaccine Alliance. 2016. Available at: http://www.gavi.org.

Global Polio Eradication Initiative. 2016. Available at: http://www.polioeradication.org/.

Nancy Leys Stepan. 2011. *Eradication: Ridding the World of Infectious Diseases Forever?* Ithaca, NY: Cornell University Press.

World Health Organization. 2013. Global Vaccine Action Plan, 2011–2020. Geneva: World Health Organization. Available at: http://www.who.int/immunization/global_vaccine_action _plan/GVAP_doc_2011_2020/en/.

33   Rethinking Global Access to Vaccines (*Excerpt*)

Dave A. Chokshi and Aaron S. Kesselheim[*]

Inadequate access to vaccines in low- and middle-income countries results in more than 2 million deaths each year.[1] Three arguments have historically dominated discussions about the cause of unequal access to vaccines in poorer countries: the primacy of healthcare infrastructure, constraints imposed by insufficient funding, and the belief that vaccine approval in high-income countries is a precondition for discussing access in other settings. Recent experiences have shown how each of these contentions is open to challenge.

Primacy of Infrastructure

Must poor healthcare infrastructure be addressed before large-scale vaccination can succeed? The claim that poor infrastructure is a more fundamental—and therefore more pressing—problem than access to vaccines must be distinguished from the claim that local logistical hurdles must be overcome to achieve equitable access. Those who agree with the former contention believe that ensuring supplies of food and clean water and building roads will do more for public health than isolated interventions such as vaccines. For example, access to rotavirus vaccination has been questioned on the grounds that it might undermine the urgency of providing clean water and sanitation for all.[2]

An exclusive focus on the primacy of basic public health interventions, however, can block the opportunity to build infrastructure through vaccination. Empirical analyses, most notably of polio eradication in the Americas, have documented how immunization programs can strengthen the infrastructure of health systems.[3] Amartya Sen describes the broader effect as an "autocatalytic process" connecting health and development, whereby improving health through direct means such as vaccines unlocks

* Originally published in *BMJ*, 2008; 336 (7647):750–753. Reprinted with permission from BMJ Publishing Group, Ltd.

the capabilities of populations to thrive economically.[4] In addition, contact between the healthcare establishment and indigent people is often sporadic and usually related to an acute health problem. Vaccines are one of the few interventions that can save lives even when healthcare infrastructure is inadequate or non-existent. Clarifying the underpinnings of this infrastructure problem permits a rigorous examination of the local obstacles that make the delivery of vaccines difficult.

Funding

Are the costs of closing the global vaccination gap out of proportion to the funding available? At the country and district levels, acceptance of the cost-funding orthodoxy has been posited as a chief reason for the slow uptake of vaccines, such as for hepatitis B vaccine in the past.[5] One reaction to this imbalance is to calculate the funding short-fall and advocate for its redress.[6] But the vaccine equation is more complicated than simply tabulating inputs and outlays. Rational policymaking depends on analysis of both costs and benefits. A recent cost-effectiveness analysis showed that a vaccination program for hepatitis B was both cost-effective and affordable in the Gambia, where the per capita gross domestic product is only $300.[7] Furthermore, vaccines can confer macroeconomic benefits such as improved labor productivity that may supersede the substantial directly measured health benefits.[8] The International Finance Facility for Immunisation (http://www.iffim.org/), which provides immediate aid from wealthier countries to GAVI, is a financial solution that represents a first step in accelerating the pace of investment in immunization.

Prior Approval

Must vaccines be developed for and approved by wealthier countries before they can be widely disseminated? Currently, availability of vaccines in low- and middle-income countries depends largely on prior evaluation by U.S. or European drug regulatory agencies.[9] Pharmaceutical manufacturers receive the vast majority of their revenues from wealthier countries, so there is less financial incentive to make a product available if it is not being sold in those markets. Also, health agencies in poorer countries often take their cues from nations with more established regulatory systems before approving new products or when removing them from the market. In 2001, after Wyeth's rotavirus vaccine Rotashield was taken off the market in the United States for a rare association with increased rates of intussusception, Wyeth stopped production, and the product was eliminated from use in low- and middle-income countries, where the higher rates of morbidity from rotavirus-associated diarrhea may have made the low risk of that side effect more tolerable.[10]

The ultimate aim of any effort to improve global access to vaccines must be to show local leaders in health care and government the benefits of vaccination.[11] Local political leadership, when combined with international financing mechanisms, can increase investment in health, prioritize disease prevention, and raise awareness about the individual benefits of vaccination.[12] The way forward—building immunity by building capacity—would help save and improve the lives of millions of patients around the world.

References

1. World Health Organization. 2005. *World Health Report 2005: Make Every Mother and Child Count.* Geneva: World Health Organization. Available at: www.who.int/whr/2005/en/index.html

2. Birn, A. E. 2005. Gates's grandest challenge: transcending technology as public health ideology. *Lancet* 366:514–519.

3. Institute of Medicine. 2002. Major efforts for disease eradication. In: Considerations for Viral Disease Eradication: Lessons Learned and Future Strategies, eds. S. Knobler, J. Lederberg, and L. Pray, 33–63. Washington, DC: Institute of Medicine. Available at: http://www.nap.edu/read/10424/chapter/4/.

4. Sen, A. K. 1999. *Development as Freedom.* New York: Knopf.

5. Clemens, J. D. 2003. Thinking downstream to accelerate the introduction of new vaccines for developing countries. *Vaccine* 21 (suppl 2):S114–S115.

6. Peny, J. M., O. Gleizes and J. P. Covilard. 2005. Financial requirements of immunisation programmes in developing countries: A 2004–2014 perspective. *Vaccine* 23:4610–4618.

7. Kim, S.-Y., J. A. Salomon and S. J. Goldie. 2007. Economic evaluation of hepatitis B vaccine in low-income countries. *Bull World Health Organ* 85:821–900.

8. Bloom, D. E., D. Canning, and M. Weston. 2005. The value of vaccination. *World Economics* 6 (3):25.

9. Brooke, S., and J. Sherris. 2006. *HPV Vaccines: Regulatory Issues.* London: PATH. Available at: www.rho.org/files/StopCxCa_regulatory_2006.pdf

10. Cohen, J. 2001. Medicine: Rethinking a vaccine's risk. *Science* 293:1576–1577.

11. Buekens, P., G. Keusch, J. Belizan, and Z. A. Bhutta. 2004. Evidence-based global health. *JAMA* 291:2639–2641.

12. Mahmoud, A. 2004. The global vaccination gap. *Science* 305:147.

34 Improving Access to Vaccines through Tiered Pricing

Seth Berkley*

Immunization is now widely recognized as one of the most efficient, successful, and cost-effective health investments in history, but despite substantial effort over the past 50 years, nearly one in five deaths of children younger than 5 years of age is still caused by a vaccine-preventable disease. With more than 22 million children in the world still unimmunized against common but life-threatening diseases (as measured by a vaccine containing a third dose of diphtheria-tetanus-pertussis [DTP]), almost all in developing countries, there is clearly still a long way to go.

In addition to the traditional and inexpensive vaccines included in the expanded program on immunization, nowadays new, more expensive, and complex vaccines are available. Mainly manufactured by a few research-based vaccine companies, these vaccines target the most common causes of the diseases that kill children, such as diarrhea and pneumonia. In 2000, the GAVI Alliance was created to help reduce the delay in the introduction of these types of new vaccines in low-income countries. Since GAVI's inception, about 440 million of the world's poorest children will have been immunized with its support by the end of 2013, with 6 million future deaths averted in the process.[1] The latest estimates predict that in the period up to 2020, the vaccines that GAVI are supporting will help to avert a further 8 million deaths.[2]

GAVI has a simple business model. It supports countries with a gross national income (GNI) per head less than US$1,550 (which is adjusted annually for inflation and due to increase to $1,570 in 2014) and negotiates reduced pricing from vaccine manufacturers to be able to supply them with vaccines.[3] Because GAVI serves only the lowest-income countries, it has been able to negotiate the lowest prices from manufacturers. As part of the model, GAVI countries pay a small proportion of the vaccine costs—so that there is some form of cost sharing. As countries become wealthier, they pay an increasing

* Reprinted from *The Lancet*, Berkley, S., Improving access to vaccines through tiered pricing, 383:2265–2267. Copyright © 2014 with permission of Elsevier.

copayment until their GNI exceeds the GAVI GNI threshold, and they graduate.[4] After a transition period, countries must take on financing the full cost of the vaccines. Graduation is a way for GAVI and its financial supporters to focus their resources on the poorest countries while enabling governments with growing economies to take increasing responsibility and ownership for vaccination programs over time.

GAVI uses several means to reduce the price of the vaccines that it procures. GAVI's ordering and purchasing on behalf of countries are backed by financial commitments from donors. These commitments give manufacturers predictability for their production planning. GAVI pools demand so that it can leverage economies of scale (at present GAVI serves 58% of the global birth cohort) while companies deal mainly with only one purchaser, procured by GAVI through UNICEF Supply Division. This process reduces transaction costs, allowing for even further savings. To give a sense of the scale of procurement, in 2012, UNICEF procured more than $790 million worth of vaccines from ten manufacturers on behalf of GAVI countries. GAVI and its Alliance partners also use push and pull mechanisms to incentivize manufacturers. For example, the Bill & Melinda Gates Foundation has provided developing-country manufacturers with investments to support product development and manufacturing scale-up in return for lower vaccine prices when they begin supplying.[5] The pneumococcal Advance Market Commitment (AMC) uses donor commitments and long-term contracts to incentivize manufacturers to accelerate and expand the supply of this vaccine.

The problem, however, is that countries with GNI greater than the GAVI threshold face much higher prices for these new, more technologically advanced vaccines. In many of these countries, governments cannot afford to pay while private-sector prices are unaffordable for most families. As a result, many children living in non-GAVI-eligible middle-income countries are not being vaccinated, and uptake of new vaccines risks lagging behind many GAVI-eligible countries. Although some of GAVI's and the Alliance partners' interventions can indirectly support non-GAVI-eligible middle-income countries (e.g., incentivizing new manufacturers increases competition and benefits all markets that they serve), GAVI's focus has been on the poorest countries. However, as countries pass the threshold and graduate from GAVI support, there is concern that they could be at risk of suspending vaccination programs because they face a so-called pricing cliff, with steep increases when they no longer have access to GAVI prices.

In view of the latest population trends, this situation is particularly worrying. In 1990, more than 90% of the world's poorest people lived in countries classified as low-income countries.[6] Nowadays, 70% of the world's poorest people live in middle-income countries.[7] Consequently, the burden of vaccine-preventable disease is now about twice as great in middle-income countries as in low-income countries, with just four countries accounting for around half of the vaccine-preventable deaths in the world, or 75% of those occurring in all middle-income countries: India, Indonesia, Nigeria, and Pakistan. Although these countries still receive GAVI support, all but Pakistan are expected to graduate in the coming years.

So, what we need is a way to ensure that children who are not living in GAVI-eligible countries also have access to affordable life-saving vaccines that will ultimately increase their chances of living healthy and productive lives. For GAVI-eligible countries, as their incomes grow, we need to find a way to ensure that their immunization coverage achievements do not stop when they graduate from GAVI support because of unsustainable prices.

A solution is transparent and consistent tiered pricing for vaccines. The idea is simple enough: to have countries pay prices according to their ability to pay, as determined by their varying level of national income. To some extent, tiered pricing for vaccines already exists, with GAVI countries paying the lowest price and non-GAVI, lower middle-income and middle-income countries representing a middle tier.[8] For example, the price of pneumococcal vaccines for GAVI countries, $3.30–3.50 per dose, is less than 5% of the $102 price that is paid for pneumococcal conjugate vaccines in the United States. However, prices in these slightly higher-income countries can vary substantially on the basis of the country's size, region, and predictability of financing, and there is a lack of transparency about who is paying what because most of these countries negotiate individually with manufacturers. There is also the vaccine revolving fund of the Pan American Health Organization (PAHO) that bands together the PAHO countries in a buying group and requires companies to provide them with one offer for all countries at the lowest worldwide price. PAHO includes some low-income countries such as Haiti, which has a GNI as low as $760, but 70% of its members are middle-income or high-income countries with a GNI of more than $4,085 and ranging up to $106,000. Yet although it cuts across tiers, PAHO has nevertheless achieved large discounts through this regional buying model. Indeed GAVI has benefited from lessons learned from this fund and from their granting of a waiver to the least price clause such that the poorest countries, including those within PAHO, can receive vaccines at the lowest prices. But given that this pooling cuts across a broad range of GNIs and because of the single price principle, middle-income countries both within the PAHO region and outside might not obtain the best possible price.

Instead, I believe that country access and ultimately company interests would be better served by a more structured global framework of price tiers, each based on country income (e.g., with use of World Bank income groupings: low income, lower-middle income, upper-middle income, and high income).[4] Because growth in GNI does not always represent country investment in social development and local risk situations can vary, criteria beyond GNI could additionally be used to tier countries (e.g., burden of disease, immunization coverage, etc.). Furthermore, this approach could include banding within price tiers on the basis of factors such as volumes and certainty of demand. Public markets would of course be treated differently than private markets.[8] To help graduating countries to transition from the GAVI environment to the wider tiered model, graduating countries could have a so-called grandfathering clause, which would allow them to keep the GAVI price for up to 5 years, following the end of GAVI support, before moving to the cost structure of their new income tier.

Tiered pricing is particularly relevant for vaccines. Technically challenging product development and high fixed costs contribute to high barriers to entry. For many vaccines, to sustain more than three or four manufacturers is difficult. This factor limits competition, which ordinarily would alone be an effective lever to drive down prices. Thus, tiered pricing could apply for all GAVI vaccines but would be most crucial for new vaccines when there are particularly few manufacturers.

Because giving industry visibility on demand is crucial to help plan production, achieve appropriate scale-up, and ultimately secure lower prices, an instrument could also be put in place to support non-GAVI, lower middle-income countries through pooled procurement mechanisms to achieve the lowest available prices within a given tier. This approach would need to be supported by careful demand forecasting, and potentially some demand guarantees, to enable countries to procure at a GAVI price plus a fixed step premium for each tier.

So although it is for manufacturers to set the prices of vaccines, the tiers would act as a guide irrespective of whether they are multinational corporations or developing country vaccine manufacturers. Most countries, rich or poor, already tend to base the decision on whether to publicly fund the introduction of a new vaccine on some form of cost-effectiveness model, so to set the price in the tier according to that equation would make sense.[9] The challenge is having reliable data to make such an assessment, so in the absence of such data, GNI usually serves as a reasonable proxy.

For many middle-income countries, prices are often still too high to finance vaccines for their national programs. Furthermore, the lack of demand predictability and transaction costs that come with dealing with countries on an individual basis, together with the fear of eroding profit margins in high-income countries because of price (and therefore implied cost) transparency, have historically resulted in keeping prices high.

But since GAVI's inception, much has changed. GAVI has shown how it is possible to provide demand predictability for low-income countries and a subset of lower-middle-income countries, and to use this information to secure lower prices. There have also been significant efforts by the vaccine industry to make new vaccines more affordable, as shown by the price reductions for rotavirus, pentavalent, and human papillomavirus vaccines,[10] the latter going from open market prices in excess of $100 and lowest public sector price of $13 a dose to a GAVI price of $4.50. With expanded and more predictably stable demand, new companies—particularly from developing countries—have begun to serve these markets, thus creating supply security and healthy competition.

A balance between fair access and fair profit levels can be struck.[11] Moreover, the global health community should not be opposed to manufacturers making a profit; after all, vaccines are not a commodity market. Indeed, we should be mindful that to some extent overcapacity is needed for supply security, and that in view of the public health benefit, we should be willing to pay for it. By giving countries prices for vaccines that reflect their ability to pay, this type of approach would give countries the ability to plan programmatically and financially, which should ultimately create better predictability. In return, vaccine companies will be able to access wider markets, increase their production volumes (which will reduce their manufacturing costs),[5] and have the opportunity to do the right thing for people who need but cannot afford their vaccines today.

References

1. GAVI Alliance. 2013, October. Global level indicators. Available at: http://www.gavialliance.org/results/gavi_alliance_goal_level_indicators/.

2. Lee, L. A., F. Franzel, J. Atwell, S. D. Datta, I. K, Friberg, S. J. Goldie, et al. 2013. The estimated mortality impact of vaccinations forecast to be administered during 2011–2020 in 73 countries supported by the GAVI Alliance. *Vaccine* 31S:B61–B72.

3. GAVI Alliance. 2013. Country eligibility policy. Available at: http://www.gavialliance.org/about/governance/programme-policies/country-eligibility/.

4. GAVI Alliance. 2009, November 18. GAVI Alliance graduation policy. Available at: http://www.gavialliance.org/library/gavi-documents/policies/gavi-alliance-graduation-policy/.

5. Plahte, J. 2005. Tiered pricing of vaccines: A win-win-win situation, not a subsidy. *Lancet Infect Dis* 5:58–63.

6. The World Bank. How we classify countries. Available at: http://data.worldbank.org/about/country-classifications.

7. Glassman, A., D. Duran, and A. Sumner. 2012. *Global Health and the New Bottom Billion: How Funders Should Respond to Shifts in Global Poverty and Disease Burden.* Washington, DC: Center for

Global Development. Available at: http://www.cgdev.org/doc/full_text/BottomBillion/Glassman _Bottom_Billion.html#_ftn2.

8. Yadav, P. 2010, August. *Differential Pricing for Pharmaceuticals: Review of Current Knowledge, New Findings and Ideas for Action.* London: Department for International Development. Available at: https://www.gov.uk/government/uploads/system/uploads/attachment_data/file/67672/diff -pcing-pharma.pdf.

9. Lopert, R., D. L. Lang, S. R. Hill, and D. A. Henry. 2002. Differential pricing of drugs: A role for cost-effectiveness analysis? *Lancet* 359:2105–2107.

10. Cutts, F., S. Franceschi, S. Goldie, X. Castellsaque, S. de Sanjose, G. Garnett, et al. 2007. Human papillomavirus and HPV vaccines: A review. *Bull World Health Organ* 85:719–726.

11. Danzon, P., and A. Towse. 2003, July. Differential pricing for pharmaceuticals: Reconciling access, R&D and patents. Brookings working paper 03–7. Available at: http://regulation2point0 .org/wp-content/uploads/downloads/2010/04/phpng.pdf.

35 Ethical Considerations for Vaccination Programs in Acute Humanitarian Emergencies

Keymanthri Moodley, Kate Hardie, Michael J. Selgelid, Ronald J. Waldman, Peter Strebel, Helen Rees, and David N. Durrheim[*]

Acute humanitarian crises pose complex ethical dilemmas for policymakers, particularly in settings with inadequate healthcare services, which often become dependent on external agencies for urgently needed care.[1] These ethical dilemmas are inherent in many spheres of the response activity, including measures to mitigate infectious disease transmission, which often cause outbreaks during humanitarian crises. In the initial emergency response, interventions to reduce communicable disease transmission, such as vaccination, should be deployed along with food, water, and shelter because communicable diseases, including some that are vaccine-preventable, can spread faster and be unusually severe in the crowded, unhygienic conditions that prevail during crises. Measles, with a case-fatality rate as high as 30% during a humanitarian crisis, is a fitting example.[2]

Several factors need to be considered before a vaccine is deployed: the potential burden of disease; vaccine-related risks (usually minimal); the desirability of prevention as opposed to treatment; the duration of the protection conferred; cost; herd immunity in addition to individual protection; and the logistical feasibility of a large-scale vaccination program. Vaccination may be the only practical way to protect people against certain diseases, such as meningococcal meningitis and measles. Individuals who undergo medical or surgical treatment often need ongoing care; those who get vaccinated do not, yet they receive long-lasting benefits. However, the feasibility of a mass vaccination effort depends largely on available resources.

In a recent study on ethics in humanitarian health care, respondents pointed out the need for ethical guidance on issues such as vaccination during emergency situations.[3] The World Health Organization (WHO) and several humanitarian nongovernmental organizations have acknowledged this need. In an effort to address it, WHO's

* Originally published in *Bulletin of the World Health Organization*, 2013;91:290–297. Reprinted under the terms of a Creative Commons Intergovernmental Organization License.

Strategic Advisory Group of Experts (SAGE) on Immunization developed a framework for decision makers on the deployment and effective use of vaccines that can save lives during emergencies.[4,5] Under the framework, countries facing crises first assess the epidemiological risk posed by a potentially dangerous vaccine-preventable disease. They then explore the feasibility of a mass vaccination campaign in light of the properties of the necessary vaccine.

The conflict between individual good and the common good is at the core of the ethical issues explored in this chapter—issues pertaining to the allocation of a limited vaccine supply, the balance between benefits and harms, obtaining informed consent, and research conduct. The key ethical principles that should prevail during public health emergencies are rooted in the more general ethical principles governing clinical medicine and public health. Acute humanitarian emergencies differ widely in nature, in the threats they pose, in the background conditions in which they occur, and in the type of agencies that must respond. Hence, this chapter does not seek to provide specific, prescriptive guidance, but merely highlights the ethical issues that policymakers need to consider when deciding to conduct mass vaccination during any emergency response.

Beneficence and Human Rights

The international community and national governments have a collective duty of care to ensure that effective, affordable measures for preventing unnecessary illness and death are available to those most in need. During humanitarian emergencies, the risk of communicable disease transmission is higher than usual. According to the duty of care based on the principle of beneficence, governments must make vaccines available against the most contagious diseases. In addition to the duty of care, institutions and individuals must abide by the rule of rescue, which is "the imperative [...] to rescue identifiable individuals facing avoidable death."[6,7] This is influenced by the urgency of the situation, the consequences of doing nothing, the feasibility of preventing serious consequences, and the sacrifice required of the responding individual or agency.[8] Humanitarian emergencies occur often enough for timely access to an ensured supply of vaccine to be necessary because certain vaccine-preventable diseases have serious outcomes, including death.[9,10] Global and local communities, including governments and nongovernmental organizations, are morally obligated to ensure this supply.

Some oppose vaccination and other measures that are not routinely offered in non-crisis settings. The underlying concern, based on the doctrines of developmental relief and sustainability, is that introducing such measures will result in aid dependency.

However, the argument becomes invalid if vaccination during an acute humanitarian crisis can provide immediate protection against serious illness or death.[11] A higher standard of care is needed during public health crises because of the immediate threat to life. It is ethically reasonable for the standard of preventive care to revert to pre-existing levels after the heightened threat has subsided. After an acute emergency, some medical interventions call for ongoing care or rehabilitation. Vaccination does not, yet it provides long-lasting benefits.

Humanitarian assistance has traditionally been seen as charity, in keeping with the principle of beneficence, but owing to the growing human rights focus, it has come to be viewed as an obligation. Those who are able to help are obligated to ensure that the rights of affected individuals and populations are respected and promoted.[12] The Sphere Project's Humanitarian Charter "defines the legal responsibilities of states and parties to guarantee the right to assistance and protection."[13] The charter draws on the Universal Declaration of Human Rights, international humanitarian law (the Geneva Conventions), and the Convention relating to the Status of Refugees to establish a legal framework for humanitarian action.[14]

From a human rights perspective, vaccination equitably promotes and protects public health. Article 25 of the Universal Declaration of Human Rights states that:

Everyone has the right to a standard of living adequate for the health and well-being of himself and his family, including food, clothing, and medical care ... [and that] every individual and every organ of society ... shall strive ... by progressive measures, national and international, to secure [its] universal and effective recognition.[15]

Irrespective of the principles underlying humanitarian assistance, vaccine donations can ensure timely access to vaccines during emergencies. Although WHO and the United Nations Children's Fund (UNICEF) have agreed on five requirements for "good donations practice" (i.e., suitability, sustainability, informed key persons, supply, and licensing), they acknowledge that in exceptional circumstances, including emergencies, these requirements can be overlooked.[16]

Non-maleficence

All decisions made during humanitarian crises involve seeking a balance between beneficence (doing good) and non-maleficence (avoiding or minimizing harm). Only vaccines that have proved effective and safe in routine use are likely to be considered for mass administration during the acute phase of a humanitarian crisis. Such vaccines not only protect people against specific diseases, but when administered on a large scale, they confer additional benefit through herd immunity, which reduces disease transmission above specific vaccination coverage thresholds.

Vaccines are generally administered before people are exposed to the pathogen causing the targeted disease. Unnecessary vaccination entails opportunity costs and puts people at risk of side effects. The risk of contagion must justify vaccination. Four variables determine risk magnitude: the nature of the illness and attendant local epidemiological and environmental characteristics, the probability of transmission, disease severity, and disease duration.[17] If a disaster occurs where vaccination coverage is already high or the risk of an outbreak is low, additional emergency vaccination may be of minimal benefit. For example, following the earthquake in Sichuan Province in China in 2008, mass measles vaccination would have been inappropriate because a province-wide measles vaccination campaign with high coverage had just been completed.[18]

Vaccines produce benefits but can also cause individual or social harm. Side effects are an example of individual harm. These range from mild, common reactions, such as inflammation and pain at the injection site, to more severe but extremely rare events. Established vaccines, which are normally used during humanitarian emergencies, have well-known side-effect profiles, but much less is known about adverse events that can occur in ill or malnourished people during a humanitarian emergency.[19] Children in this category tend to be biologically more susceptible to vaccine-preventable diseases than others, and when their parents refuse to have them vaccinated, they may be causing them individual harm. However, vaccination is sometimes contraindicated or inappropriate. A child, for instance, can be too young to receive a certain vaccine.

Parents' refusal to get vaccinated or to vaccinate their children can cause collective harm by incrementing the pool of unprotected, susceptible individuals in a community. With herd immunity compromised, devastating disease outbreaks can occur. In these settings, individuals are morally obligated to accept vaccination to prevent harm to others.[20] Harm may result from errors of omission or commission. Failure to provide a vaccine that is indicated in a specific humanitarian emergency violates the principle of non-maleficence because it places vulnerable populations and individuals at risk of contracting a vaccine-preventable disease.

Distributive Justice

Distributive justice requires the fair allocation of scarce basic resources, such as shelter, food, potable water, and vaccines in short supply. A small supply of vaccine could be equitably distributed through a lottery, but prioritizing particularly susceptible groups and individuals, or those most likely to spread the disease, would not be possible. Different rules govern decision making and priority setting during acute crises. Resource distribution during a crisis is often suboptimal because those engaged in humanitarian assistance can only do the "best they can" in the context of imperfect information, exceptional circumstances, and needs far outweighing the available resources.[9]

When resources, especially staff, are scarce, decision makers often choose among interventions—implicitly or explicitly—on the basis of cost-effectiveness because they are seeking to maximize benefits. Vaccination is highly cost-effective, and in emergencies it can mitigate the risk of serious infectious disease. Furthermore, large numbers of people can be vaccinated quickly. Other factors to consider are how urgent and intense the need is for vaccination; how much faster vaccination can be delivered than other interventions; and how groups at high risk or with high transmission rates can be targeted in situations where other interventions, such as safe water and sanitation, cannot be rapidly deployed.

All countries, regardless of their socioeconomic status or experience with humanitarian emergencies, need to decide how to allocate resources. All societies have a shared vulnerability to emergencies, although poor societies are more severely devastated because poverty undermines resilience. When allocating resources, a balance must be sought between utility—maximizing the common good and ensuring smooth economic and social functioning—and equality and fairness. This balance is essential to garner people's trust in vaccination programs during crises. In keeping with egalitarian considerations, resource allocation should not be discriminatory; everyone should have a fair chance of being vaccinated.[21] Furthermore, resources should be allocated with the aim of achieving "the greatest good for the greatest number." Utility can conflict with equality or fairness. You can, for example, save the most lives or avert the most disability affected life years (DALYs) by allocating vaccines to urban rather than rural areas because urban areas have greater population density,[21] but doing so systematically would be inequitable. In conflict zones, threats to the physical safety of health workers often determine which populations they can and cannot vaccinate.

Efforts to maximize utility can conflict with the egalitarian goal of helping the neediest. When limited supplies are allocated to the most vulnerable, overall health utility is sometimes suboptimal (e.g., less aggregate well-being, fewer lives saved, and/or fewer DALYs averted). From the perspective of value pluralism, balancing utility and equality should be the goal, rather than prioritizing one or the other. When it comes to vaccination, utility is fortunately often greatest when the most socially disadvantaged groups are targeted.

The fair distribution of limited vaccine supplies was an important issue during preparations for the 2009 pandemic influenza. People in certain categories were prioritized: those at greatest risk of infection (e.g., school children and healthcare workers), those most likely to become severely ill if infected (e.g., immunosuppressed individuals and chronic disease patients), and those most likely to spread infection (e.g., children and emergency service providers).[22] During humanitarian emergencies in which populations are displaced, neighboring communities also require attention. In most circumstances, host communities and refugees should be given access to each other's services.[23] Refugee or displaced populations should not be treated as separate from the host community, and assistance programs, including vaccination, should support everyone in the area as a whole.[24] The guiding principle should be to provide equitable access to vaccination to equalize risk. From an inclusive perspective, there is efficiency in covering two communities with all the resources available. Fair and equitable approaches result in less hostility and rivalry between the host and the displaced communities.[13]

From the point of view of utility and equity, in many cases, children should be prioritized because they are generally more vulnerable than older people to vaccine-preventable diseases. In addition, saving a child's life will result in a larger reduction in disease burden because more years of healthy life are lost when a child dies.[21] Parents and caregivers often prioritize children's needs over their own. However, some communities may place greater value on the social roles of the elderly and pregnant women and may prioritize their access to health care during emergencies.

From a utilitarian perspective, protecting frontline health workers against disease will indirectly benefit the health of the community. Under the principle of reciprocity, it is fair to prioritize the vaccination of healthcare workers, who are often more exposed than others to the risk of contagion because they are committed to caring for society. In addition, because healthcare workers come into contact with susceptible individuals, they have a moral obligation to get vaccinated to avoid placing patients at risk of infection.[25]

Procedural Justice

Procedural justice requires transparent decision making with involvement of the communities affected by the decisions.[26] To ensure procedural justice, it is useful to have guidelines or a legal framework to follow. Guidelines are especially valuable in certain situations: when large numbers of people need to be treated or protected against disease, when delayed or suboptimal measures could lead to poor outcomes, and when inadequate management could result in high mortality or a large-scale epidemic. Although guidelines do not have mandatory status, if they are evidence-based and contextually appropriate, they should be considered normative practice and a benchmark for judging the actions of health officials and practitioners.

National legal systems should guide the implementation of vaccination programs in individual nation states, but they seldom accommodate humanitarian emergencies. When national legislative frameworks are absent or dysfunctional, international human rights law dictates a duty of care to protect people needing assistance, and in such cases, implementation should follow international health guidelines. WHO Member States can legitimately follow WHO vaccination guidelines, which were developed on the strength of the evidence and which take many factors into account, including the epidemiologic and clinical features of the target disease, vaccine characteristics, costs, health system infrastructure, social impact, legal and ethical considerations, and the local context.[27,28]

Efforts to improve accountability during humanitarian emergencies have resulted in the Sphere Project, the Humanitarian Accountability Partnership, and the Active Learning Network for Accountability and Performance in Humanitarian Action.[29] All three seek to involve beneficiaries in the planning and implementation of aid programs, establish codes of conduct for responding agencies, promote technical standards, and encourage the use of performance indicators and impact assessments.

Observing appropriate rules of conduct during humanitarian crises is often difficult.[10] In certain political contexts, healthcare workers may find that following guidance from their governments or humanitarian organizations is in conflict with their commitment to promote individuals' best interests. Affected populations are often disenfranchised and unable to defend their own interests. All factors considered before the introduction of a vaccination program should be well documented and publicly available to donors, community leaders, local staff, and governments. Channels should also be established for affected communities to express their concerns directly to responding agencies.

Consent

Obtaining valid consent from individuals before a medical intervention is an obligation under the principle of respect for the autonomy of persons. In non-emergency circumstances, the consent process needs to be thorough and takes time. During emergencies, it has to be modified. If time permits, information on the risks and benefits of vaccination should be communicated to target populations in sufficient depth to allow individuals to make informed decisions, while bearing in mind that many will lack a basic understanding of germ theory and immunology. During emergencies, vaccination often takes place while people are too desperate for food and other basic necessities to recognize its importance. Furthermore, in some developing countries, people defer to decision makers at the expense of individual autonomy.

The amount of information provided to the public needs to be weighed against the risk of delaying action. However, any questions raised by the community should be thoroughly addressed. For example, vaccinators should be prepared to answer common questions about the diseases targeted, the benefits of vaccination, potential side effects, follow-up, and alternative options. They should also know where to refer undecided individuals who have other questions, although this may not always be feasible. Visual aids and other media can be used to convey important information to the public in a time-efficient manner.

Vaccination should be voluntary unless it becomes critical to "prevent a concrete and serious harm."[30] The degree of risk to communities will determine the extent to which individual rights may be restricted. Where the threat of widespread, serious infectious disease is imminent, individual liberties may be justifiably curtailed.[31] The Siracusa Principles endorsed by the United Nations Economic and Social Council state that: "Public health may be invoked as a ground for limiting certain rights in order to allow a State to take measures dealing with a serious threat to the health of the population or individual members of the population. These measures must be specifically aimed at preventing disease or injury or providing care for the sick and injured."[32] It may thus be permissible for those in authority to restrict individual autonomy to prevent harm to others. Although this approach has been limited to immediate or direct threat under traditional public health law, it should arguably be extended to what is "reasonably foreseeable" based on epidemiology and historical occurrence.[33] If the risk to health is extremely high, individuals should not be allowed to compromise group protection and communal rights.[34-36] When personal liberty is restricted to protect public health, the measures applied must be effective, the least restrictive (i.e., least liberty-infringing), proportional to the risk, equitable and non-discriminatory, minimally burdensome, and in line with due process. Those whose liberty is violated should, when appropriate, be compensated, particularly if they experience vaccine-associated side effects.[37,38] In addition, individual rights should be restricted only with utmost respect for the dignity of persons.

Children are at particularly high risk of contracting communicable diseases during humanitarian crises. In most emergencies, mortality in children under the age of 5 years is generally two to three times higher than crude mortality.[39] Vaccinating children could reduce mortality in all age groups because epidemics often arise and spread among children.[40] Parents' refusal to have their children vaccinated should be respected if the risk of disease is low or the disease is mild. However, if the risk of harm to the child is high, parental authority may be overruled to protect the child's best interests.[20,41] In emergency settings, a parent or guardian may not be available, and healthcare workers should be empowered to rapidly decide whether to vaccinate a child if done in the child and community's best interests.

Research

Opportunities for health and health service research abound during humanitarian crises.[42,43] However, in resource-limited settings, medical care and service delivery must always take precedence over research.[44] In disaster settings, research is often conducted by the same people who provide aid and thus "rightly takes second place to the pro-vision of life-saving assistance."[45] If specific personnel were assigned exclusively to research, critical human resources would not be diverted away from care.[45] Nonethe-less, such personnel should only be allowed to conduct research after a local research ethics committee has determined that enough care personnel are available to meet demand.[46] Regional or international ethics review boards should be created in places without appropriate local expertise. In countries without functioning research gover-nance structures, researchers must rely on international ethics review boards.

Research must be distinguished from disease and program surveillance.[47] Surveil-lance is essential for assessing vaccination coverage, informing program planning, eval-uating vaccine effectiveness, and monitoring safety in the population as a whole and in certain subgroups.[48] Surveillance also allows the rapid detection of cases that may signal program failure requiring remediation. Because surveillance activities have an opportunity cost, the data collected must be analyzed and used to direct public health action.[49]

Under the principle of justice, communities where research is conducted must stand to benefit. Research protocols should be relevant, methodologically sound, and explicit about the benefits and potential harms to study participants. They should also clearly explain how the findings will be delivered to study participants if they are relocated after the humanitarian crisis.[50] Research should not undermine the provision of health services and should be carried to completion.

Although most non-medical research conducted during disasters is observational, it is subject to ethics review to ensure that individual and social benefits outweigh any risks. The level of review should be proportional to the risk associated with a specific intervention. An expedited review is admissible if the risk to participants is low, whereas a full committee review is warranted when the research involves a higher risk. If the research is urgent and important, it can proceed without ethics committee approval, but retrospective review should be sought as soon as possible. Whenever the nature of the research to be conducted during a humanitarian emergency can be anticipated, a full review of the generic protocols should be planned and discussed in advance with local research ethics committees. Provision should be made for counseling or debriefing should participants find the research interviews traumatic or distressing.[51]

Potential research participants may have impaired ability to make decisions or provide voluntary individual informed consent following an acute humanitarian emergency, especially in "vulnerable communities," as defined by the Joint United Nations Programme on HIV/AIDS. Empirical research in developing countries has shown that obtaining informed consent from study participants is not easy, even under non-emergency circumstances. Acute humanitarian crises add a layer of complexity, and decisional capacity must be carefully assessed.[52-56] In acute crises in which medical care is needed, patients often assume that a research intervention is known to be therapeutic or effective. During the consent process, study participants need to be made aware that they are consenting to research only, not to special or additional care.

Conclusion

Ethical considerations are vital to decision-making about the deployment of vaccines in acute humanitarian emergencies. Commitment to human rights and the rule of rescue place an onus on wealthy countries to ensure that life-saving vaccines are made available to the poorer countries during crises. Justice and ethics obligate those who are better off to assist those who are worse off and to allocate resources accordingly.[57] National health authorities are morally obligated to do all that they reasonably can to implement evidence-based guidelines to avert preventable harm.[58]

The allocation of a limited supply of vaccine calls for a fine balance between utility and equality and fairness. Accountability demands that decision making be explicit, documented, and open to public review.

In emergencies, the informed consent process may be reasonably modified to avoid delaying protection for vulnerable communities. Autonomy is not absolute. In situations that threaten the health and well-being of others, authorities may be required to mandate vaccination and intervene on behalf of minors against parental wishes. Finally, emergency health-care workers should be trained in ethics to improve their decision-making skills during acute humanitarian emergencies.[59]

References

1. Levine, C. 2004. The concept of vulnerability in disaster research. *J Trauma Stress* 17:395–402.

2. Shears, P., A. M. Berry, R. Murphy, and M. A. Nabil. 1987. Epidemiological assessment of the health and nutrition of Ethiopian refugees in emergency camps in Sudan, 1985. *BMJ* 295:314–318.

3. Feudtner, C., and E. K. Marcuse. 2001. Ethics and immunization policy: Promoting dialogue to sustain consensus. *Pediatrics* 107:1158–1164.

4. Schwartz, L., M. Hunt, C. Sinding, L. Elit, L. Redwood-Campbell, N. Adelson, et al. 2012. Models for humanitarian health care ethics. *Public Health Ethics* 5:81–90.

5. SAGE Working Group on Vaccination in Humanitarian Emergencies. 2012. *SAGE Working Group on Vaccination in Humanitarian Emergencies: A Framework for Decision-Making.* Geneva: World Health Organization.

6. Jonsen, A. R. 1986. Bentham in a box: Technology assessment and health care allocation. *Law Med Health Care* 14:172–174.

7. Murphy, L. 2001. Beneficence, law and liberty: The case of required rescue. *Georgetown Law J* 3:605–665.

8. Akabayashi, A., Y. Takimoto, and Y. Hayashi. 2012. Physician obligation to provide care during disasters: Should physicians have been required to go to Fukushima? *J Med Ethics* 38:697–698.

9. Kenny, C. 2012. Disaster risk reduction in developing countries: Costs, benefits and institutions. *Disasters* 36:559–588.

10. Hurst, S. A., N. Mezger, and A. Mauron. 2009. Allocating resources in humanitarian medicine. *Public Health Ethics* 2:89–99.

11. Bradbury, M. 1998. Normalising the crisis in Africa. *Disasters* 22:328–338.

12. United Nations Economic, Scientific and Cultural Organization. 2005. *Universal Declaration on Bioethics and Human Rights.* Paris: United Nations Economic, Scientific and Cultural Organization.

13. Sphere Project. 2011. *The Sphere Project: Humanitarian Charter and Minimum Standards in Humanitarian Response. Bourton on Dunsmore*: Practical Action Publishing.

14. United Nations High Commissioner for Refugees. 1967. *Convention and Protocol Relating to the Status of Refugees.* Geneva: United Nations High Commissioner for Refugees.

15. United Nations. 1948. *The Universal Declaration of Human Rights.* New York: United Nations.

16. World Health Organization & United Nations Children's Fund. 2010. *Vaccine Donations: WHO—UNICEF Joint Statement.* Geneva: World Health Organization & United Nations Children's Fund.

17. Rhodes, R. S., G. L. Telford, W. J. Hierholzer, and M. Barnes. 1995. Bloodborne pathogen transmission from healthcare worker to patients: Legal issues and provider perspectives. *Surg Clin North Am* 75:1205–1217.

18. Shu, M., Q. Liu, J. Wang, R. Ao, C. Yang, G. Fang, et al. 2011. Measles vaccine adverse events reported in the mass vaccination campaign of Sichuan province, China from 2007 to 2008. *Vaccine* 29:3507–3510.

19. Savy, M., K. Edmond, P. E. M. Fine, A. Hall, B. J. Hennig, S. E. Moore, et al. 2009. Landscape analysis of interactions between nutrition and vaccine responses in children. *J Nutr* 139: 2154S–2218S.

20. Dawson, A. 2011. Vaccination ethics. In: *Public health ethics*, ed. A. Dawson, 143–153. Cambridge: Cambridge University Press.

21. Verweij, M. 2009. Moral principles for allocating scarce medical resources in an influenza pandemic. *J Bioeth Inq* 6:159–169.

22. Selgelid, M. J. 2009. Pandethics. *Public Health* 123 (3):255–259.

23. United Nations High Commissioner for Refugees. 2011. *Guiding Principles 2008–2012*. Geneva: United Nations High Commissioner for Refugees.

24. Hanquet, G., ed. 1997. *Médecins Sans Frontières. Refugee Health: An Approach to Emergency Situations*. New York: Macmillan.

25. van Delden, J. J. M., R. Ashcroft, A. Dawson, G. Marckmann, R. Upshur, and M. F. Verweij. 2008. The ethics of mandatory vaccination against influenza for health care workers. *Vaccine* 26:5562–5566.

26. Daniels, N. 1985. *Just Health Care*. Cambridge: Cambridge University Press.

27. World Health Organization. 2011. *Draft guidelines for WHO and SAGE development of evidence-based vaccine related recommendations*. Geneva: World Health Organization.

28. Duclos, P., D. Durrheim, A. Reingold, Z. Bhutta, K. Vannice, and H. Rees. 2012. Developing evidence-based vaccine recommendations and GRADE. *Vaccine* 31:12–19.

29. Humanitarian Practice Network. 2011. Humanitarian accountability. *Humanitarian Exchange Magazine* 52. Available at: http://www.odihpn.org/humanitarian-exchange-magazine/issue-52/humanitarian-accountability. Accessed January 24, 2013.

30. Verweij, M., and A. Dawson. 2004. Ethical principles for collective immunisation programmes. *Vaccine* 22:3122–3126.

31. Gostin, L. O. 2009. Influenza A (H1N1) and pandemic preparedness under the rule of international law. *JAMA* 301:2376–2378.

32. United Nations Commission on Human Rights. 1984. *The Siracusa principles on the limitation and derogation provisions in the International Covenant on Civil and Political Rights*. Geneva: United Nations Commission on Human Rights.

33. Gostin, L. O. 1995. The resurgent tuberculosis epidemic in the era of AIDS: Reflections on public health, law, and society. *MD Law Rev* 54:1–131.

34. Diekema, D., and E. Marcuse. 1998. *Ethical Issues in the Vaccination of Children: Primum Non Nocere Today*. New York: Elsevier.

35. Harris, J., and S. Holm. 1995. Is there a moral obligation not to infect others? *BMJ* 311:1215–1217.

36. Simons, K. W. 1999. Negligence. *Soc Philos Policy* 16:52–93.

37. Isaacs, D., H. Kilham, J. Leask, and B. Tobin. 2009. Ethical issues in immunisation. *Vaccine* 27:615–618.

38. Selgelid, M. J. 2009. A moderate pluralist approach to public health policy and ethics. *Public Health Ethics* 2:195–205.

39. Toole, M. J., and R. J. Waldman. 1990. Prevention of excess mortality in refugee and displaced populations in developing countries. *JAMA* 263:3296–3302.

40. Galvani, A. P., J. Medlock, G. B. Chapman. 2006. The ethics of influenza vaccination. *Science* 313:758–760.

41. Finn, A., and J. Savulescu. 2011. Is immunisation child protection? *Lancet* 378:465–468.

42. Collogan, L. K., F. Tuma, R. Dolan-Sewell, S. Borja, and A. R. Fleischman. 2004. Ethical issues pertaining to research in the aftermath of disaster. *J Trauma Stress* 17:363–372.

43. Kilpatrick, D. G. 2004. The ethics of disaster research: A special section. *J Trauma Stress* 17:361–362.

44. World Medical Association. 2006. WMA Statement on Medical Ethics in the Event of Disasters. Ferney-Voltaire: World Medical Association. Available at: http://www.wma.net/en/30publications/10policies/d7/index.html. Accessed September 24, 2012.

45. Ford, N., E. J. Mills, R. Zachariah, and R. Upshur. 2009. Ethics of conducting research in conflict settings. *Confl Health* 3:7.

46. Siriwardhana, D. C. 2007, February 13. Disaster research ethics: A luxury or a necessity for developing countries? *Asian Tribune*.

47. World Health Organization. 2009. *Research ethics in international epidemic response*. Geneva: World Health Organization. Available at: http://www.who.int/ethics/gip_research_ethics_.pdf. Accessed January 24, 2012.

48. Fottrell, E., and P. Byass. 2009. Identifying humanitarian crises in population surveillance field sites: Simple procedures and ethical imperatives. *Public Health* 123:151–155.

49. Carrel, M. 2008. Demographic and health surveillance: Longitudinal ethical considerations. *Bull World Health Organ* 86:612–616.

50. World Medical Association. 2013. *Declaration of Helsinki: Ethical Principles for Medical Research Involving Human Subjects*. Available at: http://www.wma.net/en/30publications/10policies/b3/.

51. Wallis, L., and W. Smith, eds. *Disaster Medicine*. Johannesburg: Juta.

52. Abdool Karim, Q., S. S. Abdool Karim, M. H. Coovadia, and M. Susser. 1998. Informed consent for HIV testing in a South African hospital: Is it truly informed and truly voluntary? *Am J Public Health* 88:637–640.

53. Joubert, G., H. Steinberg, E. van der Ryst, and P. Chikobvu. 2003. Consent for participation in the Bloemfontein Vitamin A Trial: How informed and voluntary? *Am J Public Health* 93:582–584.

54. Moodley, K., M. Pather, and L. Myer. 2005. Informed consent and participant perceptions of influenza vaccine trials in South Africa. *J Med Ethics* 31:727–732.

55. Molyneux, C. S., N. Peshu, and K. Marsh. 2004. Understanding of informed consent in a low-income setting: Three case studies from the Kenyan Coast. *Soc Sci Med* 59:2547–2559.

56. Frimpong-Mansoh, A. 2008. Culture and voluntary informed consent in African health care systems. *Developing World Bioeth* 8:104–114.

57. Rawls, J. 1971. *A Theory of Justice. Cambridge, MA*: Harvard University Press.

58. Emerson, C. I., and P. A. Singer. 2010. Is there an ethical obligation to complete polio eradication? *Lancet* 375:1340–1341.

59. Hunt, M. R., L. Schwartz, and L. Elit. 2012. Experience of ethics training and support for health care professionals in international aid work. *Public Health Ethics* 5:91–99.

36 Lessons from the Eradication of Smallpox: An Interview with D. A. Henderson (*Excerpt*)

D. A. Henderson and Petra Klepac*

Before smallpox eradication was attempted, four other eradication efforts had failed[1-3]: hookworm, yellow fever, yaws, and malaria. The malaria eradication campaign was particularly extensive and intensive in terms of both manpower and financial resources (more than $2.5 billion expended from 1957 to 1975).[4] These failures eventually led many in the global health community to shift their focus from targeted disease-eradication attempts to less explicitly defined programs such as providing basic health services. There was a perception that eradication programs, referred to as "vertical programs," could have a particularly deleterious impact in inhibiting the development of the basic health services (so-called "horizontal" or "integrated" programs). Thus, a proposal to undertake a global smallpox eradication campaign was a divisive and politically charged issue, further complicated by the fact that the World Health Organization (WHO) was reluctant to support another eradication campaign. However, in 1966, the World Health Assembly (WHA) passed a resolution approving an annual budget of $2.4 million to support a 10-year smallpox eradication plan by the narrow margin of two votes (fifty-eight were needed for approval, it received sixty).[1]

Interview

How did the smallpox eradication program start, and how was it received?

During the 1960s, expenditure for the malaria program represented 20% or more of all funds available to WHO, thus constraining other control programs. By the late 1960s, it became apparent that the program would be far more costly and take far longer than many anticipated. An increasingly prevalent view was that disease eradication was not

* Originally published in *Philosophical Transactions of the Royal Society B*, 2013, 368 (1623):20130113. Reprinted under the terms of a Creative Commons Attribution License.

possible (see Rene Dubos' book *Man Adapting*[5]). This was the view of the Director General of WHO, Marcelino Candau, in 1966.

Principal direction of the malaria program had been provided by an internationally recruited WHO staff of some 500 to 600 specialists. National malaria staff operated entirely separately from in-country basic health services. The heads of national malaria programs reported to the heads of state, not to the Ministries of Health (MoH). Those who worked in the malaria program were usually paid somewhat more than those in the basic health services, which enabled the recruitment of some of the best people into the malaria program. Understandably, this had substantial negative repercussions on the development of health services in countries where the malaria program was operating.

With the growing problems in the malaria eradication program, it would seem unlikely that a proposal to undertake the eradication of a second disease would be well received. However, the proposal to eradicate smallpox originated from an unexpected source—the Soviet Union. The Soviet Union and several of its allies returned to participation in WHO (and other United Nations agencies) after years of absence. One of its first acts, in 1958, was to propose that WHO undertake a smallpox program. Victor Zhdanov, a virologist and deputy minister of health for Russia, called on the WHA to undertake the global eradication of smallpox, even quoting the favorable views of Thomas Jefferson while doing so. At the subsequent Assembly, the proposal was approved by acclamation. Other countries were pleased that the Soviet Union had decided to return to full participation in WHO and were anxious to exhibit a sense of solidarity. However, over the next 7 years, little progress was made. WHO allocated limited funds, and voluntary contributions by countries were sparse. In 1966, at the request of the Assembly, the Director General drew up and presented a 10-year plan. It had two components: (1) systematic vaccination, and (2) a new concept—surveillance and containment. The latter called for weekly reports of cases from all health facilities and containment of outbreaks by special containment teams. It called for a WHO budget contribution of $2.4 million per year; voluntary contributions were expected to supplement this. Many countries doubted that eradication was possible, and others were reluctant to agree to increasing their budgetary assessment by the amounts that would be required. The eradication plan was put to a vote. The Assembly, which normally reaches decisions fairly quickly and by acclamation, debated for 3 days on this proposal and in the end put it to a vote. The resolution was passed by the narrow margin of two votes.

How did the United States get involved in the smallpox eradication efforts when it was initially opposed to it?

The United States got involved indirectly. In the 1960s, I was at the U.S. Centers for Disease Control (CDC) in charge of the surveillance section, mainly for viral diseases, smallpox, measles, flu, and so forth. I had approximately forty staff members; some were stationed at our Atlanta headquarters; others were in state and local health departments. In the early 1960s, the National Institutes of Health (NIH) staff and Merck became interested in the possible use of a new Merck measles vaccine in African countries where measles was an often fatal disease. In the United States, measles vaccine was given together with gamma-globulin to diminish the possibility of high fever sometimes associated with administration of measles vaccine. Use of gamma-globulin with the vaccine would not be feasible for countries with limited health services. Thus, they wanted to undertake a study of the effects of vaccine without immunoglobulin. An NIH-led study in Upper Volta (now Burkina Faso) showed that measles vaccine worked well without immunoglobulin and had few adverse reactions.[6,7] The government in Upper Volta supported the study in return for enough vaccine for all of its children, and U.S. Agency for International Development (USAID) indicated its willingness to cover the costs. Upper Volta was a member of L'Organisation de Coordination et de Coopération pour la Lutte contre les Grandes Endémies (OCCGE), a consortium of nine former French colonies in western Africa that collaborated in providing preventive and health services. This organization pressed USAID and Merck to make measles vaccine available for all children in these countries during the course of a 4-year program. It would require training national teams from each country. Because the focus of NIH was research, and not field operations, the CDC was asked to assume this role.

I thought the program was a bad idea. The program was expected to vaccinate 25% of the children each year, after which the countries would be expected to bear the costs for continuing vaccination. At that time, the measles vaccine cost $1.75 a dose, but the countries could not even afford 10 cents per dose for yellow fever vaccine. Starting and then stopping a vaccination program in this manner was bad public health practice. It occurred to us that if a smallpox vaccination program were instituted, it could be sustained, as smallpox vaccine cost only 1 or 2 cents a dose. Thus, we decided to propose a combined smallpox eradication—measles control vaccination program. This would at least leave some structure and sustainable activity for smallpox control as a legacy.

We believed we could stop smallpox transmission in particular countries, but with the many nomads moving through West Africa, a region-wide program would be necessary for effective smallpox control and perhaps to stop transmission. Thus, we suggested to USAID that the proposed program be extended to eighteen countries. This would have to include Nigeria, which constituted 67% of the population of the whole area. The budget we proposed, $35 million over a 5-year period, was substantially greater than the $7 million that USAID had expected to spend. Much to our surprise, the proposal was accepted in full by President Johnson as a special U.S. contribution to a United Nations initiative called "International Cooperation Year."

We were only 6 months into this program when I was called to Geneva to help WHO draw up the Director General's plans for the global smallpox program, which was to be presented months later at the May 1966 World Health Assembly. With full support now of the eighteen West African countries, a positive decision for WHO to proceed with the global plan became a certainty. Subsequently, the Director General decided that an American should direct the entire program. Thus, in less than a year, I had moved from director of a CDC surveillance program to director of an eighteen-country smallpox eradication—measles control effort and finally to the position of Chief Medical Officer for the global smallpox eradication program.

At what point did it become clear that you would make the 10-year goal to eradicate smallpox?

Initially, the 10-year plan was little more than a theoretical hope. We had little to work with in the planning—the data on reported cases were incomplete, and we had almost no information on what countries were doing already as there had been few reports provided to WHO. Hope gradually transitioned to expectation, but confidence that eradication could be achieved was not there until 1975.

About 4 to 5 years into the program, we had begun thinking that eradication within another 3 to 4 years might be feasible. The West African program had proceeded so well and so rapidly that it stunned everyone. This group of countries included those with the highest incidence of smallpox in the world but, at the same time, had the least developed communications and transportation systems and the least sophisticated health services. The plans that we had made were substantially more successful than we had anticipated. Most of East Africa also became smallpox free only a few years later. From 1967 to 1973, the number of smallpox endemic countries dropped dramatically—from thirty-one to only five—India, Pakistan, Bangladesh, Nepal, and Ethiopia. South Asia was a formidable problem and a heavily populated area. Significant changes had to be made in the strategy; resources had to be augmented—both in cash and people. The concluding barriers—Ethiopia and Somalia—posed other problems. Ethiopia was engulfed in civil war; teams in Somalia were handicapped by government officials refusing to report cases until they became epidemics. But finally, on October 26, 1977, the world's last case of smallpox was discovered in Merka, Somalia.

In India, the surveillance-containment system had to be modified—how and why?

A basic component for smallpox surveillance was a weekly report from each health center or hospital regarding each case of smallpox seen or a report stating that there were no cases. A team of two or three was then to go to the area, vaccinate all those in the immediate area, and in the process search to see whether there were other cases. India provided for reporting from health units, but the reports progressed through a hierarchy of offices, usually being delayed at each stop and sometimes changed. With a highly mobile population of 550 to 600 million, cases were usually reported too late for containment, if reported at all. More timely detection was essential. Accordingly, surveillance in India was augmented to focus on routine, repetitive active searches for cases—130,000 health personnel periodically swept through states searching every village and eventually every house during a 10-day period. The aim was to search 90% of houses every 2 months to discover outbreaks and for containment vaccination teams to follow. Initially, the searches discovered tens or even hundreds of cases where none was being reported. With time, however, performance improved; the last case in India was discovered little more than 18 months after the first search was undertaken.[8]

You mentioned that in more sparsely populated areas, special search programs were important for the surveillance-containment program. What was the nature of these?

In low-density areas, one has the particular problem of having few or no health personnel. However, as we discovered, there are always well-demarcated places where people regularly come together, such as markets or religious centers. In Ethiopia, people came to markets once a week, walking 10 to 15 miles to reach them. In Indonesia, we discovered the importance of schools—that it was possible for one worker to obtain a list of outbreaks over a wide area by going to schools and holding up a card showing a child with the typical rash of smallpox.[9] The children then told the questioner which villages, indeed which houses, had smallpox. We came to learn that children between 8 and 12 years of age know almost everything that is going on in their own village, and they are happy to share that information.

What do you see as being other benefits of the smallpox eradication program?

First was the realization by health administrators in many countries that major improvements in the health status of its people could be effected even with small budgets and a paucity of well-trained health staff if goals were clear and steps were taken to involve local residents in the program. Many weak, poorly managed primary healthcare programs benefited from the smallpox program, focusing as it did on greatly neglected vaccination initiatives. To achieve surveillance goals, weekly reports that provided feedback to field staff demonstrated a national interest in otherwise routine reports and improved morale of many in isolated primary care units. For example, the weekly smallpox surveillance program in Brazil led to the creation of the Brazil Weekly Epidemiological Report, a report that continues to be published today. Finally, the smallpox program provided the base and impetus for the launch of the follow-on Expanded Program on Immunisation (EPI), whose genesis dates back to a first exploratory WHO meeting we helped convene in 1970.

Is there any other disease that you would foresee being eradicated?

No. Not at this time, given presently available relevant technologies, our understanding of the epidemiology of the infectious diseases, and pilot programs of national disease elimination programs. The one exception is guinea worm disease. A program to eradicate it is progressing well, albeit it is in its 27th year, 13 years beyond the target date that had been set. Civil strife, however, continues to hamper it.

I believe that this is essentially the same answer that Frank Fenner, the world-renowned Australian virologist, and I provided in August 1980 at a meeting on eradication called at the Fogarty Center in Washington, DC. The meeting was held only 3 months after the WHA meeting in Geneva had declared officially that smallpox had been eradicated. The mood of the 1980 meeting was a surprise to us both. We were well aware of the realities that we had encountered in smallpox eradication and the heroic efforts made by our own and national staff to achieve eradication. It was difficult to conceive of another disease problem that could similarly be addressed. However, the meeting theme was basically to decide *what next* should be slated for eradication. Frank Fenner and I were the keynote speakers, and both of us said we did not think that at this point in time there was any candidate disease. Not surprisingly, the message was not welcomed. Subsequently, neither of us was invited to any of the many following meetings on eradication that have been conducted.

Why were you skeptical about polio/other eradication efforts?

A simple answer is to point out that I had spent 11 years of my life endeavoring to eradicate smallpox, and I knew well the diverse array of problems that a program has to navigate. Smallpox eradication proved to be infinitely more difficult than I or anyone else had imagined it would be. Indeed, it is all but a certainty that any of a number of obstacles could have blocked its completion at various points in the program, but fortunately, in each case, unexpected events or special measures intervened to resolve problems.

Little had I appreciated the magnitude or number of other imponderables—floods, wars and famines, hundreds of thousands of refugees, national bureaucracies and constraints that rivalled the United States in number and complexity, a difficult USAID program (an unwilling but a significant contributor), and a sclerotic WHO administration that often thwarted or actively impeded what appeared to be logical initiatives.

There were other unexpected events—changes in governments, fortuitous laboratory discoveries, unexpected successes in launching vaccine production operations in developing country laboratories, and the emergence of needed leadership and courage by national and international staff at numerous critical points. The program was ultimately successful, but success hung in the balance on many occasions.

From my examination of the characteristics and needs for eradicating other diseases, each has prominent features that makes it far more difficult than smallpox. With smallpox, we had a vaccine so heat stable that teams traveled in the field without refrigeration devices. We had a vaccine that provided long-term protection with one dose. One could ascertain whether vaccination was successful by determining whether a pustule had developed at the vaccination site. There were no patients with subclinical infections. Thus, we could readily identify infected areas and contain the outbreaks. Cases were so typical and readily identified that special diagnostic laboratories were unnecessary.

There are few eradication enthusiasts who have had real-world practical experience in executing a successful component of an eradication program at the local or national level, and there are even fewer who have had the opportunity (or taxing challenge) of dealing with the practical and political complexities of a targeted program at national and international levels. Prospects for eradication appear far more optimistic from the vantage point of a laboratory or an office in a university ivory tower.

Why do you think eradication programs are so popular?

There is a belief that unless eradication is set as a goal, governments will not be willing to contribute the necessary resources for infectious disease control. To me, this seems like a weak excuse for inadequate efforts on the part of public health staff to educate and persuade.

Final Words

Whatever the outcome, experiences with eradication programs to date should be cautionary to any who contemplate an eradication effort. Disease control and elimination programs can be varied in intensity and duration. Their success or failure is usually of limited importance to other countries. Eradication is a different story. It represents a global commitment from which it is problematic for countries to withdraw however unimportant the disease may be nationally. As investments in a program grow, the penalty for failure is perceived to be ever greater. How much should be expended and at what cost financially and to other programs? The polio program is now in the 25th year of what was intended to be a 12-year effort.

From experiences to date with eradication programs, it seems apparent that at least four factors should be in place before a launch: a reasonably thorough plan, an established research program, success in a significantly large demonstration site, and a firm commitment by a majority of countries with definitive concerns and resources to support a program. In light of the fact that there has been only one success among the seven global eradication programs launched to date, the implications of possible failure should be clearly stated as well.

References

1. Fenner, F., D. A. Henderson, I. Arita, Z. Jezek, and I. D. Ladnyi. 1988. The development of the global smallpox eradication program, 1958–1966. In *Smallpox and Its Eradication*, 365–420. Geneva, Switzerland: World Health Organization.

2. Henderson, D. A. 1998. Eradication: Lessons from the past. *Bull World Health Organ* 76 (Suppl 2):17–21.

3. Soper, F. L. 1963. The elimination of urban yellow fever in the Americas through the eradication of *Aedes aegypti*. *Am J Public Health Nations Health* 53:7–16.

4. Jeffery, G. M. 1976. Malaria control in the twentieth century. *Am J Trop Med Hyg* 25:361–371.

5. Dubos, R. 1965. *Man Adapting*. New Haven, CT: Yale University Press.

6. Fenner, F., D. A. Henderson, I. Arita, Z. Jezek, and I. D. Ladnyi. 1988. Western and Central Africa. In *Smallpox and Its Eradication*, 849–910. Geneva, Switzerland: World Health Organization.

7. Meyer, H. M. J., D. D. J. Hostetler, N. G. Rogers, P. Lambin, A. Chassary, and J. E. Smadel. 1964. Response of Volta children to live attenuated measles virus vaccine. *Bull World Health Organ* 30:769–781.

8. Fenner, F., D. A. Henderson, I. Arita, Z. Jezek, and I. D. Ladnyi. 1988. India and the Himalayan area. In *Smallpox and Its Eradication*, 711–805. Geneva, Switzerland: World Health Organization.

9. Fenner, F., D. A. Henderson, I. Arita, Z. Jezek, and I. D. Ladnyi. 1988. Indonesia. In *Smallpox and Its Eradication*, 627–658. Geneva, Switzerland: World Health Organization.

37 Intimidation, Coercion, and Resistance in the Final Stages of the South Asian Smallpox Eradication Campaign (*Excerpt*)

Paul Greenough[*]

Most people worldwide actively seek, or can be persuaded to accept, official measures of mass vaccination that aim to control or eradicate disease. Instances of opposition are uncommon in the literature, which tends to merge expressions of resistance into the broader phenomenon of "non-compliance."[1] Resistance in the sense of overt acts of refusal appears less common in the present than in the past, when vaccination campaigns triggered both street riots and sustained struggles to overturn compulsory vaccination laws in nineteenth-century America and Europe. Yet the potential for resistance is always present because encounters with government vaccinators are never about immunization alone. Public health measures derive their authority from the police powers of the state, and people do not lightly offer themselves (or their immune systems) to government, even when its authority is legitimate.

In this chapter, I review occasions during 1973 to 1975 when physician-epidemiologists in South Asia, working under the auspices of the World Health Organization (WHO), intimidated local health officials and resorted to coercive vaccination in the final stages of the Smallpox Eradication Programme (SEP). Both intimidation and coercion evoked resistance and therefore interfered with the smooth functioning of public health immunization. These physician-epidemiologists were all Americans who had been recruited by the U.S. Centers for Disease Control and Prevention (CDC). All of them have subsequently pursued public health careers, but only one has maintained a professional link to South Asia. Several now express regret over their participation in patterned acts of intimidation and coercion. Evidence for these statements comes from interviews, published statements, and journals kept at the time.

* Reprinted from *Social Science and Medicine*, Greenough, P., Intimidation, coercion, and resistance in the final stages of the South Asian smallpox eradication campaign, 41:633–645. Copyright © 1995 with permission of Elsevier.

I am aware that in raising such issues, I may be giving them undeserved prominence. The extent of intimidation, coercion, and resistance in South Asia in 1973 to 1975 cannot be documented quantitatively and may have been negligible, although I doubt this was the case.[2,3] I might also be said to be diverting attention from the great efforts made by CDC personnel on behalf of South Asians during those years. An ancient, deadly, often blinding disease, normally prevalent in numbers measured in tens of thousands of cases per year, was eliminated as a result of SEP personnel's hard work supported by brilliant epidemiological analysis and innovative organizational measures. Nothing I write can detract from this remarkable record of success, and my motive here is simply to document the fact that heavy-handed methods were sometimes relied on in the final stages of the eradication campaign in India and Bangladesh. Although successful in the short-run, these methods underlined the divide between foreign and host-country health professionals and may have widened the gap between the latter and the public. Thus, the long-term effects may have been negative for other health campaigns that require official, professional, and popular cooperation for success.

The Smallpox Eradication Programs in India and Bangladesh

Beginning in mid-1973, an intensified eradication campaign was launched in both India and Bangladesh under the general guidance of WHO, which set up technical units and appointed expatriate epidemiologists from several countries to work in close coordination with national SEP authorities. The reporting systems were improved, but active surveillance—aggressively seeking out cases instead of waiting for them to be reported through written notification systems—became the key measure. Surveillance teams were equipped with jeeps and motorcycles so they could roam near and far searching markets, schools, pilgrimage sites, tea-shops, and bustis (slum settlements) for cases. Repeated village-to-village and then house-to-house searches were launched in both countries. Cash rewards for pinpointing hidden cases were offered, first to the public and then to the health workers as well. At the same time, ever more rigorous containment measures were instituted. Motorized teams rushed to the scene of outbreaks to backstop local vaccination personnel. When active cases were located, the patients were either confined to their homes with guards or put into secure isolation hospitals to prevent additional contacts; local vaccinators were hired to immunize co-villagers regardless of their prior immune status. A huge monitoring effort was made to track all known cases and contacts, and supervision was exercised at every level of the SEP hierarchy.

The Context of Coercion and the Logic of Resistance

Coercion arose during containment operations, when expatriate epidemiologists accompanied by vaccination teams went into villages after surveillance had detected smallpox outbreaks. Coercion was justified by containment, but the containment concept was modified at least twice. Initially it simply meant vaccinating the known contacts of active smallpox cases; the names of contacts were elicited from patients by trained interviewers—classic public health contact tracing. These interviewers also determined the immune status of the contacts, who would be excused from vaccination if they could demonstrate prior successful smallpox immunization (e.g., by showing a characteristic scar). These interviews could be slow and were obviously hampered when smallpox patients were too ill to speak or died. In time, WHO epidemiologists, few of whom spoke local languages and were dependent on others, disparaged the interview method, arguing that even when it was well done, it was not foolproof. Containment was thus redefined in 1973 to mean that everyone in a village where active cases of smallpox had been detected had to be vaccinated, regardless of his or her prior immune status. This put an end to dilatory interviews and indeed to the need to converse with villagers at all. The turn from an interactional to a purely locational definition of containment has been described by Stanley Music, a senior WHO physician-epidemiologist from CDC assigned to the Bangladesh SEP during 1973–1975.

In the last phase of the eradication campaign, containment was again defined to mean the vaccination of everyone living within a 1- to 1.5-km radius of an outbreak. The actual application of containment so defined, however, often produced chaos in the affected villages. In Music's words,

The initial stage in the evolution of a coherent containment policy was marked by an almost military style attack on infected villages. ... In the hit-and-run excitement of such a campaign, women and children were often pulled out from under beds, from behind doors, from within latrines, etc. People were chased and, when caught, vaccinated. Many misunderstandings arose and tempers often flared in these heated situations. ... Known infected villages were revisited—often repeatedly—to check for new cases and left-outs. Almost invariably a chase or forcible vaccination ensued in such circumstances. ... We considered the villagers to have an understandable though irrational fear of vaccination. ... We just couldn't let people get smallpox and die needlessly. We went from door to door and vaccinated. When they ran, we chased. When they locked their doors, we broke down their doors and vaccinated them.[4,5]

Containment teams generally had their way, and sustained resistance (other than flight) was infrequent. When resistance did occur, it took various forms, ranging from mild avoidance to violent protest. The teams, always fearful that new outbreaks would undo their hard work, met resistance with coercion. The following accounts document a range of coercive encounters involving American WHO advisers in Bangladesh and India between 1973 and 1975.

Case 2: Bangladesh, 1973

In a second case, resistance took on a more active quality. Again, the narrator is Music, and the scene is rural Bangladesh during 1973.

[She was] an old woman who wore a dirty grey plain cotton sari over her gaunt and emaciated body. The [Sanitary Inspector] said that she wanted food and would not take vaccination unless someone gave her food. She was a beggar by "profession" but the times had been hard and she was frankly starving. I entered her house—a jute-stick and mud hut with thatch roof in poor repair—and asked her to take vaccination. She asked if I had brought her any food. I said no. She refused vaccination. She said that if I didn't care whether or not she died of starvation, why should I care if she got smallpox! After explaining that she was a risk to others in villages where she might beg, I told her that I had no choice but to vaccinate her with or without her consent. I promised to arrange some food for her and then vaccinated her myself. ... I felt it was important to get 100% vaccination and drive home the point that there could be no exceptions. With an eye to how the SI [Sanitary Inspector] and his staff would regard this situation, I felt compelled to vaccinate her there and then with or without her consent.[4]

Here the woman verbalizes her reason for refusing vaccination: if you don't care whether I die of starvation, why should I care about smallpox? Her argument represents a common response to narrowly sectoral disease campaigns among the poor.

Case 3: Bangladesh, 1973

A third case based also on Music's experience in a Bangladesh village in 1973 reveals a much higher level of coercion in response to forthright resistance.

[A man refused] to let anyone into his house or to come out to be vaccinated. When he left his house he locked the women and children inside with a padlock. When he came home he barred it from within. The [Sanitary Inspector] had tried three times to convince the family to take vaccination. I waited for the man to come home and when he did I told him that he had to take vaccination and to let his wife and children be vaccinated. He refused, went inside and barred the door. I broke the door down and vaccinated—with a struggle—every member of his family, including the man. He was very angry and told me he was going to initiate a case against me. Approximately three months later I was told by the local magistrate that a case had been registered against me but that it had been thrown out of court.[4]

Blazing anger distinguishes this response from the previous two; unlike the TB patient and the beggar widow, this man felt himself empowered to resist. He not only contested the WHO adviser personally but on behalf of others, especially his female dependents.[2,3] Locking up his dependents was a mechanical approach to a jurisdictional conflict: patriarchal authority was being pitted against the state.

Case 4: Bihar, India 1975

The fourth case refers to an unusually violent encounter in eastern India in 1975 in an aboriginal village in the Jharkhand region of Bihar. The narrator, Lawrence Brilliant, was a WHO physician-epidemiologist who had married an Indian woman and was fluent in Hindi.[6]

In the middle of the night an intruder burst through the door of the simple adobe hut. He was a government vaccinator, under orders to break resistance against smallpox vaccination. Lakshmi Singh awoke screaming and scrambled to hide herself. Her husband leaped out of bed, grabbed an axe, and chased the intruder into the courtyard. Outside, a squad of doctors and policemen quickly overpowered Mohan Singh. The instant he was pinned to the ground, a second vaccinator jabbed smallpox vaccine into his arm. Mohan Singh, a wiry 40-year-old leader of the Ho tribe, squirmed away from the needle, causing the vaccination site to bleed. The government team held him until they had injected enough vaccine; then they seized his wife. Pausing only to suck out some vaccine, Mohan Singh pulled a bamboo pole from the roof and attacked the strangers holding his wife. While two policemen rebuffed him, the rest of the team overpowered the whole family and vaccinated each in turn. Lakshmi Singh bit deep into one doctor's hand, but to no avail.[7]

Brilliant admits to being troubled by the attack on Mohan Singh's house.[8] At the time, it was justified on epidemiological grounds. A serious outbreak of smallpox had occurred in the nearby industrial city of Jamshedpur, and one case had been traced to the Ho village.[9] The containment rules were clear. The village was thus forcibly vaccinated in a military-style operation. This display of force—massed policemen and jeeps at midnight—gives the account a peculiar vividness, but there is no difference in principle between this and earlier cases: local norms have no standing and are swept away.

Discussion

As noted at the beginning of this chapter, most people worldwide actively welcome, or can be persuaded to accept, measures of mass immunization that aim to eradicate or control disease. This was true for the smallpox eradication program in the 1970s, and it is true still for the polio eradication and EPI campaigns in the 1990s. Why then raise the issues of coercion and intimidation? Hasn't smallpox eradication justified itself over and over by saving hundreds of thousands of lives and by averting blindness among nearly 5% of the survivors? Don't these results, and the substantial sums saved by dismantling a 175-year-old worldwide vaccination program, justify a limited number of obscure acts of zeal in India? By and large, they do. Yet I believe there are three reasons for stirring up the embers of the South Asian eradication program today. In the first place, the success achieved in the South Asian campaign has been highly influential and has demonstrated the technical feasibility of disease eradication as a significant public health strategy.[10] Second, coercion can leave behind a residue of resentment that sours public attitudes toward the next vaccination campaign. Third and finally, it would be an ethical error to hold that consent to immunization is less important in villages of Bihar and Bangladesh than it is in Birmingham or Buffalo—unless one accepts the ethical partition of the world. No one in the WHO leadership argued for a partition in so many words, yet coercion against resistant villagers in South Asia was tacitly accepted as necessary because it "worked," it "got the job done."

We are thus left with the question of whether expatriate epidemiologists in South Asia in the mid-1970s felt that coercion and intimidation were necessary to achieve "victory." It may be that there is a defensible case to be made for coercion and intimidation—some officials clearly believe these methods must be kept in reserve—but let the case for strong methods at least be made openly.

Notes and References

1. For a global survey of compliance, see K. Heggenhougen and J. Clements. 1987, Summer. *Acceptability of Childhood Immunisation: Social Science Perspectives, Evaluation and Planning Centre for Health Care*, Publication No. 14, 11–15, 33. London: London School of Hygiene and Tropical Medicine, and associated references in the bibliography.

2. R. N. Basu, Z. Jezek, and N. A. Ward. 1979. *The Eradication of Smallpox from India*. WHO Series History of International Public Health, No. 2. New Delhi: WHO South-east Asia Regional Office.

3. A. K. Joarder, D. Tarantola, and J. Tulloch. 1980. *The Eradication of Smallpox from Bangladesh*. WHO Regional Publication, South-east Asia Series, No. 8. New Delhi: WHO South-east Asia Regional Office.

4. S. I. Music. 1976, June. Smallpox eradication in Bangladesh: Reflections of an epidemiologist. Unpublished DTPH dissertation, London School of Hygiene and Tropical Medicine.

5. Music makes it clear that this degree of chaos was incompatible with long-term SEP methods, and that in a subsequent development, the Bangladesh program began to hire temporary male and female vaccinators in the affected villages rather than launching military-style containment raids. The definition of containment continued to rest on "focally intense ring vaccination," but the vaccinators were locals, which greatly lessened the coercive aspect.

6. Brilliant, an American, was not a CDC epidemiologist. His unusual path of recruitment into the South Asian WHO-SEP has been narrated in Ram Dass. 1991. *Miracle of Love: Stories about Neem Karoli Baba*. New York: Arkana-Penguin.

7. L. Brilliant and G. Brilliant. 1978, May–June. Death for a killer disease. *Quest.*

8. July 1992 telephone interview with Dr. Brilliant, now associated with the SEVA Foundation, San Francisco. Brilliant pointed out that Mohan Singh spoke Hindi, which Brilliant transcribed himself.

9. Singhbhum district in Bihar was a sore spot for the SEP; in spring 1964, it was called "the world's greatest exporter of smallpox," and it continued to harry WHO-SEP staff.

10. In the recent World Development Report: Investing in Health (1993), the World Bank notes that, "in many ways the Intensified Smallpox Eradication Programme exemplifies the potential of today's medicine" (p. 17), and it celebrates its status as a model of what technology can accomplish. This is a familiar position found in numerous articles and documents over the last 15 years.

38   Is Disease Eradication Ethical?

Arthur L. Caplan[*]

For many in the field of public health, the eradication of smallpox was one of the greatest triumphs of twentieth-century medicine. This astounding achievement has influenced national and international organizations to mount or consider efforts to eradicate many other infectious diseases, including measles, Guinea worm disease, Chagas' disease, polio, and malaria. Eradication may well be public health's greatest rhetorical weapon in the battle against dread diseases. Indeed, the ability to command funding, popular support, the attention of politicians, and positive media coverage by talk of disease eradication is unparalleled. As WHO's Director-General Margaret Chan told an audience of Rotarians, who have for many years made polio eradication their sole cause at the group's international convention, last year: "We have to prove the power of public health. The international community has so very few opportunities to improve this world in genuine and lasting ways. Polio eradication is one."

It may seem churlish to wonder in the face of a public health triumph that saved untold numbers from death and disability whether disease eradication is ethical. Nevertheless, there are sound reasons for wondering whether the pursuit of eradication—as opposed to aggressive and effective disease management—is the right thing to do for other infectious diseases. In questioning whether disease eradication is a desirable public health and policy goal, it is important to be clear about the meaning of eradication. In 1997, a justly famous meeting—the 81st Dahlem Conference—was held in Berlin, Germany, to examine the challenge of disease eradication. At that meeting, F. Fenner, A. J. Hall, and W. R. Dowdle presented a seminal paper on the philosophy of medicine and public health, "What Is Eradication?" They set themselves the task of cleaning up decades of confusion about what is meant by disease eradication as distinct from disease elimination, reduction, and extinction. The term *eradication*, they rightly argued,

* Reprinted from *The Lancet*, Caplan, A., Is disease eradication ethical? 373:2192–2193. Copyright © 2009 with permission of Elsevier.

should be used to describe deliberate efforts to reduce the worldwide incidence of an infectious disease to zero. This achievement would have multiple benefits. If accomplished, not only would many people be freed of the risk of acquiring a particular disease, but success would also permit the abandonment or relaxation of preventive and prophylactic measures that are often expensive, intensive, or both. Extinction is different. It is, Fenner, Hall, and Dowdle noted, a tool to achieve eradication. Extinction sometimes can be achieved by the complete destruction of all disease pathogens, or it can be achieved by the destruction of all possible vectors that permit the transmission of a disease. Elimination connotes a different goal. It captures the fact that a disease is not occurring at any given time in a particular area or population. Disease reduction is precisely that—less disease but acknowledging that some degree of disease is likely to or will continue to be present in an area or a population.

If eradication is the goal behind various past and current public heath campaigns, and if it is to be the goal of future efforts, it is important to realize exactly what target is being set by the use of this term. The stakes involved in aiming for eradication are enormous; talk of eradication portends relief forever from a disease as well as the ability to relax humanity's guard against that disease.

There are many reasons to doubt the desirability of seeking to eradicate all infectious diseases. Some have to do with the certainty with which eradication can be ascertained. Some have to do with the cost and reliability of achieving eradication. Both problems are troubling because of what happens after eradication is certified as having been achieved. If eradication is claimed to have been achieved for a disease, then efforts to prevent its recurrence will most probably cease. This occurred with respect to routine smallpox vaccination in the United States and many other nations in the 1970s. Spending money and devoting resources to a disease that cannot recur makes little sense in a world in which there is fierce competition for healthcare resources. Indeed, it is precisely the ability to capture back the costs of contending with a disease that forms the economic argument in favor of pursuing eradication.

In addition to ending prophylactic efforts, a claim of eradication will also probably stop or greatly reduce efforts at training health workers to recognize and treat the eradicated disease given other pressing educational needs. Efforts to undertake intense surveillance and further research involving the eradicated disease and its causal agents will also rapidly diminish. Eradication, in other words, means replacing prophylaxis and vigilance with indifference and trust. But are those consequences too risky in today's world? Should humanity strive to replace vigilance with indifference regarding polio, malaria, measles, HIV/AIDS, and other infectious diseases? There are reasons to think not.

Efforts at polio eradication have led to great success: polio was endemic in fifty nations in 1998 and is now believed to be present in only a small handful of nations. But the cost of eliminating these final pockets is high. Polio eradication remains a controversial goal. K. M. Thompson and R. J. Tebbens argued in an influential study that continued efforts at polio eradication made economic sense. The resources made available from permanently wiping out polio in terms of recovered cost that could be used to combat other infectious diseases or other health problems are great. But is it realistic to think that after 20 years of eradication efforts that eradication is achievable?

Surveillance to establish eradication is a huge challenge. Political and military events do not make access possible in some parts of the world for either surveillance or pro-phylaxis. Moreover, it is not clear that all polio cases can be detected because there is a significant incidence of subclinical cases. Climate change may shift the geographical areas in which polio is likely to endure or recur. Some parts of the world have proven especially challenging for confirming polio eradication. Somalia is widely acknowl-edged to be a failed state. It has no real central government, and as a result warlords and piracy are flourishing. Somalia also still has polio. It is hard to imagine an effective health campaign that can be certified as achieving eradication in such circumstances. There are other nations, such as North Korea and parts of some nations like Burma (Myanmar), where it is difficult to monitor rates of infectious diseases or gain access to all of the population to certify eradication.

Chasing down the last cases of polio is costly. In western India, Afghanistan, and Pakistan, fragile healthcare infrastructure and community support are being strained by the eradication effort. In striving to reach eradication, children are exposed to the risk of multiple vaccinations because record-keeping in these areas is so poor. Govern-ment budgets and resources in poor nations are diverted from other far more pressing local problems to try and capture the last marginal cases. It is also simply a fact of human nature that it is difficult to command continued enthusiasm for a goal whose achievement begins to stretch across decades.

These problems are compounded when it comes to mounting other efforts to eradicate infectious diseases. Many nations lack the surveillance capacities to know whether a disease has recurred in wild-type form or whether it is present in forms in animal populations that can spread back to human beings. Some nations, such as Indonesia, have made it clear that they are willing to withhold information on the inci-dence of infectious disease as a bargaining chip to help secure the requisite resources to combat outbreaks of pandemic infectious diseases.

In other parts of the world, the emergence of respect for a patient's right to choose has created problems for those seeking to eradicate diseases such as measles or rubella.

There are many people in the United States, United Kingdom, and Canada who oppose all form of vaccination and make every effort to ensure that they and their families are not vaccinated. Rates of refusal for measles vaccination are not high, but they are significant enough in some parts of some nations to guarantee reservoirs of disease that can lead to the continuous recurrence of disease. Modern air and road transportation allow for the rapid spread of disease back to populations, putting people at risk when prophylactic vaccination campaigns have been allowed to lag due to the promise of eradication. There are no substantive public policy efforts underway that would override patients' rights in favor of the goal of eradication of these diseases. Even the outbreak of H1N1 pandemic influenza has not led to the enactment of vaccine mandates for any particular group or population.

Bioterrorism continues to be an all too real possibility. This fact may mean that for some diseases, no trust should be placed in claims of eradication. Although bioterror is at present beyond the means of those lacking sophisticated training, it is not beyond the capacity of nations who tolerate terrorism and have the requisite expertise on hand to carry it through. Added to this threat is the emergence of synthetic biology that permits the creation of the genomes of various viruses and microbes. The polio and smallpox genomes have both been mapped, and information about them is readily available to anyone seeking it. The reality of this new form of applied genomic biology further undercuts the desirability of setting the goal of eradication for every disease.

For some diseases, eradication may make sense. But for other diseases, such as polio, measles, mumps, and malaria, the dream of eradication may not be one that can be relied on. The best that may be done is to seek elimination or control rather than eradication and to hope that politics, war, climate change, economics, and ethics allow us to get that far. I would contend it is crucial that all parties now involved in efforts or plans involving eradication rethink their rhetoric and their goals lest the world's faith in the possibility of eradication be misplaced with disastrous consequences.

Further Reading

Bazin, H. 2000. *The Eradication of Smallpox: Edward Jenner and the First and Only Eradication of a Human Infectious Disease*. San Diego, CA: Academic Press.

Fenner, F., A. J. Hall, and W. R. Dowdle. 1998. What is eradication? In: *The Eradication of Infectious Diseases*, eds. W. R. Dowdle and D. R. Hopkins, 3–18. Chichester: Wiley.

Thompson, K. M., and R. J. Tebbens. 2007. Eradication versus control for poliomyelitis: An economic analysis. *Lancet* 369:1363–1371.

Caplan, A. L., and D. Curry. 2007. Leveraging genetic resources or moral blackmail? Indonesia and avian flu virus sample sharing. *Am J Bioeth* 7:1–2.

39   Is There an Ethical Obligation to Complete Polio Eradication?

Claudia I. Emerson and Peter A. Singer*

In May 2010, the World Health Assembly (WHA) is expected to endorse the aggressive new strategy of the Global Polio Eradication Initiative (GPEI) to stop polio transmission. Earlier this year, the Executive Board of the WHA expressed strong support for finishing the job of polio eradication. They were encouraged by the Independent Evaluation of Major Barriers to Interrupting Poliovirus Transmission, which concluded in November 2009 that "if the managerial, security, and technical issues can be addressed, polio eradication can be achieved." To supporters of the GPEI, this renewed commitment must surely come as a relief—after more than 20 years of effort, the initiative has come under fire for failing to achieve eradication and support for adopting an "effective control" strategy has gained traction.

Those who favor "effective control" (maintaining fewer than 500 polio cases per year indefinitely) question the wisdom of pursuing eradication for diseases such as polio and malaria, given the technical and sociopolitical challenges, costs, and uncertainty in ascertaining eradication. Although the ethical case against eradication has been articulated, we were surprised to find no explicit ethical justification in support of polio eradication. Ethics discussions about mass immunization programs, and polio eradication more specifically, have focused on analyses of risks and benefits, informed consent, transparency, and the tension between the individual and collective good. However, there have been no claims about an ethical obligation to eradicate polio. Why is an ethical argument for disease eradication needed? Because ethical motivation can be compelling: moral obligations are weighty concerns that cannot be easily dismissed, even in the face of sound non-moral arguments. Acts and omissions having a moral dimension can be praiseworthy or blameworthy, giving strong reasons

* Reprinted from *The Lancet*, Emerson, C. I., and P. A. Singer, Is there an ethical obligation to complete polio eradication? 375:1340–1341. Copyright © 2010 with permission of Elsevier.

to consider the implications of one's actions. This is particularly pressing in contexts where action outcomes have large-scale impact, such as the case of polio eradication where millions of lives are affected.

There are compelling moral reasons to continue the pursuit of polio eradication. First, failing to pursue eradication results in harm, and there is a moral obligation to avert preventable harm. We have the means to avert harm in the case of polio; thus, we can argue that we have a duty to pursue eradication. This duty may be more precisely characterized as a duty to rescue: a moral duty to rescue someone in distress provided one has the ability to do so, and doing so would not require excessive sacrifice. Three conditions must be satisfied to invoke a duty to rescue: there must be opportunity and capability, and the burden must not be so taxing as to make the circumstance before rescue preferable to the circumstance after rescue. The commitment from the GPEI and the availability of effective vaccines satisfy the first two conditions, but one can distinguish between "hard rescues" and "easy rescues," and on the third condition it could be argued that completing polio eradication amounts to a "hard rescue" that imposes excessive burden. However, this line of argument is unconvincing because the burden may be distributed so that it is not excessively taxing for any particular actor, and on balance the benefits of completing the rescue outweigh the collective burden. When the three conditions for rescue are met, failing to act represents an omission for which the actor, in this case the global health community, can be morally blamed. In the context of polio, under an "effective control" regime, the alternative to eradication, WHO projects that we would fail to rescue 4 million children in the next 20 years. How can we ethically justify this course of action when the opportunity and means to rescue are available? Generally, forward-looking analyses of completing polio eradication have focused on the economic aspects, overlooking an important moral calculation: the human cost of failing to eradicate. This is the cost of lives not saved, the lives afflicted by polio (including those family members who care for paralyzed children), and the impact of those lives on the future of the broader community.

Second, completing eradication spares future generations the harms associated with polio. Obligations to future generations are difficult to define and may be limited, but if preventing harm is a moral duty, there may be a chain of obligation that persists through generations and applies to circumstances where present generations could have meaningful impact—such as disease eradication. There is a parallel argument in guarding against environmental degradation to preserve the environment for those who will inherit it. Hans Jonas' influential theory of responsibility claimed that the present generation has a responsibility to ensure its conduct does not result in consequences that could threaten the existence of future human beings. As a corollary, one might argue that the pursuit of polio eradication safeguards the existence of future generations, to whom our ethical obligations go beyond simply tallying the costs and benefits in the immediate future.

Third, there is already a recognized moral commitment to the pursuit of public health as a global public good. The reduction in the global burden of disability and death is of benefit to all. Take, for example, the eradication of smallpox, which was effectively wiped out in the late 1970s. As a result, up to 2 million lives are saved, 10 to 15 million smallpox infections are prevented annually, and no one is further threatened by this disease. The eradication of polio would similarly achieve global public good. The GPEI has already made strides in this direction: since its launch in 1988, more than 2 billion children have been immunized, and a 99% reduction in polio has been achieved. Arguably, those who enjoy the benefits of public goods should be motivated to act in pursuit of such goods. Thus, the onus is on the global community to continue supporting polio eradication efforts.

The preceding arguments suggest a strong ethical case for pursuing polio eradication. However, the success of eradication and maintaining a polio-free world post-eradication may depend on the global coordination of switching from oral polio vaccine to the more costly inactivated polio vaccine that resource-poor countries cannot afford. Although the global health community has yet to reach consensus on this point, many experts agree that this switch in vaccines is required to reduce the risk of harm caused by circulating vaccine-derived polioviruses once wild poliovirus transmission has been interrupted globally. Who should pay for the cost of this switch? Wealthy nations have strong moral reasons to subsidize the cost of switching from oral to inactivated polio vaccine. Self-interest may be the strongest reason. Although polio has been absent from the developed world for more than 30 years, the threat of re-emergence looms in a world where people and viruses easily cross international borders. Polio remains endemic in four countries—India, Pakistan, Afghanistan, and Nigeria—and over the years has been exported to previously polio-free countries in sub-Saharan Africa and elsewhere. Moreover, subsidizing the switch will relieve burdened healthcare systems as more lives are saved; once polio is eradicated, resources that would be spent on control strategies can be applied to other health needs—including other infectious diseases. Self-preservation is a powerful motivator, but there are also less selfish reasons to subsidize the switch—especially solidarity with the global community. Unlike altruism, solidarity recognizes that people are capable of responding sympathetically to others or empathizing with a condition afflicting them because they can identify with a common feature or hold shared values, and they can see themselves experiencing that fate. We can all imagine being affected by polio.

Another approach is for the developing world, including polio-affected countries, to take ownership of the switch through affordable innovation and manufacture of inactivated polio vaccine. The GAVI Alliance recently reported a price drop in the life-saving pentavalent vaccine, a direct consequence of increased market competition from developing world manufacturers. Affordable innovation is a strategy compatible with the recurring theme of "ownership at all levels" that the WHA Executive Board urged should be taken by polio-affected countries.

In a world of limited and finite resources, there have to be trade-offs. Pursuing the eradication of one disease will inevitably raise questions. Why eradicate polio and not focus resources toward something else? Are moral duties absolute in a world of fixed resources? Are there easier rescues? These are legitimate questions. It need not be the case, however, that disease prevention, detection, and treatment should be selected at the expense of eradication of specific diseases, or vice versa. These are what philosopher Joseph Raz would consider incommensurable goods: neither one is better than the other. Disease eradication is qualitatively different from other investments; as a long-term strategy, it generates future health benefits and a revenue stream that can be applied to short-term goals—it is an annuity that keeps on paying. The global benefit—cost ratio of the eradication of smallpox has exceeded 400:1, with the United States alone recouping its total investment of US$32 million every 26 days. Moreover, the evocative power of eradication should not be underestimated. This year, rinderpest, a viral disease of ruminants related to human measles, is likely to be declared eradicated. Guinea worm disease is the next probable candidate, having just missed its 2009 target for eradication. Failure to complete polio eradication now could undermine plans to target other infectious diseases in the future. We are on the last kilometer of a marathon; surely it is worth crossing the finish line.

Further Reading

Caplan, A. L. 2009. Is disease eradication ethical? *Lancet* 373:2192–2193.

Chan, M. *The Case for Completing Polio Eradication*. Geneva: World Health Organization.

Editorial. 2010. Eradicating infectious diseases in 2010. *Nat Rev Microbiol* 8:2.

Jonas, H. 1984. *The Imperative of Responsibility: In Search of an Ethics for the Technological Age*. Chicago: The University of Chicago Press.

Mohamed, A. J., P. Ndumbe, A. Hall, V. Tangcharoensathien, M. J. Toole, and P. Wright. 2009, October 20. Independent evaluation of major barriers to interrupting poliovirus transmission. Executive Summary. Available at: http://www.polioeradication.org/content/general/Polio_Evaluation_PAK.pdf. Accessed March 29, 2010.

40   Letter from Public Health Deans Regarding Fictional Vaccination Campaigns in the Search for Osama Bin Laden and Response from The White House

January 6, 2013

Dear President Obama,

In the first years of the Peace Corps, its director, Sargent Shriver, discovered that the Central Intelligence Agency (CIA) was infiltrating his efforts and programs for covert purposes. Mr. Shriver forcefully expressed the unacceptability of this to the President. His action, and the repeated vigilance and actions of future directors, has preserved the Peace Corps as a vehicle of service for our country's most idealistic citizens. It also protects our Peace Corps volunteers from unwarranted suspicion, and it provides opportunities for the Peace Corps to operate in areas of great need that otherwise would be closed off to them.

In September, Save the Children was forced by the Government of Pakistan (GoP) to withdraw all foreign national staff. This action was apparently the result of the CIA having used the cover of a fictional vaccination campaign to gather information about the whereabouts of Osama Bin Laden. In fact, Save the Children never employed the Pakistani physician serving the CIA, yet in the eyes of the GoP, he was associated with the organization. This past month, eight or more United Nations health workers who were vaccinating Pakistani children against polio were gunned down in unforgivable acts of terrorism. While political and security agendas may by necessity induce collateral damage, we as an open society set boundaries on these damages, and we believe this sham vaccination campaign exceeded those boundaries.

As an example of the gravity of the situation, today we are on the verge of completely eradicating polio. With your leadership, the U.S. is the largest bilateral donor to the Global Polio Eradication Initiative and has provided strong direction and technical assistance as well. Polio particularly threatens young children in the most disadvantaged communities and today has been isolated to just three countries: Afghanistan, Nigeria, and Pakistan. Now, because of these assassinations of vaccination workers, the UN has been forced to suspend polio eradication efforts in Pakistan. This is only one example and illustrates why, as a general principle, public health programs should not be used as cover for covert operations.

Independent of the Geneva Conventions of 1949, contaminating humanitarian and public health programs with covert activities threatens the present participants and future potential of much of what we undertake internationally to improve health and provide humanitarian assistance. As public health academic leaders, we hereby urge you to assure the public that this type of practice will not be repeated.

International public health work builds peace and is one of the most constructive means by which our past, present, and future public health students can pursue a life of fulfillment and service. Please do not allow that outlet of common good to be closed to them because of political and/ or security interests that ignore the type of unintended negative public health impacts we are witnessing in Pakistan.

Sincerely,

Pierre M. Buekens, M.D., M.P.H., Ph.D. Dean, Tulane University School of Public Health and Tropical Medicine

James W. Curran, M.D., M.P.H. Dean, Rollins School of Public Health, Emory University

John R. Finnegan, Jr., Ph.D. Professor and Dean, University of Minnesota School of Public Health; Chair of the Board, Association of Schools of Public Health

Julio Frenk, M.D., M.P.H., Ph.D. Dean and T&G Angelopoulos Professor of Public Health and International Development Harvard School of Public Health

Linda P. Fried, M.D., M.P.H. Dean, Mailman School of Public Health, Columbia University

Howard Frumkin, M.D., Dr.P.H. Dean, School of Public Health, University of Washington

Lynn R. Goldman, M.D., M.P.H. Professor and Dean, School of Public Health and Health Services, George Washington University

Jody Heymann, M.D., M.P.P., Ph.D. Dean, UCLA Fielding School of Public Health

Michael J. Klag, M.D., M.P.H. Dean, Johns Hopkins Bloomberg School of Public Health

Martin Philbert, Ph.D. Dean, School of Public Health, University of Michigan

Barbara K. Rimer, Dr.P.H. Dean and Alumni Distinguished Professor UNC Gillings School of Global Public Health

Stephen M. Shortell, Ph.D. Dean, School of Public Health, University of California Berkeley

●

The White House, Washington

Dear Deans:

The United States strongly supports the Global Polio Eradication Initiative and efforts to end the spread of polio virus forever.

In response to your January 2013 letter to the President expressing concern about the safety of vaccination workers, I wanted to inform you that the Director of the Central Intelligence Agency (CIA) directed in August 2013 that the Agency make no operational use of vaccination programs, which includes vaccination workers. Similarly, the Agency will not seek to obtain or exploit DNA or other genetic material acquired through such programs. This CIA policy applies worldwide and to U.S. and non-U.S. persons alike. Please feel free to share this information with whomever you deem appropriate.

Your tireless efforts to improve global health are inspiring. Thank you for the work you do.

Sincerely,

Lisa O. Monaco

Assistant to the President for Homeland Security and Counterterrorism

VII Frontiers in Vaccination

As we have seen, vaccination has a remarkable history of public health achievements, a wide range of ongoing activities around the world, and a broad base of enthusiastic supporters in government, public health and the other health professions, industry, and civil society committed to building and sustaining vaccination programs. From this enthusiasm and commitment has come attention in recent years to novel strategies that seek to apply the foundational principles and technologies of vaccination to a range of new infectious and non-infectious targets. In this final section, we introduce some of these ongoing areas of interest and research attention that represent the cutting edge of the global vaccination enterprise. As work proceeds on these new directions in vaccine science, we can expect corresponding attention to the interconnected policy and ethical considerations emerging from them, some of which are already receiving attention.

Building on our discussion of global vaccination issues in part VI, Peter Hotez begins this section with an appeal for greater research attention to potential "antipoverty" vaccines, as he calls them in his chapter. The diseases on which he focuses cause considerable illness and death, but because they occur mainly in very poor regions that offer little prospect of large commercial markets, the traditional incentives for vaccine research and development by the major manufacturers are not present. New models for collaboration and new incentives are needed to stimulate attention to potential vaccines against these diseases, Hotez explains.

Vaccine strategies are no longer limited to traditional infectious targets such as viruses or bacteria, as the next two chapters discuss. Ongoing research has sought to develop safe and effective vaccines against drugs of addiction such as cocaine and methamphetamine, as the chapter by Thomas Kosten and colleagues discusses. Approved vaccines against these substances—or others like nicotine, also in development—could revolutionize approaches to addiction prevention and treatment, but their potential use raises vexing questions of public policy and ethics regarding when, how, and to whom they would be administered.

Vaccines against hepatitis B and HPV are sometimes referred to as "cancer vaccines" because they prevent viral infections that are capable of causing liver and cervical cancer, respectively. There is also research in progress that seeks to develop *therapeutic* cancer vaccines, as Justin Liu writes. These vaccine strategies attempt to target cancer cells or their unique cellular components, using patients' own immune systems. This class of new vaccines would offer important new tools for cancer therapy but, in so doing, would transform public understandings of vaccines and vaccination. The implications of this expansion of the concept of "vaccination" are just beginning to be considered.

The frontiers of vaccination include not only attention to new disease targets but also the development of novel technologies that could dramatically reshape existing vaccination programs. A particularly promising focus of such efforts is influenza vaccines, as the need for annual revaccination against seasonal influenza and the months required to produce novel vaccines in the event of an outbreak or a pandemic are both problematic. Development of a "universal" influenza vaccine is a major research focus to address the first concern, and as Philip Dormitzer and colleagues write, advances in synthetic biology may permit their rapid development. This would dramatically shorten the time needed for novel vaccines to be available following the emergence of a new strain capable of causing a pandemic, for example.

We conclude with chapters discussing aspects of vaccine development against two major global health threats—malaria and Ebola—which, despite their many differences in geographic spread, mode of transmission, and overall disease burden, are leading targets for vaccine development. Amed Ouattara and Matthew Laurens summarize the state of vaccine development against malaria, a disease for which Bill Gates and other influential voices in global health have endorsed eradication as a feasible long-term target.

More urgent calls for accelerated vaccine research followed the outbreak of Ebola centered in West Africa in 2013. As efforts unfolded to respond to an urgent global health crisis while identifying effective therapies or vaccines against the virus, an ethical debate emerged over whether randomized controlled trials were appropriate in Ebola-affected regions. Clement Adebamowo and colleagues argue that alternative approaches were better equipped to provide rapid information in the context of what at the time was an unprecedented unfolding health crisis. Edward Cox, Luciana Borio, and Robert Temple from the U.S. Food and Drug Administration (FDA) similarly recognize the urgent need to help affected populations but discuss why randomized controlled trials are essential for providing valid evidence of whether a vaccine or other therapy is effective now or would be in future Ebola outbreaks. Proceeding with those trials was both ethically and scientifically sound, they conclude.

Further Reading

Bill Gates. 2014. We Can Eradicate Malaria—Within a Generation. *GatesNotes*. Available at: https://www.gatesnotes.com/Health/Eradicating-Malaria-in-a-Generation.

U.S. National Cancer Institute. 2016. "Cancer Vaccines." Available at: http://www.cancer.gov/about-cancer/causes-prevention/vaccines-fact-sheet.

World Health Organization. 2014. Ethical Considerations for Use of Unregistered Interventions for Ebola Virus Disease: Report of an Advisory Panel to WHO. Available at: http://www.who.int/csr/resources/publications/ebola/ethical-considerations/en/.

Michael J. Young, et al. 2012. Immune to Addiction: The Ethical Dimensions of Vaccines against Substance Abuse. *Nature Immunology* 13 (6):521–524.

41 A Handful of "Antipoverty" Vaccines Exist for Neglected Diseases, but the World's Poorest Billion People Need More

Peter Hotez[*]

A full year has passed since the launch of the "Decade of Vaccines," which was articulated when the Bill & Melinda Gates Foundation made a 10-year commitment to ensuring the development and delivery of new vaccines for the poorest people living in the world's low- and middle-income countries. Since then, enormous progress has been made in increasing global access to vaccines that combat the great childhood killer diseases, such as pneumococcal pneumonia, rotavirus, *Hemophilus influenzae* type b, and measles.

That progress was made possible through enhanced cooperation among the GAVI Alliance, the multinational pharmaceutical companies, and organizations supported by the Bill & Melinda Gates Foundation, such as the Program for Appropriate Technology in Health (PATH). New financial incentives, including a $1.5 billion advance market commitment, have also contributed to the progress.[1]

Lagging far behind these global efforts against the major killer childhood diseases are parallel activities to produce and deliver a new generation of vaccines for so-called neglected diseases (these are sometimes known as neglected tropical diseases).[2] These neglected diseases are the most common infections of the world's poor, and almost all of the "bottom billion"—the 1.4 billion people who live below the poverty level defined by the World Bank—suffer from one or more of the neglected diseases.[3-5]

The World Health Organization (WHO) now identifies seventeen conditions as "neglected tropical diseases."[6] The most common neglected diseases are caused by parasitic worms, including hookworm infection, ascariasis (intestinal roundworm), trichuriasis (whipworm), schistosomiasis (bilharzia), lymphatic filariasis (elephantiasis), and onchocerciasis (river blindness); by parasitic protozoa, including Chagas disease and leishmaniasis (kala-azar); or by bacterial and viral infections, such as trachoma, leprosy, and dengue.[6]

Although the neglected diseases are caused by a wide variety of pathogens, they overlap geographically and have functional similarities. This has led to a common global health policy framework for these conditions.[3,5] In areas of extreme poverty, it is common to find multiple neglected diseases occurring in the same place or whole populations infected simultaneously with more than one disease.[3-5] Four of the neglected diseases listed above occur in at least 400 million people.

Chronic neglected diseases in children, especially hookworm infection and schistosomiasis, impair physical and intellectual development, and ultimately future wage earning. Neglected diseases in adults can cause chronic disabilities such as blindness and disfigurement, which reduce productive capacity and work productivity.[3-5] The neglected diseases disproportionately affect girls and women through their adverse effects on pregnancy and their ability to cause disfigurement, which is highly stigmatizing.[7] In addition, tens of millions—and possibly hundreds of millions—of women in Africa suffer from a form of schistosomiasis that causes ulcers on their cervix, uterus, and lower genital tract, which increases susceptibility to HIV/AIDS.[8] Such links between the neglected diseases and the "big three" infectious diseases—HIV/AIDS, tuberculosis, and malaria—have only been recognized recently.[8-11]

Through their chronic and disabling effects, neglected diseases represent an important contribution to poverty among the world's poor.[4] Yet despite their public health, social, intellectual, and economic importance, global efforts to develop vaccines for the neglected diseases have not benefited from the coordinated efforts by many of the organizations that have joined forces to develop new vaccines for the other major childhood infectious diseases. Indeed, only the dengue and rabies vaccine are currently being developed by any of the multinational pharmaceutical companies.[12]

Conspicuous by Their Absence

Overall, there are three important reasons for this absence of interest in neglected disease vaccines by the multinational pharmaceutical companies.

High-Morbidity, Low-Mortality Conditions
Although the neglected diseases produce an enormous amount of disability, they are usually not killer diseases in and of themselves. It is estimated that 217,000 to 608,000 people die annually from all of the neglected diseases combined, which is a relatively small percentage of the 6 million children who die each year. The low mortality rates

from the neglected diseases could lead some in the global public health community to erroneously conclude that the diseases are not of sufficient public health importance to warrant investment in vaccine research and development. By one estimate, the neglected diseases result in up to 112 million disability-adjusted life-years lost annually,[10,13] a number equivalent to or exceeding the global disease and disability from HIV/AIDS.[10]

Hidden in Remote Rural Areas

So-called emerging infections, such as severe acute respiratory syndrome (SARS) and avian or swine flu, appear unexpectedly, threaten wealthy countries, and strike in a dramatic fashion, often causing high rates of mortality. In sharp contrast, the neglected diseases are ancient conditions that have afflicted humankind for centuries.[14,15] These diseases occur predominantly in rural areas, which often are remote and not easily accessible by tourists or visitors.[3-5]

Expensive Research and Development

The seventeen neglected diseases occur almost exclusively in the poorest countries of Africa, Asia, and Latin America. Moreover, the neglected diseases generally affect only people living in extreme poverty, often in remote areas of these countries. As a result, there are no commercial markets for vaccines against these diseases.[16-19] Without any hope of recovering their financial investments in research and development, multinational corporations that develop vaccines have—so far—been unwilling to invest the tens of millions or possibly hundreds of millions of dollars that would be required to develop and test new vaccines for neglected diseases.

In addition, developing vaccines for parasitic worms (helminths) and other complicated pathogens presents formidable scientific challenges because they are complicated organisms.

A New Generation of Antipoverty Vaccines for Neglected Diseases

Vaccines for the neglected diseases fall into at least three different categories.

Category 1: No Vaccine Required

There are five neglected diseases in this category. Dracunculiasis has been nearly eradicated through environmental control and the substitution of safe drinking water for unsafe water. Ascariasis, lymphatic filariasis, trachoma, and trichuriasis are being controlled, and in some cases eliminated, through mass administration of antibiotics and other drugs often administered annually or twice a year.[3-5]

Category 2: Veterinary Vaccines and Transmission-Blocking Vaccines

The neglected diseases cysticercosis and echinococcosis are larval tapeworm infections and are considered both important veterinary and human public health problems. In addition, a form of human African trypanosomiasis, which occurs in East Africa, as well as a form of human schistosomiasis, which occurs in Asia, are infections transmitted from animals to humans.

For these diseases, it is believed that human infection may be preventable by immunizing the animal populations that harbor the infection, such as pigs in the case of cysticercosis, sheep for echinococcosis, and cattle for East African human trypanosomiasis and Asian schistosomiasis. These diseases adversely affect livestock, so there is a potential commercial market for these veterinary vaccines. At the same time, expanded use of the vaccines could interrupt zoonotic transmission to humans.[19] There are modest but bona fide markets for veterinary vaccines affecting commercial livestock, and several so-called ag-vet companies could develop and test such products.

Category 3: Human Antipoverty Vaccines

Vaccines for neglected diseases affecting humans are sometimes referred to as antipoverty vaccines because of their potential impact to both improve human health and promote economic development.[2] The antipoverty vaccines present the greatest economic hurdles and disincentives. With the exception of rabies and dengue, none of the multinational pharmaceutical companies has undertaken research and development efforts for any of the diseases.

The lack of interest by multinational corporations is occurring despite the introduction of new "pull mechanisms" meant to create incentives for commercial development. So-called priority review vouchers, designed as incentives for multinational pharmaceutical companies to invest in vaccines and treatments for diseases affecting poor countries, have not attracted sufficient interest on the part of those companies to make vaccines for the neglected diseases, nor are there advance market commitments in place for antipoverty vaccines. In this sense, not all neglected diseases are the same, and those diseases characterized as neglected "tropical" diseases find themselves in a special category of neglect apart from malaria, tuberculosis, and the childhood killer diseases.

The reasons for the absence of interest in antipoverty vaccines among pharmaceutical corporations need to be fully explored. Among the possibilities is the fact that at least some prospect of profitable commercialization is still required by industry to make a case for investment or to meet shareholders' expectations. Most of the neglected diseases are not endemic in North America, Europe, or Japan. Chagas disease is a possible exception because it occurs in the United States, but even this disease occurs overwhelmingly among poor immigrant populations living along the border with Mexico.[20,21]

Vaccine Development through Partnerships

Today, several vaccines for bona fide neglected diseases are being developed through unique collaborations among product development partnerships, university laboratories, and public-sector manufacturers in middle-income countries. New human vaccines for the hookworm infections leishmaniasis and schistosomiasis are entering Phase I or Phase II clinical trials, while human vaccines for Chagas disease, foodborne trematode infections, and onchocerciasis, or river blindness, are at an earlier preclinical stage of development.

Two of the major nonprofit product development partnerships for new human neglected disease vaccines are initiatives by the Sabin Vaccine Institute and the Infectious Disease Research Institute.

Sabin Vaccine Institute

The vaccine development arm of Sabin is a nonprofit partnership and one of the only such enterprises embedded in an academic laboratory. In August 2011, Sabin's laboratory was scheduled to relocate to Texas Children's Hospital and Baylor College of Medicine in Houston. Sabin's goal is to develop the neglected disease vaccines that the major multinational pharmaceutical companies cannot or will not produce. In the lab, Sabin scientists discover and isolate vaccine antigens and develop processes for manufacturing a vaccine at a scale suitable for pilot production. Following development of these processes (as well as some unique tests for ensuring the quality of the product), the technology is transferred to contract organizations that can manufacture the vaccine under current good manufacturing practices.

Sabin works with public-sector vaccine manufacturers located in Brazil and Mexico. In the Latin America and Caribbean region, five public-sector vaccine manufacturers are members of the Developing Countries Vaccine Manufacturers Network.[22] These organizations were built by, and are maintained with, public funds from their respective federal governments. In the case of the Brazilian biomedical research center Instituto Butantan, additional substantive and large-scale funding is provided by the state of São Paulo in Brazil. Together, Argentina, Brazil, Cuba, and Mexico are known as innovative development countries with a high level of sophistication with respect to biotechnology and investments in biotechnology, yet with high levels of poverty and endemic neglected diseases.[23]

The Sabin Vaccine Institute has produced new vaccines for hookworm infection and intestinal schistosomiasis. Together with its Brazilian vaccine manufacturing partners (Instituto Butantan and the Oswaldo Cruz Foundation, known as FIOCRUZ), Sabin will soon begin preliminary clinical testing in a rural area of Brazil where hookworm infections occur in 32 million people and intestinal schistosomiasis occurs in 2 to 7 million people.[16,24] In addition, Sabin is beginning to develop new vaccines for Chagas disease and leishmaniasis, together with the Autonomous University of Yucatan, Centro de Investigación y de Estudios Avanzados del Instituto Politécnico Nacional, the U.S. National Institutes of Health, and the public-sector vaccine manufacturer Birmex, for product and clinical development in Mexico.

Infectious Disease Research Institute

At the same time, the Seattle-based Infectious Disease Research Institute has partnered with Instituto Butantan to produce a new leishmaniasis vaccine for both human and veterinary use. Clinical testing is underway in Brazil, Peru, and elsewhere in Latin America.[25-27]

To date, long-term financing of these activities is occurring through support from the Bill & Melinda Gates Foundation, the Carlos Slim Institute of Health, and other private support, as well as public funds from the Dutch Ministry of Foreign Affairs and the U.S. National Institutes of Health. The Brazilian government has now made major contributions to support product and clinical development for these vaccines.

Outside Latin America and the Caribbean

Outside of Latin America, India and China could also become major contributors to producing vaccines for neglected diseases. For instance, although meningococcal A meningitis occurs in both developed and developing countries[28] and is not categorized as a "neglected tropical disease," it disproportionately occurs in sub-Saharan Africa.[29,30] PATH, an international nonprofit organization dedicated to improving global health, together with the Serum Institute of India, a private for-profit vaccine manufacturer, have successfully produced and registered a new meningococcal A vaccine.[30]

A vaccine for urogenital schistosomiasis is also under development by the French government research agency Institut National de la Santé et de la Recherche Médicale (INSERM) and Institut Pasteur. Clinical testing of this vaccine is in progress in sub-Saharan Africa.[31]

Conclusion

An alliance of public-sector vaccine manufacturers in the Latin America and Caribbean region, together with non-profit product development partnerships and university laboratories, represents an exciting new mechanism for expanding the clinical pipeline of vaccines for neglected diseases. Greater cooperation, especially between vaccine manufacturers in developing countries and the public sector, could further promote knowledge sharing and cost savings.

Today, sub-Saharan Africa and Latin America share most of the seventeen neglected diseases with the exception of dracunculiasis and human African trypanosomiasis (sleeping sickness), which do not occur in Latin America, and Chagas disease, which does not occur in Africa.[24,32] This affords an opportunity for the major Latin American public-sector vaccine manufacturers to look beyond the Western Hemisphere for joint vaccine development in the African region. For instance, FIOCRUZ has recently established an office in the Portuguese-speaking nation of Mozambique. Through such South–South partnerships, it may be possible to conduct multicenter Phase III clinical trials for vaccines against hookworm, schistosomiasis, and other neglected diseases in both South America and Africa.

There will be an urgent need to identify financial mechanisms to support a new alliance between public-sector vaccine manufacturers, product development partnerships, and university laboratories to support antipoverty vaccine development for Latin America and Africa. Such a push to develop new vaccines would stimulate innovation and indirectly provide economic return. Thus, some of the larger banking enterprises, such as the Brazilian Development Bank, the Inter-American Development Bank, and the African Development Bank, might represent potential sources of support.

It would be especially attractive to consider establishing a pooled innovation fund for the Americas and Africa, possibly supported by several of the so-called Group of 20 developing nations to specifically address diseases of the poorest people in these regions. There are also enormous, yet largely untapped, sources of private wealth, especially in Latin America, that could be pooled together and centralized for supporting vaccine research and development, much as the recent End Neglected Diseases fund has been established for fighting disease through broad drug distribution in sub-Saharan Africa.

Beyond Latin America, additional partnerships may be possible with research organizations in the Middle East. Almost one-half (46%) of the world's neglected diseases occurs in member nations of the Organisation of the Islamic Conference, particularly in Africa and Asia.[33]

Additionally, several new and advanced research institutes located in the wealthy oil-producing nations of the Middle East could be enlisted to cooperate on joint vaccine development and manufacturing activities. Such activities represent an innovative means to inculcate neglected disease vaccine development into global diplomacy and foreign policy.[33]

Ultimately, developing a new generation of antipoverty vaccines represents a highly innovative and meaningful approach to eliminating the world's neglected diseases, lifting the bottom billion out of poverty, and promoting international diplomacy.

References

1. Advance Market Commitments for Vaccines. 2011, April 8. *The Pneumococcal AMC: Ready to Save Lives.* Geneva: Advance Market Commitments for Vaccines. Available at: http://www .vaccineamc.org/pneu_amc.html

2. Hotez, P. J., and M. Ferris. 2006. The antipoverty vaccines. *Vaccine* 24:5787–5799.

3. Hotez, P. J., D. H. Molyneux, A. Fenwick, J. Kumaresan, S. E. Sachs, J. D. Sachs, et al. 2007. Control of neglected tropical diseases. *N Engl J Med* 357:1018–1027.

4. Hotez, P. J., A. Fenwick, L. Savioli, and D. H. Molyneux. 2009. Rescuing the bottom billion through control of neglected tropical diseases. *Lancet* 73:1570–1575.

5. Musgrove, P., P J. Hotez. 2009. Turning neglected tropical diseases to forgotten maladies. *Health Aff (Millwood)* 28 (6):1691–1706.

6. World Health Organization. 2010. *Working to Overcome the Global Impact of Neglected Tropical Diseases.* Geneva: World Health Organization. Available at: http://www.who.int/neglected _diseases/2010report/en/index.html

7. Hotez, P. J. 2009. Empowering women and improving female reproductive health through control of the neglected tropical diseases. *PLoS Negl Trop Dis* 3:e559.

8. Hotez, P. J., A. Fenwick, and E. F. Kjetland. 2009. Africa's 32 cents solution for HIV/AIDS. *PLoS Negl Trop Dis* 3:e430.

9. Brooker, S., W. Akhwale, R. Pullan, B. Estambale, S. E. Clarke, R. W. Snow, et al. 2007. Epidemiology of plasmodium-helminth co-infection in Africa: Populations at risk, potential impact on anemia, and prospects for combining control. *Am J Trop Med Hyg* 77:88–98.

10. Hotez, P. J., D. H. Molyneux, A. Fenwick, E. Ottesen, S. E. Sachs, and J. D. Sachs. 2006. Incorporating a rapid-impact package for neglected tropical diseases with programs for HIV/AIDS, tuberculosis, and malaria. *PLoS Med* 3:e102.

11. Hotez, P. J., M. Neeraj, J. Rubinstein, and D. J. Sachs. 2011. Integrating neglected tropical diseases into AIDS, tuberculosis, and malaria control. *N Engl J Med.* Forthcoming.

12. Mahoney, R., L. Chocarro, J. Southern, D. P. Francis, J. Vose, and H. Margolis. 2011. Dengue vaccines regulatory pathways: A report on two meetings with regulators of developing countries. *PLoS Med* 8:e10000418.

13. King, C. H. 2010. Parasites and poverty: The case of schistosomiasis. *Acta Trop* 113:95–104.

14. Hotez, P. J., E. Ottesen, A. Fenwick, and D. Molyneux. 2006. The neglected tropical diseases: The ancient afflictions of stigma and poverty and the prospects for their control and elimination. *Adv Exp Med Biol* 582:23–33.

15. Hotez, P. J. 2006. The "biblical diseases" and US vaccine diplomacy. *Brown World Affairs J.* 12:247–258.

16. Hotez, P. J., J. M. Bethony, D. J. Diemert, M. Pearson, and A. Loukas. 2010. Developing vaccines to combat hookworm infection and intestinal schistosomiasis. *Nat Rev Microbiol* 8: 814–826.

17. Hotez, P. J., and A. S. Brown. 2009. Neglected tropical disease vaccines. *Biologicals* 37:160–164.

18. Hotez, P. J., and B. Pecoul. 2010. "Manifesto" for the control and elimination of the neglected tropical diseases. *PLoS Negl Trop Dis* 4:e718.

19. Bethony, J. M., R. N. Coler, X. Guo, S. Kamhawi, M. Lightowlers, A. Loukas, et al. 2011. Vaccines to combat the neglected tropical diseases. *Immunol Rev* 239:37–270.

20. Hotez, P. J. 2011. America's most distressed areas and their neglected infections: The United States Gulf Coast and the District of Columbia. *PLoS Negl Trop Dis* 5:e843.

21. Hotez, P. J. 2009. Neglected diseases amid wealth in the United States and Europe. *Health Aff (Millwood)* 28 (6):1720–1725.

22. Jadhav, S., M. Datia, H. Kreeftenberg, and J. Hendriks. 2008. The Developing Countries Vaccine Manufacturers' Network (DCVMN) is a critical constituency to ensure access to vaccines in developing countries. *Vaccine* 26:1611–1615.

23. Morel, C. M., T. Acharya, D. Broun, A. Dangi, C. Elias, N. K. Ganguly, et al. 2005. Health innovation: The neglected capacity of developing countries to address neglected diseases. *Science* 309:401–404.

24. Hotez, P. J., M. E. Bottazzi, C. Franco-Paredes, S. K. Ault, and M. Roses Periago. 2008. The neglected tropical diseases of Latin America and the Caribbean: Review of estimated disease burden and distribution and a roadmap for control and elimination. *PLoS Negl Trop Dis* 2:e300.

25. Vélez, I. D., K. Gilchrist, S. Martinez, J. R. Ramírez-Pineda, J. A. Ashman, F. P. Alves, et al. 2009. Safety and immunogenicity of a defined vaccine for the prevention of cutaneous leishmaniasis. *Vaccine* 28:329–337.

26. Llanos-Cuentas, A., W. Calderón, M. Cruz, J. A. Ashman, F. P. Alves, R. N. Coler, et al. 2010. A clinical trial to evaluate the safety and immunogenicity of the LEISH-F1+MPL-SE vaccine when

used in combination with sodium stibogluconate for the treatment of mucosal leishmaniasis. *Vaccine* 28:7427–7435.

27. Nascimento, E., D. F. Fernandes, E. P. Vieira, A. Campos-Neto, J. A. Ashman, F. P. Alves, et al. 2010. A clinical trial to evaluate the safety and immunogenicity of the LEISH-F1+MPL-SE vaccine when used in combination with meglumine antimoniate for the treatment of cutaneous leish-maniasis. *Vaccine* 28:6581–6587.

28. Harrison, L. H. 2010. Epidemiological profile of meningococcal disease in the United States. *Clin Infect Dis* 56 (Suppl 2):537–544.

29. Khatami, A., and A. J. Pollard. 2010. The epidemiology of meningococcal disease and the impact of vaccines. *Expert Rev Vaccines* 9:285–298.

30. PATH. 2011, February 20. *Meningitis Vaccine Project*. Seattle, WA: PATH. Available at: http://www.path.org/menafrivac/

31. Institut national de la santé et de la recherche médicale. 2011. Bilhvax. Paris: Institut national de la santé et de la recherche médical. Available at: http://www.bilhvax.inserm.fr/

32. Hotez, P. J., and A. Kamath. 2009. Neglected tropical diseases in sub-Saharan Africa: Review of their prevalence, distribution, and disease burden. *PLoS Negl Trop Dis* 3:e412.

33. Hotez, P. J. 2010. Peace through vaccine diplomacy. *Science* 327:1301.

42 Vaccines against Stimulants: Cocaine and Methamphetamine (*Excerpt*)

Thomas Kosten, Coreen Domingo, Frank Orson, and Berma Kinsey[*]

Worldwide, the United Nations Office on Drugs and Crime (UNDOC) estimates between 0.3% to 0.4% of the adult population, between 15 and 19 million people, have used cocaine at least once in the previous year. Still, the highest prevalence of cocaine use remains in North America, affecting approximately 2% of adults ages 15–64 years.[1] To date, although there are no FDA-approved pharmacotherapies for treating cocaine dependence, of those that are in use, there are multiple limitations. Of these limitations, the most significantly problematic include cost, availability, medication compliance, dependence, diversion of some to illicit use, and relapse to addiction after discontinuing their use. Here, immunotherapies using either passive monoclonal antibodies or active vaccines have distinctly different mechanisms and therapeutic utility from small molecule approaches to treatment and have shown distinct promise with demonstrated potential to help the patient achieve and sustain abstinence and have few of the limitations associated with anti-addiction medications.

Immunotherapy for addictions also has been steadily growing as an area for new ideas and technologies, although human studies of these therapies have been limited to active vaccines against nicotine and cocaine, and no monoclonals for passive immunization have been tested in humans. Therefore, this chapter will focus on vaccines rather than monoclonals, and it will focus on the human vaccine issues for cocaine, because a cocaine vaccine has progressed to late phase 2 clinical trials in humans. This chapter also will cover the pre-clinical vaccine design issues for methamphetamine (MA) because many technical innovations are being deployed for MA vaccines that will be highly relevant to second-generation cocaine vaccines.

* Originally published in *British Journal of Clinical Pharmacology*, 2014; 77 (2):368–374. Reprinted with permission of John Wiley and Sons.

Antibody Actions in Blocking Abused Drugs

Drugs of abuse lead to reward and reinforcement by rapidly entering the brain and attaching to neuronal receptors on specific brain pathways, and antibodies prevent those drugs from accessing these brain pathways. Specifically, both cocaine and MA bind to the three monoamine transporters (dopamine, norepinephrine, and serotonin), preventing these transporters from removing these neurotransmitters from the synapse.

Antibodies capture the abused drug before it can cross the blood–brain barrier, thereby preventing activation of the brain's reinforcement pathways, but they also have an additional pharmacokinetic effect of buffering against rapid transit of abused drugs into the brain.[2,3] Antibodies in the circulation have a similar kinetic way of slowing drug entry into the brain and reducing the reinforcing effects of the drug.

The fundamental concept in creating anti-drug antibodies is to create a new macromolecular compound, which the body will recognize as a foreign antigen that requires an immune response. Drugs of abuse by themselves are far too small to elicit such immune responses from the antibody generating B and T white blood cells, so their presentation to the immune processes must be changed through a conjugate vaccine. A conjugate vaccine chemically links the abused drug to a large immunogenic protein such as inactivated tetanus or cholera toxin.[4] Both of these proteins are widely used vaccines, and the concept of linking them to small molecules called haptens to produce an antibody response was pioneered in the 1970s as a treatment for digitalis toxicity and as an anti-morphine vaccine.[5-7]

Cocaine Vaccine in Clinical Trials

An ongoing multi-site, phase IIb clinical trial has followed the success of this first cocaine vaccine clinical trial of TA-CD.[8] This 4-month, double-blind, randomized, placebo-controlled, multi-center study includes 300 treatment-seeking, cocaine-dependent individuals receiving five vaccinations. Based on the success of this vaccine in the earlier clinical trials, this cocaine vaccine may be one of the first anti-addiction vaccines. The full clinical registration path for FDA approval of this vaccine will require another multisite phase 3 study replication, if this current study can demonstrate a significantly greater proportion of subjects becoming cocaine-abstinent for at least 3 weeks on the vaccine compared with the placebo. However, it does not appear that a full 1,000 vaccinated subjects will be required for a safety assessment because the CTB carrier has an outstanding safety record, and the clinical trials for this nor-cocaine hap-tenated conjugate vaccine have been remarkably free of adverse events.

The behavioral challenges for any successful vaccination program start with the need to have 2 to 3 months where the patient can be brought to a treatment site for the series of vaccinations. While continued drug abuse during the 3 months of vacci-nation does not interfere with the vaccine's ability to stimulate the required antibody production, the patient needs to get these vaccinations at appropriate times over the 3 months (e.g., 2, 4, 8, and 12 weeks after the initial vaccination), and continued drug abuse may increase the risk of failure to appear for these follow-up visits. Thus, counsel-ing or other treatment efforts will be critical to ensure compliance with the schedule of vaccinations. Such interventions could vary from residential substance abuse care to outpatient contingency management, in which patients are paid to come for the vac-cinations with an escalating pay schedule for each vaccination obtained.

Future Clinical Developments

In addition to the clinical trials being conducted on vaccines for cocaine, preclinical development of second-generation vaccines for MA and cocaine are ongoing. Future vaccine trials will use more potent adjuvants than alum and include more effective carriers such as OMPC, which have adjuvant properties due to their lipopolysaccaride content. Several outstanding adjuvants are commercially available, and nicotine vac-cines are the most likely to first benefit from these new adjuvants due to the already ongoing interest in these vaccines of major pharmaceutical companies such as Novartis and GSK, which control these novel adjuvants. Another likely focus will be on using booster injections with different adjuvants from the original vaccine that might only use alum. Shifting adjuvants during a series of vaccinations could prolong antibody durations and perhaps strengthen the development of high affinity in the polyclonal antibodies. Some work is also expected outside the United States, in China in particu-lar, for commercializing these vaccines. Chinese companies have the capital needed, as well as the required government support, for moving these vaccines rapidly into the public health sectors where they are most needed.

References

1. United Nations Office on Drugs and Crime. 2010. World Drug Report. Available at: http://www.unodc.org/documents/wdr/WDR_2010/2.3_Coca-cocaine.pdf. Accessed March 8, 2012.

2. Kosten, T., and S. M. Owens. 2005. Immunotherapy for the treatment of drug abuse. *Pharmacol Ther* 108:76–85.

3. Orson, F. M., B. M. Kinsey, R. A. Singh, Y. Wu, T. Gardner, and T. R. Kosten. 2008. Substance abuse vaccines. *Ann N Y Acad Sci* 1141:257–269.

4. Plotkin, S. A., ed. 2008. *History of Vaccine Development.* New York, Dordrecht, Heidelberg, and London: Springer.

5. Curd, J., T. W. Smith, J. C. Jaton, and E. Haber. 1971. The isolation of digoxin-specific antibody and its use in reversing the effects of digoxin. *Proc Natl Acad Sci USA* 68:2401–2406.

6. Berkowitz, B., and S. Spector. 1972. Evidence for active immunity to morphine in mice. *Science* 178:1290–1292.

7. Bonese, K. F., B. H. Wainer, F. W. Fitch, R. M. Rothberg, and C. R. Schuster. 1974. Changes in heroin self-administration by a rhesus monkey after morphine immunization. *Nature* 252:708–710.

8. Martell, B. A., F. M. Orson, J. Poling, E. Mitchell, R. D. Rossen, T. Gardner, and T. R. Kosten. 2009. Cocaine vaccine for the treatment of cocaine dependence in methadone-maintained patients: A randomized, double blind, placebo-controlled efficacy trial. *Arch Gen Psychiatry* 66:1116–1123.

43 Anti-Cancer Vaccines—A One-Hit Wonder? (*Excerpt*)

Justin H. K. Liu[*]

Since the 1950s, the idea of a vaccination against cancer has developed from a fanciful hypothesis into a hard-lined reality that has captivated generations of cancer researchers with its ever-increasingly vast potential.[1] Arguably, one of the most attractive aspects of this branch of cancer immunotherapy, compared with all other treatments currently available for cancer (e.g., surgery, chemotherapy, radiotherapy, small molecule inhibitors, monoclonal antibodies, etc.), is that, in theory, it is something that can be administered just once or over a short course with booster vaccinations (much like current vaccination programs against bacterial or viral infections) with minimal invasiveness and can potentially protect an individual against cancer for life.[2]

In the past 60 years, a better understanding of the role of the immune system against cancer along with improving strategies for vaccine development have allowed for the creation of many potential vaccines against specific cancers, a few of which have been licensed for use in clinical practice, with many more currently in phase II/III clinical trials.[3] Of the handful of anti-cancer vaccines currently being used in clinical practice, perhaps the most famous of these is a prophylactic vaccine that targets a subset of the human papilloma virus (HPV), which causes cervical cancer. For its discovery and development, Harald zur Hausen was awarded the 2008 Nobel Prize in Physiology and Medicine, serving as a breakthrough moment and underlining the credibility of vaccination as a means of treating and preventing cancer.[4]

Broadly speaking, anti-cancer vaccines can be divided into two types: therapeutic and preventive. Therapeutic vaccines are used to treat patients who already have cancer, whereas preventive vaccines (such as the HPV vaccine) are used to prevent cancer from occurring.[5] This chapter will explore examples of both therapeutic and preventive vaccines and will discuss the state of some of the new potential anti-cancer vaccines

* Originally published in *Yale Journal of Biology and Medicine*, 2014; 87 (4):481–489. Reprinted with permission.

currently in development and some of the scientific and economic drawbacks of their use.

Therapeutic Anti-Cancer Vaccines

Rapid advancements in the understanding of the immune system and its role in cancer have allowed for the development of therapeutic vaccines that utilize the host's own immune system to essentially prime it to specifically target, attack, and kill tumor cells.[6]

To date, the only therapeutic anti-cancer vaccine that has been licensed for use in clinical practice is sipuleucel-T (Provenge), which is used for the treatment of prostate cancer. It was first licensed by the U.S. Food and Drug Administration (FDA) in 2010 for use in the treatment of asymptomatic/minimally symptomatic metastatic castration-resistant prostate cancer (mCRPC).[7] The milestone that sipuleucel-T has provided in the timeline of anti-cancer vaccine development should not be underestimated and provides hope for further therapeutic anti-cancer vaccines reaching clinical practice in the future. With exciting new tools in biomedical research, such as next-generation sequencing, additional potential TSA and TAA candidates are now being identified, with anti-cancer vaccines currently in various stages of clinical trial development and testing. Therefore, the question is: Can any of these new developments reach the milestone-setting heights of sipuleucel-T?

Preventive Anti-Cancer Vaccines

The other major type of anti-cancer vaccine aims to prevent cancer from developing in the first place and is therefore prophylactic in nature. Currently, all of the licensed preventive anti-cancer vaccines used in clinical practice target virus-causing cancers (oncoviruses).[8] Most common is the HPV vaccine, which was first licensed by the FDA in 2006 and recommended for use in females between the ages of 9 and 26 for the prevention of cervical cancer along with various other HPV-associated cancers (e.g., vaginal cancers, vulvar cancers, anal cancers, HPV-induced oral cancers, etc.).[9] Unlike sipuleucel-T, the HPV vaccine relies primarily on generating an antibody response to prevent initial HPV infection.[10] Data from phase III clinical trials indicate that the HPV vaccine protects against more than 90% of HPV infection caused by HPV 16 or 18 for females who had received three doses of the vaccine.[11] However, because the vaccine is not fully protective against all cases of cervical cancer, cervical screening still remains a vital tool for the detection and diagnosis of cervical cancer.[12]

Viruses are the underlying cause in approximately 10% of all cases of cancer and are therefore an attractive therapeutic target for cancer prevention. Previous success with vaccines used to treat and prevent infectious diseases caused by viruses has provided a platform for identifying oncoviruses and utilizing the host immune system to effectively target and eliminate them. The biggest challenges currently facing preventive anti-cancer vaccines are clinical, social, and economic in nature. Debates are currently ongoing, and key decisions are still yet to be made with regard to how preventive anti-cancer vaccines can be delivered to a general population in an ethical and cost-effective manner (see discussion below).

Promising Anti-Cancer Vaccines Currently in Development

Although only a handful of anti-cancer vaccines are currently available in clinical practice, over the years, many more have been put through clinical trials, each with varying degrees of success and failure. One of the most advanced anti-cancer vaccines currently in development is the gp100 melanoma vaccine. This therapeutic vaccine contains an enhanced version of a TAA, gp100, which is expressed on the surface of melanoma tumor cells.

Another promising anti-cancer vaccine that has recently generated considerable interest is L-BLP25 (Stimuvax). This therapeutic vaccine contains both CD4 and CD8 epitopes for a proteoglycan, mucin 1 (MUC-1), expressed on the cell surface of several tumor types.[13] Creating an anti-cancer vaccine that has a common target for various different cancers is clearly advantageous, not least from both a practical and cost-effectiveness point of view. Currently, two large ongoing phase III clinical trials (START and INSPIRE) are testing L-PLP25 for the treatment of non-small cell lung cancer.[14]

Along with sipuleucel-T, another anti-cancer vaccine, Prostvac, is being developed as a potential treatment against prostate cancer. The target epitope is an enhanced form of prostate-specific antigen (PSA), a commonly used clinical biomarker for prostate cancer. Several phase II clinical trials concluded that Prostvac improved median overall survival rates and saw a significant reduction in the death rate in patients with mCRPC,[15,16] with a phase III randomized trial still ongoing.[3] Several clinical trials have given Prostvac in combination with various chemotherapeutic or hormonal agents with promising results.[17,18]

Conclusion

The notion of a vaccine that could be used to treat and offer lifelong protection against cancer has traveled a long path since it was first proposed. Along the way, many obstacles have had to be overcome, and although many hurdles are still in the way, the first few anti-cancer vaccines recently have reached clinical practice. Of this small handful, one is a therapeutic vaccine (sipuleucel-T) used to treat prostate cancer, whereas the others are preventive vaccines against virus-causing cancers. The licensing and approval of these vaccines have forged the way for other vaccines currently being developed and in various stages of clinical testing. There are currently many clinical trials looking at different anti-cancer vaccines against other targets, each with their own merits and flaws. A popular trend currently being trialed is combining anti-cancer vaccines with other chemotherapeutic agents and small molecule inhibitors, thus highlighting the huge strides that have been made in the development of new cancer treatments in this era of personalized therapy. With current advances in genetic sequencing and biomedical research, effort is now being directed toward the translation of the results obtained from laboratory experiments and clinical trials into developing more advanced and specialized drug targets for cancer treatment in clinical practice.

However, this does not come without new and additional obstacles that have yet to be overcome. For example, an increased perspective of the tumor microenvironment and how tumor cells evade the host immune system to survive and metastasize, along with a greater understanding of how the immune system is kept in check through negative regulation, poses additional questions for anti-cancer vaccines in the future. Also, the issue of side effects has to seriously be considered. Finally, from an economic standpoint, there is the issue of cost-effectiveness and the use of preventive vaccines to prevent specific cancers from occurring in the general population.

Overall, the state of anti-cancer vaccines looks promising. With a few anti-cancer vaccines currently in clinical practice and several more currently in phase III clinical trials, the future certainly looks bright for the once much-maligned concept. The question, however, still remains: Has a revolution truly begun or are anti-cancer vaccines just a one-hit wonder?

References

1. Gilboa, E. 2004. The promise of cancer vaccines. *Nat Rev Cancer* 4 (5):401–411.

2. Lollini, P. L., F. Cavallo, P. Nanni, and G. Forni. 2006. Vaccines for tumour prevention. *Nat Rev Cancer* 6 (3):204–216.

3. Schlom, J. 2012. Therapeutic cancer vaccines: Current status and moving forward. *J Natl Cancer Inst* 104 (8):599–613.

4. Nour, N. M. 2009. Cervical cancer: A preventable death. *Rev Obstet Gynecol* 2 (4): 240–244.

5. Finn, O. J. 2003. Cancer vaccines: Between the idea and reality. *Nat Rev Immunol* 3 (8):630–641.

6. Guo, C., M. H. Manjili, J. R. Subjeck, D. Sarkar, P. B. Fisher, and X. Y. Wang. 2013. Therapeutic cancer vaccines: Past, present and future. *Adv Cancer Res* 119:421–475.

7. Cheever, M. A., and C. S. Higano. 2011. PROVENGE (Sipuleucel-T) in prostate cancer: The first FDA-approved therapeutic cancer vaccine. *Clin Cancer Res* 17 (11):3520–3526.

8. Schiller, J. T., and D. R. Lowy. 2010. Vaccines to prevent infections by oncoviruses. *Annu Rev Microbiol* 64:23–41.

9. Garland, S. M., and J. S. Smith. 2010. Human papillomavirus vaccines: Current status and future prospects. *Drugs* 70 (9):1079–1098.

10. Stanley, M. 2007. Prophylactic HPV vaccines. *J Clin Pathol* 60 (9):961–965.

11. Cutts, F. T., S. Franceschi, S. Goldie, X. Castellsague, S. de Sanjose, G. Garnett, et al. 2007. Human papillomavirus and HPV vaccines: A review. *Bull World Health Organ* 85 (9):719–726.

12. Kitchener, H. C., K. Denton, K. Soldan, and E. J. Crosbie. 2013. Developing role of HPV in cervical cancer protection. *BMJ* 347:f4781.

13. Finn, O. J., K. R. Gantt, A. J. Lepisto, S. Pejawar-Gaddy, J. Xue, and P. L. Beatty. 2011. Importance of MUC-1 and spontaneous mouse tumour models for understanding the immunobiology of human adenocarcinomas. *Immunol Res* 50 (2–3):261–268.

14. Mellstedt, H., J. Vansteenkiste, and N. Thatcher. 2011. Vaccines for the treatment of non-small cell lung cancer: Investigational approaches and clinical experience. *Lung Cancer* 73 (1):11–17.

15. Gulley, J. L., P. M. Arlen, R. A. Madan, K. Y. Tsang, M. P. Pazdur, L. Skarupa, et al. 2010. Immunologic and prognostic factors associated with overall survival employing a poxviral-based PSA vaccine in metastatic castrate-resistant prostate cancer. *Cancer Immunol Immunother* 59 (5):663–674.

16. Kantoff, P. W., T. J. Schuetz, B. A. Blumenstein, L. M. Glode, D. L. Bilhartz, M. Wyand, et al. 2010. Overall survival analysis of a phase II randomised controlled trial of a poxviral-based PSA-targeted immunotherapy in metastatic castration-resistant prostate cancer. *J Clin Oncol* 28 (7):1099–1105.

17. Arlen, P. M., J. L. Gulley, C. Parker, L. Skarupa, M. Pazdur, D. Panicali, et al. 2006. A randomised phase II trial of concurrent docetaxel plus vaccine versus vaccine alone in metastatic androgen-independent prostate cancer. *Clin Cancer Res* 12 (4):1260–1269.

18. Madan, R. A., J. L. Gulley, J. Schlom, S. M. Steinberg, D. J. Liewehr, W. L. Dahut, et al. 2008. Analysis of overall survival in patients with nonmetastatic castration-resistant prostate cancer treated with vaccine, nilumatide and combination therapy. *Clin Cancer Res* 14 (14):4526–4531.

44   Synthetic Generation of Influenza Vaccine Viruses for Rapid Response to Pandemics (*Excerpt*)

Philip R. Dormitzer, Pirada Suphaphiphat, and colleagues*

The response to the 2009 H1N1 influenza pandemic was the fastest global vaccine development effort in history. Within 6 months of the pandemic declaration, vaccine companies had developed, produced, and distributed hundreds of millions of doses of licensed pandemic vaccines. Unfortunately, the response was not fast enough. Substantial vaccine quantities were available only after the second pandemic wave had peaked.[1] Manufacture of influenza virus subunit vaccines requires a vaccine virus that grows well enough in eggs or cultured mammalian cells to produce sufficient amounts of the essential vaccine antigen, hemagglutinin (HA), to meet vaccine needs. Late availability of a high-yielding vaccine virus contributed to the delay in vaccine supply.

In parallel with other efforts,[2,3] Novartis Vaccine and Diagnostics (NV&D) used recombinant DNA methods to generate a potential vaccine virus on a standard [A/ Puerto Rico/8/1934 (H1N1) (PR8)] vaccine backbone on May 11, 2009, 11 days after receiving influenza strain A/California/04/2009 (H1N1) viral RNA from the U.S. Centers for Disease Control (CDC). In contrast, NV&D first received a conventional reassortant vaccine virus (X179A) from a World Health Organization (WHO) Collaborating Center at one of its vaccine manufacturing facilities on May 29, 18 days after we had generated our potential vaccine virus with recombinant methods. Adaptation of the research-based process of recombinant vaccine virus generation to one that used a manufacturing-qualified cell line and good manufacturing practice (GMP) standards was completed at the Philipps-Universität Marburg on June 1, 2009, 3 days after receipt of X179A.[4,5] Our recombinant vaccine virus was not used to produce the vaccines distributed to the public in the 2009 pandemic response because the regulatory hurdles for using a new process to produce an urgently needed vaccine were too great. Instead,

* From Dormitzer, P. R., et al. 2014. Synthetic generation of influenza vaccine viruses for rapid response to pandemics. *Science Translational Medicine* 5:185ra68. Reprinted with permission from AAAS.

although the yield of HA from X179A was only 30% to 50% of the yield from H1N1 vaccine viruses typically used for seasonal vaccine manufacture,[2] the pandemic vaccine manufacturing campaign was initiated with an X179A-derived vaccine seed virus.

This experience with the 2009 H1N1 virus provided lessons for the next pandemic vaccine response: (1) Synthetic genomics techniques to produce influenza genome segments rapidly, accurately, and reliably are needed, so that instantaneous exchange of electronic sequence data followed by local gene synthesis can replace the isolation of viruses, preparation of high-growth reassortant vaccine viruses, and shipment of viruses and nucleic acids between geographically dispersed sites where vaccines are manufactured. (2) A reverse genetics system that uses these synthesized genes to generate viruses that are suitable for use in GMP-compliant vaccine manufacturing should be in place. (3) To increase the reliability of generating high-yielding, antigenically correct vaccine viruses, a greater variety of influenza HA and neuraminidase (NA) variants should be rescued in the context of multiple combinations of other influenza genome segments. (4) The use of synthetic and reverse genetic technologies for pandemic responses in seasonal influenza vaccine manufacture could establish regulatory and public acceptance and familiarity to allow reliable application of these approaches during a public health emergency.

On the basis of these lessons and the U.S. government's interest in improving the influenza vaccine manufacturing enterprise, NV&D, the J. Craig Venter Institute (JCVI), Synthetic Genomics Vaccines Inc. (SGVI), and the Biomedical Advanced Research and Development Authority (BARDA), the U.S. Department of Health and Human Services, initiated a collaboration to develop a rapid process for synthetic vaccine virus generation. We addressed three major technical barriers to more rapid and reliable pandemic responses: the speed of synthesizing DNA cassettes to drive production of influenza RNA genome segments, the accuracy of rapid gene synthesis, and the yield of HA from vaccine viruses.

•

We have demonstrated that an enzymatic system of gene assembly with error correction lowers error rates sufficiently to allow HA and NA gene cassettes, assembled from chemically synthesized oligonucleotides, to be used to rescue influenza vaccine viruses with prespecified HA and NA sequences and backbones without the need to pause for cloning in E. coli and sequencing before transfection. The improved fidelity decreased the time from obtaining a sequence to transfecting cells with synthetic HA and NA genes from 4.5 to 5.5 days to less than 1 day. The reliability of influenza virus rescue in a vaccine manufacturing cell line and yields of HA were increased through the use of improved vaccine backbones. A timed test of vaccine virus synthesis in response to a simulated H7N9 influenza outbreak demonstrated that this process can generate vaccine viruses rapidly, and the use of this system to rescue diverse synthetic influenza viruses demonstrated the system's robustness. The antigenic equivalence, based on two-way HI testing with ferret infection sera, of a synthetic H7N9 vaccine virus and the wild-type H7N9 virus from which the sequence data for synthesis were obtained confirms that the synthetic viral antigens are immunogenic and supports the expectation that vaccines made using synthetic or conventional influenza vaccine viruses will be equivalently protective.

A fast, straightforward, and accurate method of synthesizing higher-yielding influenza vaccine viruses, as described here, could enable more rapid pandemic responses and a more reliable supply of better matched seasonal and pandemic vaccines than available at present. In addition to increasing the speed of gene synthesis and virus rescue, this method also alleviates the need to ship viruses and clinical specimens between laboratories, as well as the requirement for a separate set of viral manipulations, classic reassortment (the "mating" of influenza viruses with stochastic exchange of genome segments during co-infection), to generate high-yielding vaccine strains.

Today, more than 120 National Influenza Centers conduct influenza surveillance and periodically ship clinical specimens to WHO Collaborating Centers, which propagate wild-type viruses in MDCK cells, assess their antigenicity and sequence, reisolate selected viruses in chicken eggs, and reassort them with high-growth backbones. High-growth reassortants recommended by the WHO are then shipped to vaccine manufacturers for further adaptation to make vaccine seed viruses. A system that uses synthetic gene generation could be more efficient. National Influenza Centers could sequence HA and NA genomic RNAs in clinical specimens and post the data on publicly accessible Web sites for immediate download by manufacturers, public health agencies, and researchers worldwide. Continuous comparison of newly posted sequences to databases of sequence and HI data by algorithms now under development could identify the emerging viruses most likely to differ antigenically from current vaccine strains.[6] Efficient synthetic virus rescue with a panel of high-growth backbones (or alternatively with native backbones, if additional influenza genome segment sequences were provided) could generate simultaneously viruses for antigenic testing and the best vaccine virus candidates for antigenically distinct strains. The speed and accuracy of gene synthesis by cell-free, enzymatic techniques could also enable more rapid production of the strain-specific genetic constructs used to manufacture recombinant alternatives to conventional influenza vaccines.[7] Today, vaccine viruses are only shipped to manufacturers after a regimen of testing at WHO-associated laboratories, which often takes longer than actually generating the vaccine strains. Decentralized generation of synthetic viruses could allow manufacturers to undertake scale-up and process development with strains that they generate immediately after the National Influenza Centers post sequences. Carrying out manufacturing activities simultaneously with seed testing could cut additional weeks from pandemic response times. Maintenance of libraries of synthetic influenza genes could further accelerate pandemic responses if they contain presynthesized genes that match future pandemic strains.

Technical and nontechnical hurdles must be overcome to realize fully the potential benefits of synthetic vaccine viruses for pandemic responses. Research protocols must be translated into performance-tested, at-scale manufacturing processes that have been approved by regulatory authorities. More prompt and open sequence and antigen data sharing is needed, as are biosafety standards for virus synthesis that ensure safety without unduly slowing vaccine production. The efficiency of testing synthetic vaccine viruses must increase. In particular, panels of post-infection ferret sera that react against previous reference viral strains are needed for initial antigenic screening of vaccine viruses, and procedures must be established for decentralized generation of ferret sera against selected synthetic strains for definitive antigenic testing. The current potency assay for vaccine release, which requires a lengthy immunization protocol to generate strain-specific sheep antisera, must be replaced by a more rapid, non–serum-requiring release assay, potentially one based on the physical characteristics of properly folded, immunogenic HA.

Further, the regulatory pathway for strain changes in licensed influenza vaccines must be adapted for synthetic vaccine viruses. Automation could enable access to the technologies needed for a global pandemic response system based on sequencing HA and NA genes in clinical specimens and rapidly synthesizing vaccine viruses.

On April 17, 2009, a new influenza virus strain that caused outbreaks in Mexico was detected in Southern California.[8,9] An initial qualified vaccine virus (X179A) was not received at one of our manufacturing facilities until May 29th, and a vaccine virus (NIBRG-121xp) with ordinary HA yield (10 to 15 mg of HA per 100 eggs) was not received until August 21st, too late to manufacture vaccines for the primary pandemic response.[2] If laboratory demonstrations of synthetic vaccine technology such as that reported here prove themselves in manufacturing and field implementation before the next pandemic, a high-yielding vaccine virus could be available to manufacturers for testing, scale-up, and process optimization days, not months, after a new virus is first detected.

References

1. Tizzoni, M., P. Bajardi, C. Poletto, J. J. Ramasco, D. Balcan, B. Gonçalves, et al. 2012. Real-time numerical forecast of global epidemic spreading: Case study of 2009 A/H1N1pdm. *BMC Med* 10:165.

2. Robertson, J. S., C. Nicolson, R. Harvey, R. Johnson, D. Major, K. Guilfoyle, et al. 2011. The development of vaccine viruses against pandemic A(H1N1) influenza. *Vaccine* 29:1836–1843.

3. Verity, E. E., S. Camuglia, C. T. Agius, C. Ong, R. Shaw, I. Barr, et al. 2012. Rapid generation of pandemic influenza virus vaccine candidate strains using synthetic DNA. *Influenza Other Respi Viruses* 6:101–109.

4. Strecker, T., J. Uhlendorff, S. Diederich, C. Lenz-Bauer, H. Trusheim, B. Roth, et al. 2012. Exploring synergies between academia and vaccine manufacturers: A pilot study on how to rapidly produce vaccines to combat emerging pathogens. *Clin Chem Lab Med* 50:1275–1279.

5. Doroshenko, A., and S. A. Halperin. 2009. Trivalent MDCK cell culture-derived influenza vaccine Optaflu (Novartis Vaccines). *Expert Rev Vaccines* 8:679–688.

6. Stockwell, T. B. Personal communication.

7. Dormitzer, P. R., T. F. Tsai, and G. Del Giudice. 2012. New technologies for influenza vaccines. *Hum Vaccin Immunother* 8:45–58.

8. Fraser, C., WHO Rapid Pandemic Assessment Collaboration. 2009. Pandemic potential of a strain of influenza A (H1N1): Early findings. *Science* 324:1557–1561.

9. Centers for Disease Control and Prevention. 2009. Swine influenza A (H1N1) infection in two children—Southern California, March—April 2009. *MMWR Morb Mortal Wkly Rep* 58:400–402.

45   Vaccines against Malaria (*Excerpt*)

Amed Ouattara and Matthew B. Laurens[*]

Malaria remains a significant public health threat, with approximately half of the world's population at risk of infection. The disease is caused by parasites transmitted to humans by the bite of an infected mosquito. Those residing in the poorest countries are particularly vulnerable to death from malaria illness, especially children ages <5 years in sub-Saharan Africa.[1] From 2000 to 2012, malaria mortality rates dropped by 45%, due in part to expanded funding for malaria control interventions including long-lasting insecticidal nets, indoor residual spraying programs, and access to artemisinin combination therapy.[1]

Currently, there is no licensed vaccine against malaria. A malaria vaccine would represent a public health tool that is viewed by some experts to be necessary for successful malaria elimination. The World Health Organization (WHO) recently published strategic goals to license malaria vaccines by 2030 that target Plasmodium falciparum and Plasmodium vivax, have at least 75% protective efficacy against clinical malaria, and reduce transmission to enable elimination.[2] The most advanced candidate vaccine to date, RTS,S/AS01, is currently in phase 3 testing in seven African countries; final results are expected by 2015.** Efforts to improve on the modest efficacy of RTS,S/AS01 include more than twenty malaria vaccine strategies currently in clinical testing; these include the use of candidate antigens in monovalent and multivalent formulations either alone or with other agents, viral vectors, and/or vaccine adjuvants. Here,

* Reprinted from Ouattara A, Laurens MB, "Vaccines against Malaria," *Clinical Infectious Diseases*, 2015; 60 (6):930–936, by permission of Oxford University Press.

** *Editors' Note*: The RTS,S vaccine was approved by the European Medicines Agency in July 2015, after this chapter was originally published. In October 2015, experts at the World Health Organization recommended that a series of pilot projects be conducted prior to any large-scale use of this vaccine in malaria-affected regions. Favorable results from these pilot projects could lead to the broad introduction of the vaccine in 3 to 5 years, it is estimated.

we review the history of malaria vaccine development. We then explain the malaria life cycle as a backdrop to our description of the challenges, approaches, and focus of current malaria vaccine development efforts.

Advances in Malaria Vaccine Development

Early malaria vaccine research began in the 1930s with a focus on inactivated or killed parasites that failed to generate a protective immune response. The addition of adjuvant systems demonstrated immunogenicity of malaria vaccine candidates in animal models; Jules Freund and colleagues demonstrated partial protection in ducklings.[3] Subsequent vaccine development efforts used rodent malaria models. This led to the first human malaria vaccine trial with demonstrated efficacy, a study that delivered irradiated *P. falciparum* sporozoites to vaccinees by mosquito bite.[4] This breakthrough was regarded as impractical for mass vaccination campaigns, and synthetic peptide vaccines based on immunogenic parasite proteins began to be developed in the 1980s. Because there is no biological correlate of protection for malaria, continued efforts in vaccine development were painstakingly time-consuming. A series of steps needed to be taken before phase 2 field testing in the target population of children in malaria-endemic areas could finally be performed to determine vaccine efficacy. These steps included initial development of a candidate vaccine in the laboratory, testing for safety and proof-of-concept in animal models, and age de-escalation phase 1 testing in adults and then in children for safety and reactogenicity. These multiple steps represent an arduous process, require significant funding support due to the lengthy product development timeline, and carry the risk of a negative end result. To abrogate this risk, controlled human malaria infection (CHMI), where participants are inoculated with sporozoites via the bite of infected female Anopheles mosquitoes in well-controlled settings, was used to obtain data on vaccine and drug efficacy to support or refute further clinical testing in malaria-endemic areas.[5] Early testing of the RTS,S vaccine using CHMI predicted efficacy in field studies, as well as helped to refine the choice of adjuvant and support reformulation to a lyophilized form.[6]

The first malaria immunization trials to use experimental challenge by infected mosquitoes were conducted in the mid-1970s.[4,7] However, after more than 35 years of laboratory research and field trials, the only vaccine that has progressed to phase 3 testing is the RTS,S vaccine, which showed efficacy of 30% in newborns and 50% in children ages 5–17 months in interim analyses from the ongoing phase 3 trial.[8] This limited success has called into question the likelihood of having a highly efficacious malaria vaccine available within the next few years. However, with funding agencies, the private sector, and international organizations joining forces to contain or even eradicate malaria, strategies are being scaled up to control the disease burden. In addition to effective treatment of clinical malaria and use of insecticide-impregnated barriers, malaria vaccines could play an important role in this initiative. Malaria vaccines can be divided into the following three groups based on the parasite developmental stages: pre-erythrocytic vaccines, blood-stage vaccines, and "other" vaccines, including transmission-blocking vaccines and vaccines against pregnancy-associated malaria.

Pre-Erythrocytic Malaria Vaccines

An effective immune response must act quickly to thwart *P. falciparum* sporozoites in their minutes-long journey from the skin to the liver. RTS,S is the leading pre-erythrocytic malaria vaccine. In the first phase 3 clinical trial of a malaria vaccine, efficacy against clinical malaria in children during the 18 months following dose 3 was 46% overall, waned over time, was higher in older children than in infants, and showed the highest impact in areas with the greatest malaria prevalence.[9] Continued challenges to the RTS,S vaccine developers include inducing a protective immune response to the genetically different strains found in nature and establishing a vaccine correlate of protection, obstacles considered central to all malaria vaccine development efforts.

Erythrocytic Malaria Vaccines

Clinical manifestations of malaria result from parasite blood-stage infection. Blood-stage vaccines are therefore intended to prevent disease and death without necessarily preventing infection. The gradual acquisition of natural protection against clinical disease following repeated infections in areas of malaria transmission indicates that a blood-stage malaria vaccine strategy is feasible, provided that it mimics acquired immunity to malaria in endemic areas.

In recent years, only four blood-stage antigens (AMA1, MSP1, MSP3, and GLURP) have been tested in phase 2 vaccine trials. None of the vaccines based on the four antigens tested was efficacious based on the primary endpoint of clinical malaria. However, one AMA1-based vaccine tested in Mali demonstrated significant efficacy against clinical malaria infections that shared the identical genetic sequence with the vaccine strain with respect to key immunologically relevant amino acid positions.[10] These analyses give insight into how current and potential vaccine candidate antigens can be designed to provide broad protection against diverse parasites.

Transmission-Blocking Vaccines

Recent increased interest in halting parasite spread to other persons has led to advances in transmission-blocking vaccines. These are sometimes called altruistic vaccines because there is no direct benefit to vaccinees. A successful transmission-blocking vaccine would induce neutralizing antibody responses against the malaria parasite's gametocyte and/or ookinete sexual stages, thereby blocking fertilization and halting reproduction.[11]

Conclusion

The renewed worldwide effort to eliminate malaria is underway, and experts agree that this goal cannot be achieved without new tools such as a malaria vaccine that can interrupt malaria transmission (VIMT).[12] This concept of VIMT is described as any malaria vaccine that can impact transmission, including vaccines that target the sexual and oocyte stages, but also pre-erythrocytic and erythrocytic vaccines that reduce transmission. To show promise, candidate malaria vaccines must demonstrate reduced transmission of malaria as a result of vaccination, a new challenge for malaria vaccine clinical trial design.

What are the next steps for malaria vaccine development? A vaccine with at least 75% efficacy against clinical malaria, as outlined in the malaria vaccine technology road map,[2] must be efficacious against the highly diverse strains of malaria that circulate in endemic areas. A multiantigen vaccine, similar to the approach used for vaccines against *Streptococcus pneumoniae*, may be necessary. Antigens selected for inclusion should also be highly immunogenic and provide immunity that lasts at least 2 years.[2] Alternatively, a highly efficacious, whole organism approach can potentially transcend strain-specific diversity constraints and is currently being tested in malaria-endemic areas.

If scientific and donor interest in malaria vaccine development continues at or above current levels, then the difficult task to develop a highly efficacious malaria vaccine is achievable. Modeling studies that take cost, malaria transmission, overall malaria burden of disease, and other relevant scientific evidence into account will help determine where vaccine is deployed based on public health priorities at local and national levels. Ongoing research and evaluation will help to overcome challenges of vaccine delivery and integrate insecticide-treated bed net use and other malaria control initiatives to reduce and eventually eliminate malaria burden.

References

1. World Health Organization. 2013. *World Malaria Report*. Geneva, Switzerland: World Health Organization.

2. World Health Organization. 2013. Malaria Vaccine Technology Roadmap. Geneva, Switzerland: World Health Organization. Available at: http://www.who.int/immunization/topics/malaria/vaccine_roadmap/en/.

3. Freund, J., K. J. Thomson, H. E. Sommer, A. W. Walter, and E. L. Schenkein. 1945. Immunization of rhesus monkeys against malarial infection (*P. knowlesi*) with killed parasites and adjuvants. *Science* 102:202–204.

4. Clyde, D. F., H. Most, V. C. McCarthy, and J. P. Vanderberg. 1973. Immunization of man against sporozite-induced falciparum malaria. *Am J Med Sci* 266:169–177.

5. Laurens, M. B., M. Roestenberg, and V. S. Moorthy. 2012. A consultation on the optimization of controlled human malaria infection by mosquito bite for evaluation of candidate malaria vaccines. *Vaccine* 30:5302–5304.

6. Kester, K. E., J. F. Cummings, O. Ofori-Anyinam, C. F. Ockenhouse, U. Krzych, P. Moris, et al. 2009. Randomized, double-blind, phase 2a trial of falciparum malaria vaccines RTS,S/AS01B and RTS,S/AS02A in malaria-naive adults: Safety, efficacy, and immunologic associates of protection. *J Infect Dis* 200:337–346.

7. Clyde, D. F. 1975. Immunization of man against falciparum and vivax malaria by use of attenuated sporozoites. *Am J Trop Med Hyg* 24:397–401.

8. Agnandji, S. T., B. Lell, J. F. Fernandes, B. P. Abossolo, B.G. Methogo, A. L. Kabwende, et al. 2012. A phase 3 trial of RTS,S/AS01 malaria vaccine in African infants. *N Engl J Med* 367:2284–2295.

9. Agnandji, S. T., B. Lell, J. F. Fernandes, B. P. Abossolo, B.G. Methogo, A. L. Kabwende, et al. 2014. Efficacy and safety of the RTS,S/AS01 malaria vaccine during 18 months after vaccination: A phase 3 randomized, controlled trial in children and young infants at 11 African sites. *PLoS Med* 11:e1001685.

10. Thera, M. A., O. K. Doumbo, D. Coulibaly, M. B. Laurens, A. Ouattara, A. K. Kone, et al. 2011. A field trial to assess a blood-stage malaria vaccine. *N Engl J Med* 365:1004–1013.

11. Matuschewski, K., and A. K. Mueller. 2007. Vaccines against malaria—an update. FEBS J. 274:4680–4687.

12. The malERA Consultative Group on Vaccines. 2011. A research agenda for malaria eradication: Vaccines. *PLoS Med* 8:e1000398.

46 Randomized Controlled Trials for Ebola: Practical and Ethical Issues

Clement Adebamowo, Oumou Bah-Sow, and colleagues*

Two months ago, when the numbers known to have died from Ebola in West Africa could still be counted in the hundreds, the World Health Organization (WHO) made an important statement about investigational drugs and vaccines. This crisis is so acute, WHO declared, that it is ethical to offer interventions with potential benefits but unknown efficacy and side effects, although every effort should be made to evaluate benefits and risks and share all data generated.

The need for drugs and vaccines was urgent then. With cases now rising exponentially and health systems overwhelmed, it is even greater today. Vaccine safety trials are underway in the United States and the United Kingdom and poised to roll out to Africa soon. But treatments for those with infection are required too. Besides playing a direct part in containing the epidemic, interventions that could improve outcomes for the sick would help to rebuild the confidence of affected communities in health services, a critical step if Ebola is to be overcome.

A fast-track initiative for evaluating investigational drugs was launched in September 2014.[1] Although the question of whether unproven treatments should be offered at all is now settled, the question of how they should be deployed and tested is not. Still at issue is whether such treatments should be made available only in the context of randomized controlled trials (RCTs), in which patients receive either a new intervention and conventional care, or conventional care alone or with a placebo.

Advocates of this RCT approach[2] state that as this experimental design will create the most robust evidence for the future, and is what regulators are used to, it is the only approach that should be considered. We disagree.

Although we concur that RCTs provide robust evidence and support their use where this is ethical and practical, we do not believe that either consideration is likely to be

* Reprinted from *The Lancet*, Adebamowo, C., et al., Randomized controlled trials for Ebola: Practical and ethical issues, 384:1423–1424. Copyright © 2014 with permission of Elsevier.

satisfied in the context of this epidemic. The priority must be to generate data about effectiveness and safety as swiftly as possible, so that the most useful new treatments can be identified for rapid deployment. Alternative trial designs have the potential to do this more quickly and with greatest social and ethical acceptability.

The first objection to RCTs in which investigational drugs plus conventional care are compared purely with conventional care is ethical. Such randomization is ethical when there is equipoise—when there is genuine uncertainty about whether an untested treatment has benefits or risks that exceed those of conventional care. Equipoise is a useful principle, but it can break down when conventional care offers little benefit and mortality is extremely high. This is precisely the problem with Ebola: current conventional care does not much affect clinical outcomes, and mortality is as high as 70%. When conventional care means such a high probability of death, it is problematic to insist on randomizing patients to it when the intervention arm holds out at least the possibility of benefit. Ethical arguments are not the same for all levels of risk.

No one insisted that Western medical workers offered zMapp, and other investigational products were randomized to receive the drug or conventional care plus a placebo. None of us would consent to be randomized in such circumstances. In cancers with a poor prognosis for which there are no good treatments, evidence from studies without a control group can be accepted as sufficient for deployment, and even for licensing by regulators, with fuller analysis following later. There is no need for rules to be bent or corners to be cut: the necessary procedures already exist and are used.

The second objection is practical. Even if randomization were ethically acceptable, it might not be deliverable in the context of healthcare systems, and indeed the wider social order, that are breaking down, as in Liberia, Guinea, and Sierra Leone. Populations who are terrified by the progress of the epidemic, and who lack trust in healthcare and aid workers, and in public authorities in the aftermath of civil wars, cannot be expected to offer informed consent to such randomized trials. It is also unclear that any capacity exists to impose controlled conditions during a raging epidemic. Insisting on RCTs could even worsen the epidemic by undermining trust in the Ebola treatment centers that are central to containing it.

Randomization is not, moreover, the only way to gather reliable information about the safety and effectiveness of potential Ebola therapies. Indeed, other methods might be more appropriate for achieving the key objective, which is to identify drug regimens that improve outcomes over existing methods of care quickly so that WHO can recommend their use and lives can be saved.

One viable approach would be to try different treatments in parallel and at different sites, following observational studies that document mortality under standard care. This approach could effectively triage treatments into those with great benefits that should be rolled out immediately, those with no effect that should be discarded quickly, and those with promise needing follow-up in randomized trials. These trials can be designed adaptively, meaning that patient enrollment can be altered as efficacy data emerge, minimizing the number of individuals who get ineffective treatments and increasing the numbers getting those that show benefits. This is not different from phase 2 studies as currently conducted and accepted by regulatory authorities for other diseases. It will also enable quick follow-up trials of combinations of antivirals and new treatments that have already shown evidence of activity. A different type of RCT might also become an option once more than one drug has shown efficacy—even efficacy in animal models. Then patients could ethically be randomized to one investigational drug or another. No one would receive only standard care.

We accept that RCTs can generate strong evidence in ordinary circumstances but not in the midst of the worst Ebola epidemic in history. The urgent need is to establish whether new investigational drugs offer survival benefits, and thus which, if any, should be recommended by WHO to save lives. We have innovative but proven trial designs for doing exactly that. We should be using them, rather than doggedly insisting on gold standards that were developed for different settings and purposes.

References

1. Wellcome Trust. 2014, September 23. Ebola treatment trials to be fast-tracked in West Africa. Available at: http://www.wellcome.ac.uk/News/Media-office/Press-releases/2014/WTP057419.htm. Accessed October 9, 2014.

2. Joffe, S. 2014. Evaluating novel therapies during the Ebola epidemic. *JAMA*. 312:1299(300).

47   Evaluating Ebola Therapies—The Case for RCTs

Edward Cox, Luciana Borio, and Robert Temple[*]

The worst Ebola epidemic in history is ongoing. With the number of deaths from Ebola virus disease (EVD) already in the thousands and predicted to rise to the tens of thousands,[1] the situation is tragic. No treatments have yet been shown to be safe and effective in patients with EVD. Some candidate therapies have shown benefit in animal models of infection, and others have shown activity against certain Ebola strains in cell culture, but concerns have been raised about possible toxicity of some of these agents. There is an urgent need to identify therapies that are effective and safe, and well-designed clinical trials are the fastest and most reliable way to achieve that goal.

Studying investigational therapies for EVD presents scientific, practical, and ethical challenges. Not surprisingly, there has been substantial debate about the best and most appropriate study approaches.[2,3] It is generally agreed that a trial with a concurrent control group, in which patients are randomly assigned to receive the test drug plus the best available supportive care (BASC) or to BASC alone, would be the most efficient and reliable way to evaluate the safety and effectiveness of candidate products. Some people in the healthcare community, however, have argued against such trials, urging instead use of a historical control—that is, making investigational drugs as widely available as their supply allows and then comparing mortality rates among treated patients with rates that would have been expected absent the drugs, on the basis of past experience with EVD. The desire to allow all patients access to investigational drugs is understandable, but there are strong reasons to doubt the ability of such "historically controlled" studies to distinguish effective therapies from ineffective ones.

Insofar as such studies cannot reliably identify effective treatments, their use could have tragic consequences. If historical comparisons falsely suggest a benefit or fail to detect modest but meaningful clinical effectiveness, then the investigational drug might be erroneously adopted as effective or discarded as ineffective. Possible consequences include exposure of subsequent patients to harm or to lack of effect from the mistakenly adopted treatment and failure to use a drug with a real, although modest, ability to improve survival, as well as failure to further develop an intervention that provides meaningful benefit.

Historically controlled studies compare study outcomes with outcomes in an external group that is thought to be similar to the study participants. The challenge of such trials is identifying a pertinent historical experience. If the two groups are not similar, observed differences in results may be unrelated to the therapy, instead reflecting underlying differences between the groups or differences in supportive care.

Case fatality rates in past outbreaks of EVD have ranged from less than 50% to more than 80%,[4] and even limited supportive care probably improves survival rates. Thus, the historical case fatality rates are irrelevant if current study patients receive better supportive care. Without clear knowledge of the mortality that would be expected with the study's level of supportive care, a historically controlled study cannot determine whether a treatment has helped or harmed patients.[5] In a randomized trial, by contrast, all patients would receive similar supportive care so that the effect (or lack of effect) of the added treatment could be assessed. Moreover, such a trial could detect even a small but meaningful benefit that a historically controlled trial could not credibly identify.

Randomized controlled trials (RCTs) with a BASC control group are a powerful tool for evaluating effects of an investigational therapy. Randomization ensures reasonable similarity of the test and control groups and protects against various imbalances and biases that could lead to erroneous conclusions. Properly designed RCTs that give reliable answers are critical to identifying urgently needed treatments for responding to the ongoing Ebola crisis and any future outbreaks.

The number of infected patients greatly exceeds the supply of certain investigational agents. Regardless of debates over trial design or ethics, when there are only limited supplies, most patients cannot receive specific antiviral therapy. RCTs for evaluating these agents will therefore not be depriving patients of treatment but will provide a pathway for identifying effective treatments as rapidly and reliably as possible. Even when sufficient supplies are available, RCTs will provide the definitive answer on effectiveness, in a generally quicker fashion than alternative trial designs.

When preclinical data suggest that a candidate treatment has a low likelihood of clinical effectiveness or may have substantial toxicity, RCTs including a BASC group are the most efficient and reliable way to identify benefits or harm. Given the accelerated development of Ebola drugs (which involves, for example, proceeding on the basis of only limited phase 1 data and little or no traditional phase 2 data) and preliminary data suggesting potential for adverse effects, such drugs need to be evaluated in RCTs with an appropriate control group so that any harm can be detected. Otherwise, it may not be possible to distinguish serious adverse drug effects from manifestations of EVD.

Some public health authorities are reluctant to support RCTs, which they see as traditional and slow trials.[3] However, advances in trial design can and should be incorporated into Ebola RCTs. For example, such trials should include ongoing monitoring of results (e.g., group-sequential designs), adaptive elements, and other trial efficiencies to reduce the time required to identify an effective treatment, particularly a very effective treatment. If one investigational drug clearly shows benefit, then trials should incorporate it into the new standard of care for all treatment groups thereafter. Then a regimen adding a different investigational therapy to the new standard of care could be compared with the new standard of care alone. If multiple investigational drugs are simultaneously available for clinical testing, an RCT could include more than one drug and a shared control group. Trials could be designed to assess effects on survival (recovery from disease) as the most important and measurable end point.

RCTs will yield the safety and effectiveness data that are so desperately needed and will do so ethically, giving all patients in a study an equal opportunity to receive the often limited supply of investigational drugs. So far, investigational drugs have generally been used in the few patients treated in the United States or Europe. An RCT with sites in West Africa, the United States, and Europe could result in more equitable distribution because random allocation provides a fair means of deciding who has access to limited quantities of an investigational drug.

Scientists at the National Institutes of Health, in collaboration with the U.S. Food and Drug Administration, the Biomedical Advanced Research and Development Authority, the U.S. Department of Defense, and clinicians caring for patients with EVD in the United States, are leading efforts to develop and implement such trials. They have developed a protocol for an RCT with a BASC control group that will use Bayesian analytic methods, allow for the study of more than one investigational drug using a shared control group, and permit incorporation of a therapy into the regimen for the standard-of-care group once it has been shown to be effective against Ebola. The trial will be initiated first in the United States, with an opportunity for subsequent expansion to affected countries in West Africa. Establishing such trials in those countries is likely to have additional beneficial effects, such as improving supportive care.

Conducting such trials in affected regions will be challenging. It is critical for public health leaders to articulate the rationale for conducting scientifically valid trials, work closely with local health authorities, and engage community leaders so that trials can be acceptable to the affected populations. Such efforts are essential if we are to correctly identify therapies that will benefit patients with EVD now and in the future.

References

1. WHO Ebola Response Team. 2014. Ebola virus disease in West Africa—The first 9 months of the epidemic and forward projections. *N Engl J Med* 371:1481–1495.

2. Joffe, S. 2014. Evaluating novel therapies during the Ebola epidemic. *JAMA* 312:1299–1300.

3. Adebamowo, C., O. Bah-Sow, F. Binka, R. Bruzzone, A. Caplan, J-F. Delfraissy, et al. 2014. Randomised controlled trials for Ebola: Practical and ethical issues. *Lancet* 384:1423–1424.

4. Ebola virus disease: fact sheet no. 103. Updated September 2014. Geneva: World Health Organization. Available at: http://www.who.int/mediacentre/factsheets/fs103/en).

5. Lamontagne, F., C. Clement, T. Fletcher, S. T. Jacob, W. A. Fischer II, and R. A. Fowler. 2014. Doing today's work superbly well—treating Ebola with current tools. *N Engl J Med* 371: 1565–1566.

Index

Quackery, 10
Quality control, 9
Quarantine, 19, 276

Rabies vaccine, 5, 43, 368
Randomized controlled trials
  for Ebola virus disease, 404–406
  ethical principle of equipoise, 400
  unproven treatments, 399, 400
Rational-choice economics, 156
Rationing, 26, 32, 261, 263–264, 266
Rawls's theory of justice as fairness, 157
Reasonable availability, 92, 94, 96
Recombinant technology, 67–68, 387
Recommended immunization schedules
  advisory groups on, 25, 72, 137–138
  alternative schedules, 190, 220
  enforcement of, 231
  first recommendations, 25
  recent additions to, 17, 128
Red Book, 250
Red Scare of 1919, 24
Regulations
  as barriers, 8, 387
  compulsory laws in Britain, 10
  exceptions for personal beliefs, 10
  International Health Regulations (2005), 288
  international law on resource allocation, 288–289
  pricing and, 63
  shaping vaccinology, 6
Regulatory agencies, 63, 71, 99, 283, 312–313
Religious beliefs, 17, 31–32, 199
Religious exemptions, 31–32, 209, 219, 231, 255
Research. See Clinical trials; Ethical research
Research and development, 57–58
  in academia, 62
  collaborators in, 57, 59
  costs of development, 60
  in developing countries, 62
  divestment of public agencies, 13
  effect of advanced commitments on, 81

funding sources, 60–62
incentives, 61–62, 79, 367, 370
intellectual property, 63
neglected diseases, 369, 370
new sciences, 74–75
partnerships, 371–372
patents, 63
phase 1 testing, 61, 92–93
technical feasibility, 61
in the United States, 59
Resistance, 343, 345–347
Resource allocation. See also Prioritization schemes
  distributive justice, 324–326
  guiding principles for, 283–284
  during humanitarian crises, 324–326
  international law, 288–289
  during pandemics, 269, 283–284
Right to health, 288
Rimland, Bernard, 170, 171
Rinderpest, 358
Risk
  adverse events, 47, 49, 119
  age factors, 263, 266
  benefit-risk ratios, 131, 148, 153
  communication of, 134, 211
  community risk with vaccine refusal, 221, 248
  disease transmission, 322, 324
  extent of individual rights restriction, 328
  for host countries, 110
  individual risk with vaccine refusal, 220, 247
  perception, 149
  sharing, 155, 203
  tolerance, 131
  uncertainty, 153, 156
  vaccine complications vs. disease, 132, 148–149, 206, 217
Roosevelt, Franklin, 24
Rotarians, 351
Rotashield, 312
Rotavirus, 59, 65, 66, 67, 312
Roundworm, 367

Basic Bioethics

Arthur L. Caplan, editor

Books Acquired under the Editorship of Glenn McGee and Arthur L. Caplan

Peter A. Ubel, *Pricing Life: Why It's Time for Health Care Rationing*

Mark G. Kuczewski and Ronald Polansky, eds., *Bioethics: Ancient Themes in Contemporary Issues*

Suzanne Holland, Karen Lebacqz, and Laurie Zoloth, eds., *The Human Embryonic Stem Cell Debate: Science, Ethics, and Public Policy*

Gita Sen, Asha George, and Piroska Östlin, eds., *Engendering International Health: The Challenge of Equity*

Carolyn McLeod, *Self-Trust and Reproductive Autonomy*

Lenny Moss, *What Genes Can't Do*

Jonathan D. Moreno, ed., *In the Wake of Terror: Medicine and Morality in a Time of Crisis*

Glenn McGee, ed., *Pragmatic Bioethics, 2d edition*

Timothy F. Murphy, *Case Studies in Biomedical Research Ethics*

Mark A. Rothstein, ed., *Genetics and Life Insurance: Medical Underwriting and Social Policy*

Kenneth A. Richman, *Ethics and the Metaphysics of Medicine: Reflections on Health and Beneficence*

David Lazer, ed., *DNA and the Criminal Justice System: The Technology of Justice*

Harold W. Baillie and Timothy K. Casey, eds., *Is Human Nature Obsolete? Genetics, Bioengineering, and the Future of the Human Condition*

Robert H. Blank and Janna C. Merrick, eds., *End-of-Life Decision Making: A Cross-National Study*

Norman L. Cantor, *Making Medical Decisions for the Profoundly Mentally Disabled*

Margrit Shildrick and Roxanne Mykitiuk, eds., *Ethics of the Body: Post-Conventional Challenges*

Alfred I. Tauber, *Patient Autonomy and the Ethics of Responsibility*

David H. Brendel, *Healing Psychiatry: Bridging the Science/Humanism Divide*

Jonathan Baron, *Against Bioethics*

Michael L. Gross, *Bioethics and Armed Conflict: Moral Dilemmas of Medicine and War*

Karen F. Greif and Jon F. Merz, *Current Controversies in the Biological Sciences: Case Studies of Policy Challenges from New Technologies*

Deborah Blizzard, *Looking Within: A Sociocultural Examination of Fetoscopy*

Ronald Cole-Turner, ed., *Design and Destiny: Jewish and Christian Perspectives on Human Germline Modification*

Holly Fernandez Lynch, *Conflicts of Conscience in Health Care: An Institutional Compromise*

Mark A. Bedau and Emily C. Parke, eds., *The Ethics of Protocells: Moral and Social Implications of Creating Life in the Laboratory*

Jonathan D. Moreno and Sam Berger, eds., *Progress in Bioethics: Science, Policy, and Politics*

Eric Racine, *Pragmatic Neuroethics: Improving Understanding and Treatment of the Mind-Brain*

Martha J. Farah, ed., *Neuroethics: An Introduction with Readings*

Jeremy R. Garrett, ed., *The Ethics of Animal Research: Exploring the Controversy*

Books Acquired under the Editorship of Arthur L. Caplan

Sheila Jasanoff, ed., *Reframing Rights: Bioconstitutionalism in the Genetic Age*

Christine Overall, *Why Have Children? The Ethical Debate*

Yechiel Michael Barilan, *Human Dignity, Human Rights, and Responsibility: The New Language of Global Bioethics and Bio-Law*

Tom Koch, *Thieves of Virtue: When Bioethics Stole Medicine*

Timothy F. Murphy, *Ethics, Sexual Orientation, and Choices about Children*

Daniel Callahan, *In Search of the Good: A Life in Bioethics*

Robert Blank, *Intervention in the Brain: Politics, Policy, and Ethics*

Gregory E. Kaebnick and Thomas H. Murray, eds., *Synthetic Biology and Morality: Artificial Life and the Bounds of Nature*

Dominic A. Sisti, Arthur L. Caplan, and Hila Rimon-Greenspan, eds., *Applied Ethics in Mental Healthcare: An Interdisciplinary Reader*

Barbara K. Redman, *Research Misconduct Policy in Biomedicine: Beyond the Bad-Apple Approach*

Russell Blackford, *Humanity Enhanced: Genetic Choice and the Challenge for Liberal Democracies*

Nicholas Agar, *Truly Human Enhancement: A Philosophical Defense of Limits*

Bruno Perreau, *The Politics of Adoption: Gender and the Making of French Citizenship*

Carl Schneider, *The Censor's Hand: The Misregulation of Human-Subject Research*

Lydia S. Dugdale, ed., *Dying in the Twenty-First Century: Towards a New Ethical Framework for the Art of Dying Well*

John D. Lantos and Diane S. Lauderdale, *Preterm Babies, Fetal Patients, and Childbearing Choices*

Harris Wiseman, *The Myth of the Moral Brain*

Jason L. Schwartz and Arthur L. Caplan, eds., *Vaccination Ethics and Policy: An Introduction with Readings*

DATE DUE

NOV 02 2017

PRINTED IN U.S.A.